Recent Results in Cancer Research 177

H. Riess · A. Goerke · H. Oettle (Eds.)

Pancreatic Cancer

With 48 Figures and 16 Tables

Springer

Prof. Dr. med. Hanno Riess
Andrea Goerke
Priv.-Doz. Dr. med. Helmut Oettle

Charité – Universitätsmedizin Berlin
Campus Virchow-Klinikum
Medizinische Klinik mit Schwerpunkt
Hämatologie und Onkologie
Augustenburger Platz 1
13353 Berlin
Germany

Library of Congress Control Number: 2007938498

ISSN 0080-0015
ISBN 978-3-540-71266-4 Springer Berlin Heidelberg New York

Springer is a part of Springer Science + Business Media
springer.com

Editor: Dr. Ute Heilmann, Heidelberg
Desk editor: Dörthe Mennecke-Bühler, Heidelberg
Production editor: Anne Strohbach, Leipzig
Cover design: Frido Steinen-Broo, eStudio Calamar, Spain
Typesetting: LE-TEX Jelonek, Schmidt & Vöckler GbR, Leipzig
Printed on acid-free paper SPIN 12031573 21/3100/YL – 5 4 3 2 1 0

Preface

Pancreatic cancer is one of the most frequent malignant tumor entities—with increasing incidences reported for both females and for males—and yet it still has a poor prognosis. Therefore, it is surprising that no volume in the *Recent Results in Cancer Research* series has been dedicated to this tumor entity until now. It remains speculative whether this is related to the lack of firm findings concerning the pathogenesis, to a missing breakthrough in treatment, or simply to general therapeutic frustration. We are pleased to present this volume, compiled by a team of competent authors, representing the recent achievements and the present state of the art in the management of pancreatic cancer.

The different chapters emanate rays of hope and pioneering spirit in terms of more precise diagnostics and of improved therapeutic strategies. However, the challenges we are still facing with this disease are obvious:

- Deficiencies in the understanding of pancreatic tumor biology (e.g., initiation, progression, resistance to chemo- and radiotherapy).
- Lack in achieving sustained success with standard methods of surgery, radiotherapy, and chemotherapy in contrast to the success in multimodal treatments for other solid tumors.
- Sufficiently effective drugs are missing and the testing of already existing and of new compounds and therapies in well-planned and adequately recruiting prospective clinical trials is cumbersome and time consuming.

We therefore hope that the present volume will initiate novel ideas and approaches to overcome these challenges.

It is our vision and desire that this *RRCR* volume on pancreatic cancer promotes genuine interest in this mostly incurable disease and launches promising and interdisciplinary efforts among basic researchers, surgeons, medical oncologists, radiologists, gastroenterologists, and pathologists, which lead to significant therapeutic and prognostic progress.

October 2007
P. M. Schlag, Berlin
H.-J. Senn, St. Gallen

Contents

List of Contributors

Holger Amthauer, MD
Charité – Universitätsmedizin Berlin
Campus Virchow-Klinikum
Klinik für Strahlenheilkunde
Augustenburger Platz 1
13353 Berlin
Germany

Alexander Arlt, MD
Klinik für Allgemeine Innere Medizin
Labor für Molekulare Gastroenterologie
und Hepatologie
Universitätsklinikum Schleswig-Holstein
Campus Kiel
Schittenhelmstraße 12
24105 Kiel
Germany

Marcus Bahra, MD
Charité – Universitätsmedizin Berlin
Campus Virchow-Klinikum
Klinik für Allgemein-, Visceral-
und Transplantationschirurgie
Augustenburger Platz 1
13353 Berlin
Germany

Volker Budach, MD
Charité – Universitätsmedizin Berlin
Campus Mitte
Klinik für Strahlenheilkunde
Charitéplatz 1
10117 Berlin
Germany

Timm Denecke, MD
Charité – Universitätsmedizin Berlin
Campus Virchow-Klinikum
Klinik für Strahlenheilkunde
Augustenburger Platz 1
13353 Berlin
Germany

Matthias P. A. Ebert, MD, PhD
II. Medizinische Klinik
Klinikum rechts der Isar
Technische Universität München
86175 Munich
Germany

Birgit Fischer-Blass, PhD
Antisense Pharma GmbH
Josef-Engert-Str. 9
93053 Regensburg
Germany

Andrea Goerke
Charité – Universitätsmedizin Berlin
Campus Virchow-Klinikum
Medizinische Klinik mit Schwerpunkt
Hämatologie und Onkologie
Augustenburger Platz 1
13353 Berlin
Germany

Robert Grützmann, MD
Klinik für Viszeral-, Thorax-
und Gefäßchirurgie
Universitätsklinikum Carl Gustav Carus
Technische Universität Dresden
Fetscherstr. 74
01307 Dresden
Germany

Steffen Heeger, MD, MSc
Merck Pharma GmbH
Alsfelder Str. 17
64289 Darmstadt
Germany

Volker Heinemann, PhD
Klinik Bad Trissl GmbH & Co. KG
Abt. für Strahlentherapie
Bad-Trissl-Str. 73
83080 Oberaudorf
Germany

Andreas Hilbig, MD
Charité – Universitätsmedizin Berlin
Campus Virchow-Klinikum
Medizinische Klinik mit Schwerpunkt
Hämatologie und Onkologie
Augustenburger Platz 1
13353 Berlin
Germany

Dietmar Jacob, MD
Charité – Universitätsmedizin Berlin
Campus Virchow-Klinikum
Klinik für Allgemein-, Visceral-
und Transplantationschirurgie
Augustenburger Platz 1
13353 Berlin
Germany

Andreas Kaiser, MD
Charité – Universitätsmedizin Berlin
Zentrum für Tumormedizin
Klinik für Strahlentherapie CCM
Charitéplatz 1
10117 Berlin
Germany

Thomas Kittner, MD
Chefarzt
Krankenhaus Dresden-Friedrichstadt
Städtisches Klinikum
Akademisches Lehrkrankenhaus
der Technischen Universität Dresden
Friedrichstraße 41
01067 Dresden
Germany

Enrique Lopez Hänninen, MD
Charité – Universitätsmedizin Berlin
Campus Virchow-Klinikum
Klinik für Strahlenheilkunde
Augustenburger Platz 1
13353 Berlin
Germany

Sylvia Ludwig, DVM
Antisense Pharma GmbH
Josef-Engert-Str. 9
93053 Regensburg
Germany

Ulf Neumann, MD, PhD
Charité – Universitätsmedizin Berlin
Campus Virchow-Klinikum
Klinik für Allgemein-, Visceral-
und Transplantationschirurgie
Augustenburger Platz 1
13353 Berlin
Germany

Helmut Oettle, MD
Charité – Universitätsmedizin Berlin
Campus Virchow-Klinikum
Medizinische Klinik mit Schwerpunkt
Hämatologie und Onkologie
Augustenburger Platz 1
13353 Berlin
Germany

Uwe Pelzer, MD, PhD
Charité – Universitätsmedizin Berlin
Campus Virchow-Klinikum
Medizinische Klinik mit Schwerpunkt
Hämatologie und Onkologie
Augustenburger Platz 1
13353 Berlin
Germany

Hanno Riess, MD, PhD
Charité – Universitätsmedizin Berlin
Campus Virchow-Klinikum
Medizinische Klinik mit Schwerpunkt
Hämatologie und Onkologie
Augustenburger Platz 1
13353 Berlin
Germany

Christoph Röcken, MD, PhD
Charité – Universitätsmedizin Berlin
Institut für Pathologie
Charitéplatz 1
10117 Berlin
Germany

Lars Roll, MD
Charité – Universitätsmedizin Berlin
Campus Virchow-Klinikum
Medizinische Klinik mit Schwerpunkt
Hämatologie und Onkologie
Augustenburger Platz 1
13353 Berlin
Germany

Juri Ruf, MD
Charité – Universitätsmedizin Berlin
Campus Virchow-Klinikum
Klinik für Nuklearmedizin
Augustenburger Platz 1
13353 Berlin
Germany

Heiner Schäfer, PhD
Klinik für Allgemeine Innere Medizin
Labor für Molekulare Gastroenterologie
& Hepatologie
Universitätsklinikum Schleswig-Holstein
Campus Kiel
Schittenhelmstraße 12
24105 Kiel
Germany

Karl-Hermann Schlingensiepen, MD, PhD
Antisense Pharma GmbH
Josef-Engert-Str. 9
93053 Regensburg
Germany

Susanne Schmaus, PhD
Antisense Pharma GmbH
Josef-Engert-Str. 9
93053 Regensburg
Germany

Susanne Sebens, PhD
Klinik für Allgemeine Innere Medizin
Labor für Molekulare Gastroenterologie
& Hepatologie
Universitätsklinikum Schleswig-Holstein
Campus Kiel
Schittenhelmstr. 12
24105 Kiel
Germany

Jens Stieler, MD
Charité – Universitätsmedizin Berlin
Campus Virchow-Klinikum
Medizinische Klinik mit Schwerpunkt
Hämatologie und Onkologie
Augustenburger Platz 1
13353 Berlin
Germany

Christian Stroszczynski, MD
Institut und Poliklinik für Radiologische
Diagnostik
Universitätsklinikum Carl Gustav Carus
Technische Universität Dresden
Fetscherstr. 74
01307 Dresden
Germany

Ralf Wilkowski, PhD
Klinik Bad Trissl GmbH & Co. KG
Abt. für Strahlentherapie
Bad-Trissl-Str. 73
83080 Oberaudorf
Germany

Maria Wolf, MD
Klinik Bad Trissl GmbH & Co. KG
Abt. für Strahlentherapie
Bad-Trissl-Str. 73
83080 Oberaudorf
Germany

1 Pancreatic Cancer: Step by Step Forward

H. Riess, A. Goerke, H. Oettle

Recent Results in Cancer Research, Vol. 177

With the diagnosis of pancreatic cancer, the majority of patients are faced with an unexpected tragedy. There is a persistently low rate of curability, a so-called case fatality rate of around 95%.

Complete resection is the prerequisite for curation, but only one-fifth of the patients are considered for surgical therapy. Even so, only about half of these individuals finally undergo successful, complete resection. Whereas nowadays surgery can be performed with low rates of perioperative morbidity and mortality at experienced high-volume centers, postoperative relapses are observed frequently. Neoadjuvant strategies to improve surgical resectability and the overall cure rate remain experimental, but due to the results of different trials, adjuvant treatments strategies are becoming standard worldwide. Transatlantic differences in the interpretation of study results with the use of chemoradiation probably will be overcome by the recent results of adjuvant chemotherapy in patients with adenocarcinoma of the pancreas, which have shown significant benefit in relapse-free survival, 3- and 5-year survival, and therefore—most likely—cure [1]. Ongoing studies will definitely clarify the role and kind of chemotherapy to be recommended for patients resected completely (R0) and those with microscopic involvement of the resection margin (R1).

For the majority of patients with nonresectable, locally advanced, metastasized, or relapsing pancreatic cancer, progress has been limited for several years. It took more than 10 years from the approval of gemcitabine for the treatment of advanced adenocarcinoma of the pancreas—and a great number of large-scaled phase III trials—before a second improvement in systemic therapy was implemented in patient care.

Erlotinib, a tyrosine kinase inhibitor blocking epidermal growth factor (EGF) receptor-mediated downstream signaling, succeeded in improving outcome in patients with advanced pancreatic cancer when applied in combination with gemcitabine, with a hazard ratio of 0.8 resulting in a 7% excess in 1-year survival as compared to gemcitabine plus placebo [2]. Due to this study, erlotinib obtained approval in the United States and Europe and is on the way to finding its place in routine treatment.

Confirming former nonsignificant results of gemcitabine in combination with capecitabine, it was recently demonstrated that this combination of cytotoxic drugs improved median and 1-year survival in a prospective randomized but non-placebo-controlled trial [3].

The impact of these data for standard care of patients with adenocarcinoma of the pancreas cancer needs to be defined. As adverse effects of cytotoxic drugs and targeted therapies differ, tailoring patient-specific first-line therapy has become a challenge for oncologists.

An improvement in quality of life, estimated by the clinical benefit response, occurs in a relevant proportion of patients due to first-line therapy with gemcitabine [4]. Therefore an increasing number of patients with pancreatic cancer progressing while on first-line therapy need to be considered for second-line therapy, based on their good performance status. The identification of principally active cytotoxic drugs, such as oxaliplatin (together with folinic acid and fluorouracil) or taxanes, antibodies, and small molecules, such as erlotinib and sorafenib, offer second-line treatment alternatives that have to undergo evaluation in clinical trials. Initial results favor oxaliplatin-based therapy [5, 6].

These small steps forward in the systemic therapy of pancreatic cancer give rise to some prudent optimism. In order to alter the perspectives of patients with pancreatic cancer, further understanding of the basic aspect of disease development as well as methods for screening or early diagnosis of this disease have to be developed. It is the aim of this issue of *Recent Results in Cancer Research* to compile the available knowledge concerning pancreatic cancer.

Acknowledgements

The editors recognize and acknowledge the important contributions of the various authors, all of them involved in the challenging effort of fighting this frightening cancer.

References

1. Oettle H, Post S, Neuhaus P, et al (2007) Adjuvant chemotherapy with gemcitabine versus observation in patients undergoing curative-intent resection of pancreatic cancer. A multicenter randomized controlled trial. JAMA 297:267–277
2. Moore MJ, Goldstein D, Hamm J, et al (2007) Erlotinib plus gemcitabine compared with gemcitabine alone in patients with advanced pancreatic cancer: a phase III trial of the National Cancer Institute of Canada Clinical Trials Group. J Clin Oncol 25:1960–1966
3. Cunningham D, Chau I, Stocken D, Davies C, Dunn J, Valle J, et al (2005) Phase III randomised comparison of gemcitabine (GEM) versus gemcitabine plus capecitabine (GEM-CAP) in patients with advanced pancreatic cancer. Eur J Cancer 3:4 [Suppl]
4. Burris HA 3rd, Moore MJ, Andersen J, et al (1997) Improvements in survival and clinical benefit with gemcitabine as first line therapy for patients with advanced pancreas cancer: a randomized trial. J Clin Oncol 15:2403–2413
5. Oettle H, Pelzer U, Stieler J, Hilbig A, Roll L, Schwaner I, Adler M, Detken S, Dörken B, Riess H (2005) Oxaliplatin/folinic acid/5-fluorouracil [24 h] (OFF) plus best supportive care versus best supportive care alone (BSC) in second-line therapy of gemcitabine-refractory advanced pancreatic cancer (CONKO 003). Clin Oncol 23:16S, abstr 4031
6. Riess H, Pelzer U, Stieler J, Schwaner I, Heil G, Görner M, Mölle M, Hilbig A, Dörken B, Oettle H (2007) A randomized second line trial in patients with gemcitabine refractory advanced pancreatic cancer—CONKO 003. J Clin Oncol 25:18S, abstr 4517

Part I Diagnosis

2 CT and MR Imaging of Pancreatic Cancer

C. Stroszczynski, R. Grützmann, T. Kittner

Recent Results in Cancer Research, Vol. 177

Abstract

Computed tomography (CT) and magnetic resonance imaging (MRI) are emerging noninvasive techniques for imaging of the pancreas. Based on multislice technology, CT enables multiplanar imaging of the pancreas (multislice-CT, MSCT) with a high contrast between vessels and parenchyma. In addition, MRI of the pancreas including the imaging of the lumina of the biliary tree and the pancreatic duct (magnetic resonance cholangiopancreaticography, MRCP) and the abdominal vessels (MR angiography, MRA) has become available for daily clinical practice in most hospitals. The addition of multiplanar and curved reformations may increase the sensitivity of CT and improves its agreement with surgical findings. Beyond abdominal MR imaging, techniques such as magnetic resonance cholangiopancreaticography (MRCP) and MR angiography should be integrated in the imaging protocol whenever possible.

2.1 Introduction

Pancreatic cancer is the third most common malignancy of the gastrointestinal tract, the incidence rate is estimated by 10 cases per 100,000 people per year. Surgery is the only therapy with curative intention and may result in long-term survival in those cases where the cancer is still confined to the organ itself. Surgery of the more advanced stages is being performed in some centers, but so far it has not become a routine procedure. Differentiating between pancreatic malignancy and focal chronic pancreatitis—in particular when taking into account that long-term pancreatitis is a risk factor in pancreatic cancer—is still a clinical challenge.

The main tasks of diagnostic imaging of the pancreas are the detection of pancreatic lesions and the differentiation between malignant and benign (e.g., inflammatory) changes in the pancreas. In addition, computed tomography/magnetic resonance (CT/MR) imaging should ideally be able to permit staging of pancreatic tumors including the detection of malignant infiltration of lymph nodes and distant metastases (Malka et al. 2002). When surgery is considered, resectability of the tumor is usually defined by the presence or absence of the infiltration of the portal vein, the venous confluens, or the superior mesenteric vein. Moreover, the detection of anatomic variations of the branches of the celiac trunk and the superior mesenteric artery is of crucial importance (Fuhrman et al. 1994).

CT and MRI are emerging noninvasive techniques for imaging of the pancreas. Based on multislice technology, CT enables multiplanar imaging (multislice-CT, MSCT) with a high contrast between vessels and parenchyma. In addition, MRI of the pancreas including the imaging of the lumina of the biliary tree and the pancreatic duct (magnetic resonance cholangiopancreaticography, MRCP) and the abdominal vessels (MR angiography, MRA) has become available for daily clinical practice in most hospitals. Therefore, invasive digital subtraction angiography (DSA) has lost its importance in many institutions for preoperative diagnosis of the pancreas.

2.2 Technical Aspects

2.2.1 CT of the Pancreas

CT is a well-established modality in diagnostic imaging and staging of pancreatic cancer. The introduction of fast multidetector spiral CT has made it possible to study the pancreas during different perfusion phases of the organ (Richter et al. 1996). Raw data of multislice images of the different perfusion phases may be used for the reconstructions of the parenchyma of the pancreas (usually 3–5 mm) as well as for reconstructions of the arterial and venous vessels (CT angiography, CTA) based on the thinner slices (0.5–1.0 mm; Fig. 2.1). CT scanning during the arterial phase of the perfusion is advantageous in the diagnostic workup of pancreatic cancer due to the presence of low perfused fibrotic and necrotic tissue in pancreatic cancer. For practical considerations, CT of the pancreas is mostly performed in multiple phases including at least the

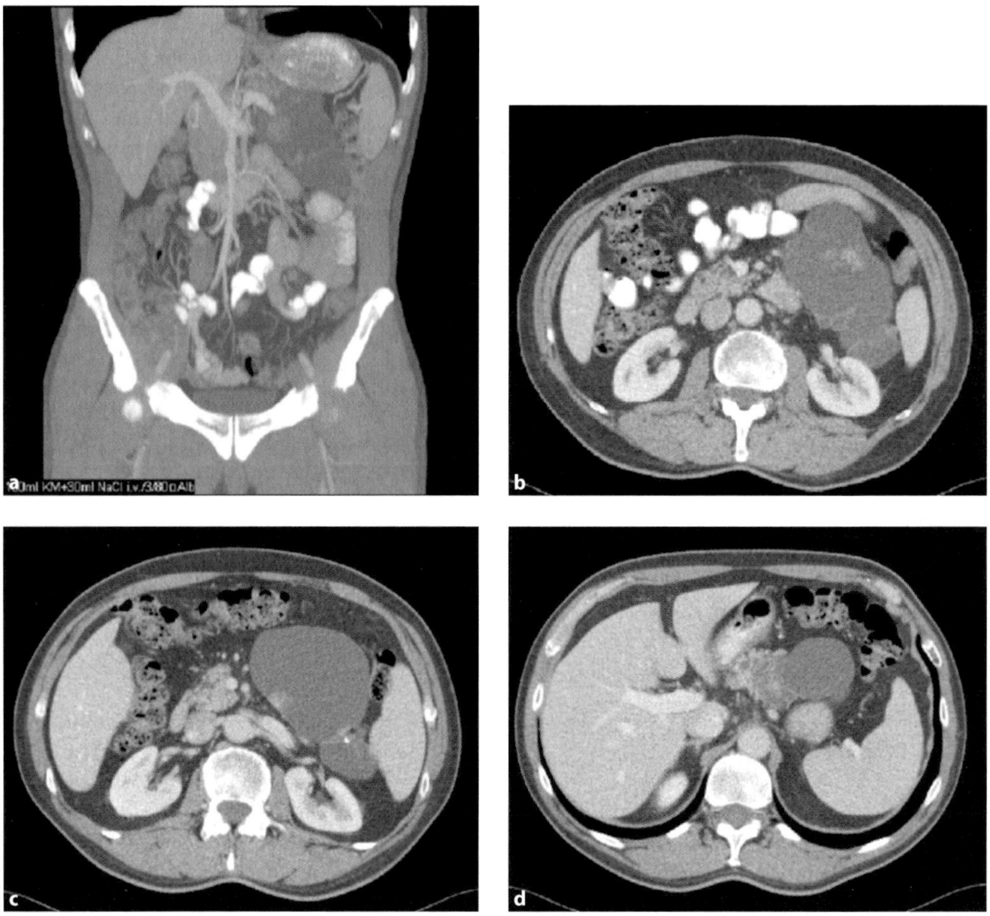

Fig. 2.1a–d Multislice CT of a patient with a cystic lesion located in the pancreatic tail. **a** Maximum intensity projection (MIP) in coronal orientation demonstrated a multilocular appearance with multiple segmentations. **b** Thin slice reconstructions showed nodular structures in the wall of the cysts, implicating a cystic neoplasm. **c** The parenchyma of the pancreatic head had a normal appearance, which is another argument against a pseudocyst lesion based on chronic pancreatitis. **d** The histology of this tumor was an intraductal papillary mucinous neoplasm (IPMN). On CT, the dilatation of the pancreatic ducts can be visualized

arterial and the portal venous phase, enabling an accurate detection of distant metastases in the liver as well as the imaging of the abdominal veins (Graf et al. 1997). Very recently, Ichikawa et al. (2006) demonstrated that there is some use for an additional parenchymal scan between the arterial and portal venous phases in combination with multiplanar reconstructions for tumor detection based on a population of 35 patients.

Hydro-CT (oral contrast enhancement with 800–1,000 ml of water) has become standard clinical practice in many institutions due to a better delineation of the pancreas from the posterior gastric wall (Baum et al. 1999; Schima and Ba-Ssalamah 1999; Richter et al. 1996).

Curved reformation techniques as recently introduced for CT imaging of the pancreatic duct may be play an important role in daily clinical practice because of a better availability due to faster reconstruction techniques (Sahani et al. 2006).

2.2.2 Magnetic Resonance Imaging of the Pancreas

While 3 T and more seems to be the new standard for imaging of the central nervous system, 1.5 T is still state-of-the-art for MRI of the abdomen. MRI of pancreatic neoplasms is optimally performed by using breath-hold acquisitions implicating that the patient should be able to stop breathing for more than 15 s. Conventional T1 weighted and T2 weighted images in transversal orientation are usually performed. In addition, dynamic, three-dimensional sequences after the administration of gadolinium-diethylenetriaminepentaacetic acid (DTPA) or other nephrotropic contrast media are obtained in arterial, portal, and delayed phases. On post-contrast images, fat suppression techniques that increase the contrast between uninvolved fat tissue and the enhancing tumor are recommended (Martin and Semelka 2000).

MRCP are usually obtained to evaluate the pancreatic duct and to exclude pancreatic cysts. Moreover, MRCP is an additional tool to increase the sensitivity of MRI for the detection of small pancreatic tumors (Fig. 2.2). Based on heavily T2 weighted sequences, MRCP sequences enable the selective imaging of fluids inside the biliary system and the pancreatic duct.

Single breath-hold MRCP techniques provide selective views of the whole pancreatic duct including the extrahepatic biliary tract without artifact using thick (2- to 8-cm) sections. Some authors prefer oral dark lumen contrast media to avoid an overlay based on adjacent organs such as stomach or duodenum. However, additional thin slice MRCP may enable a precise localization of the fluid structures. Some authors prefer secretin administration in improving pancreatic ductal details in MRCP (Petersein et al. 2002; Fulcher and Turner 1999). Based on an exog-

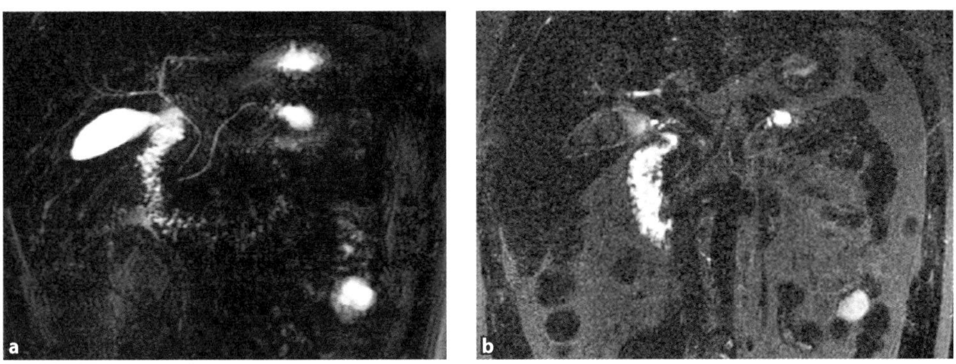

Fig. 2.2a,b MRCP of a patient without clinical signs of pancreatitis. **a** Thick slice MRCP clearly visualizes the lesion. **b** On thin slice MRCP, the pancreatic duct is visible as a small line that reaches the cystic lesion, suggesting communication with the cyst

enous administration of secretin, the secretion of pancreatic juice is stimulated, which consequently increases the volume of stationary fluid in the pancreatic ducts, which may improve diagnosis in small pancreatic tumors.

Mangafodipir trisodium (Mn-DPDP) was introduced as a tissue-specific contrast agent a couple of years ago. Some authors recommend the use of Mn-DPDP for the detection of subtle pancreatic neoplasms in equivocal cases. The mechanism of action of Mn-DPDP is that normal pancreatic parenchyma enhances following administration and becomes hyperintense on T1 weighted images whereas most of pancreatic neoplasms do not enhance (Kettritz et al. 1996; Gehl et al. 1993). It has been reported that Mn-DPDP-enhanced MRI provides better delineation of the pancreatic tumor but does not significantly improve the detection rate and staging accuracy of focal pancreatic lesions over MRI without this contrast medium (Romijn et al. 2000). However, no clinical data exist to date that underline an impact on differential diagnosis of pancreatic masses when compared with dynamic MRI based on gadopentetate dimeglumine (Gd-DTPA) or other Gd-chelates (Fig. 2.3).

MR angiography based on Gd-chelates may be used in conjunction with abdominal MRI including MRCP in one session using 3D gradient echo sequences. These so-called "all-in-one" MRI are becoming increasingly popular in clinical practice because of their versatility in patients with pancreatic tumors for the evaluation for surgical resection (Fig. 2.4). There is a slight difference between the MR sequences used for dynamic images (better soft tissue contrast due to higher signal of the pancreas, thicker slices) than for MR angiography (higher contrast between vessels and parenchyma) in theory. Morakkabati-Spitz et al. (2002) did not observe any advantages of dynamic imaging in patients with a suspicion of pancreatic cancer and concluded that the injection of contrast material should preferably be used for the performance of a contrast-enhanced MR angiography at the expense of a dynamic MR examination.

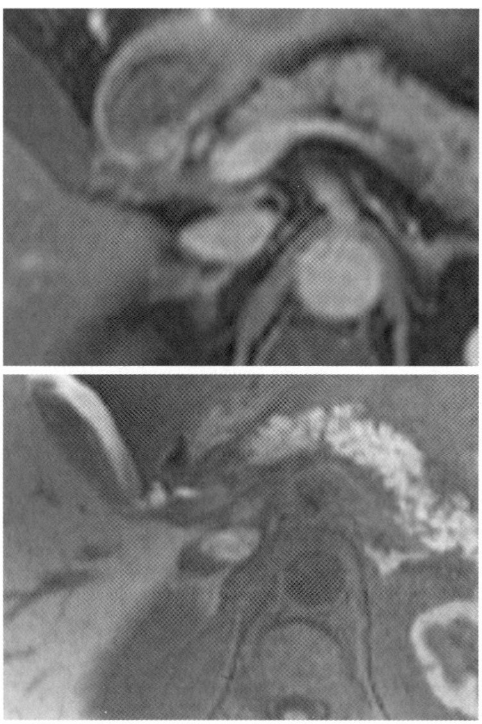

Fig. 2.3 Comparison of contrast enhanced MRI of a normal patient with two different contrast media. Please note that the pancreatic corpus shows less enhancement after Gd-chelate (*upper image*) than after Mn-DPDP (*lower image*)

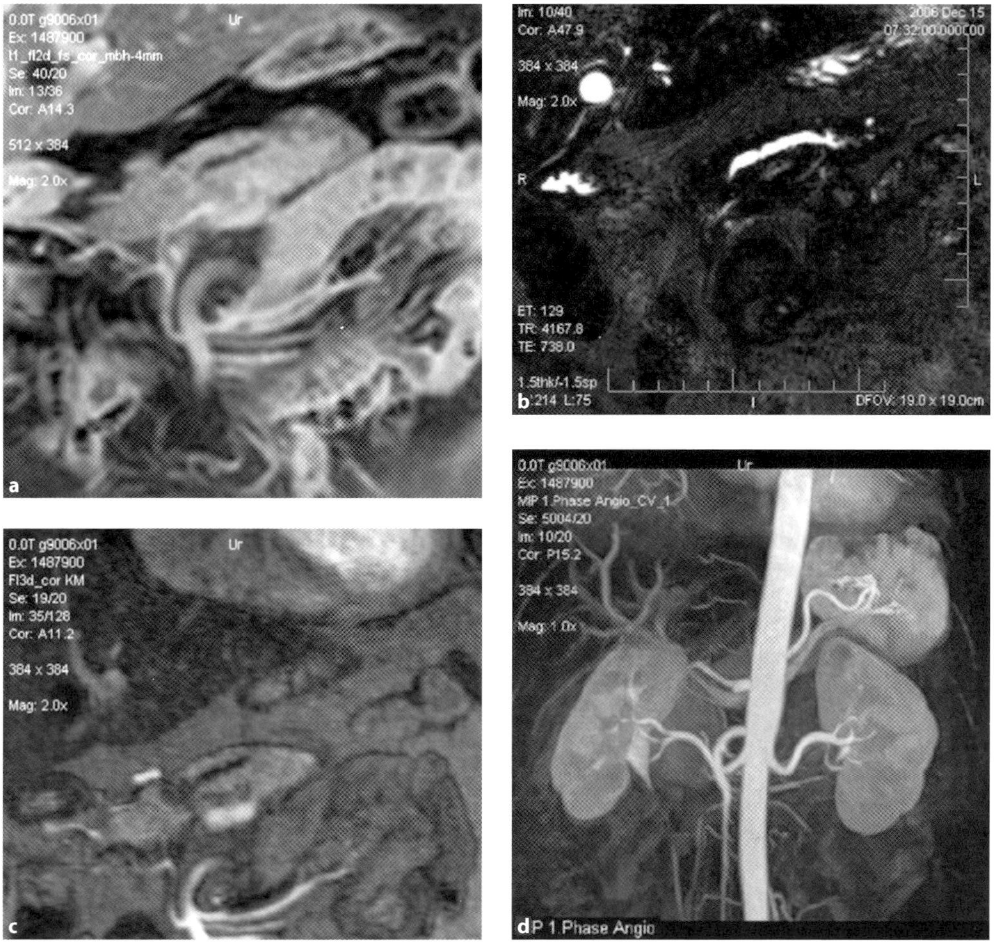

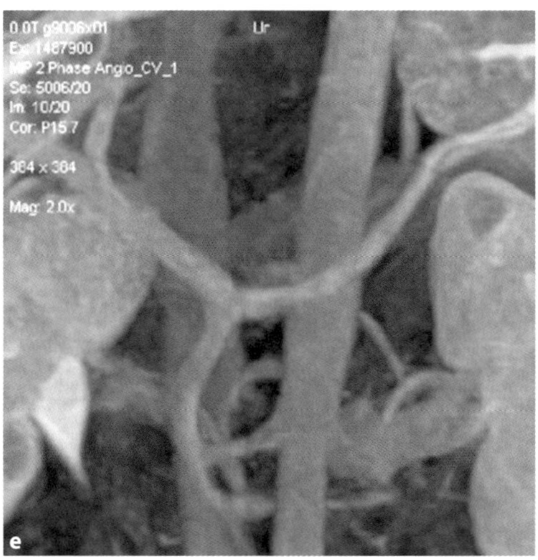

Fig. 2.4a–e All-in-one MRI in a patient with a small adenocarcinoma of the pancreas. **a** On contrast-enhanced MRI (coronal orientation), the pancreas is inhomogeneous without a defined focal lesion. The tubular structure in the center of the pancreas is interrupted, reflecting a stenosis of the pancreatic duct. **b** MRCP (single slice technique, coronal view) shows the interrupted pancreatic duct, highly suspect for a pancreatic tumor. **c** The arterial phase of dynamic MRI demonstrates a small focal lesion in the pancreatic parenchyma. **d** On this 3D reconstruction of the abdominal arteries a normal anatomy is visible. **e** Normal 3D angiography of the confluens region

2.3 Differential Diagnosis

2.3.1 Solid Tumors of the Pancreas

The accuracy of CT for the differentiation of solid tumors of the pancreas varies widely and can be explained by different techniques, different study populations, and the degree of awareness of the investigators assessing the images. In addition, it seems to be of crucial importance whether or not the investigators assessing the lesions have knowledge of the clinical picture (Lemke et al. 2004). Catalano et al. (2003) studied a total of 46 patients and reported a sensitivity of 97.0% and a specificity of 80.0%. In contrast, the sensitivity was 76.6% and the specificity was 63.9% in a study with 100 patients examined by Lemke et al. (2004) without clinical information. Most of the studies published so far do not break down the lesions according to size, but several studies have demonstrated a low specificity of CT in patients with lesions with a diameter of less than 2 cm (Taoka et al. 1999; Baum et al. 1999; Freeny 1999).

2.3.1.1 Magnetic Resonance Imaging

The vast majority of pancreatic adenocarcinomas are generally slightly hypointense relative to the pancreas on T2 weighted images. However, the tumors are difficult to visualize on plain MR images unless there is substantial necrosis.

When compared with normal pancreatic tissue, pancreatic adenocarcinomas enhance to a lesser extent than normal pancreatic tissue. This effect is often transient and may be best visualized on early post-contrast images during the arterial phase after bolus injection of nephrotropic contrast media. Many tumors, especially when substantial necrosis is apparent, demonstrate a more or less thin rim of greater enhancing pancreatic tissue and may underline the focal nature of a pancreatic lesion. Vascular encasement due to the typical perivascular growth of this malignant tumor is equivocal or better delineated by MRI when compared with dynamic contrast-enhanced CT (Martin and Semelka 2000). MR angiography with fat suppression is superior to other sequences in delineating regional vascular encasement or occlusion as well as regional vascular anatomy.

MRCP is the method of choice to visualize the characteristic features of pancreatic head adenocarcinoma including encasement and obstruction of the pancreatic duct or bile duct. The well-known "double duct sign" occurs in 77% of the cases, while biliary duct stenosis alone may be observed in about 9% as well as pancreatic duct stenosis alone (about 12%) (Fulcher et al. 1998). While the detection of even small peripancreatic lymph nodes is now possible on MRI, the accurate differentiation between malignant and reactive enlarged lymph nodes is still a diagnostic challenge that remains unresolved until today. In contrast, MR using gadolinium DTPA has greater accuracy in the detection and characterization of liver metastasis compared with helical CT (Martin and Semelka 2000; Freeny 1999).

2.3.2 Cystic Pancreas Tumor

Cystic tumors of the pancreas are rare but must be considered in every patient with cystic lesions of the pancreas. In contrast to solid tumors of the pancreas where adenocarcinomas are predominant, there is a wide variation of histologic findings, dignity, and prognosis of cystic tumors. In addition, known entities have been better classified as new ones are described. For example, many pancreatic neoplasms, including those previously termed papillary carcinomas, ductectatic mucinous cystadenomas, villous adenomas, and mucin-producing tumors of the pancreas, are now classified as intraductal papillary mucinous neoplasms (IPMN) of the pancreas. Once considered a rare tumor, now they are increasingly recognized at CT and MR imaging. Therefore, radiologic differentiation between benign and malignant lesions is important in the determination of the appropriate treatment.

The presence of mural nodules, mural thickening, and contrast enhancement is suggestive of malignancy; however, the absence of mural nodules or enhancement does not indicate that the tumor is benign (Fig. 2.5). A maximum main pancreatic duct diameter of greater than 15 mm and diffuse dilatation of the main pancreatic duct are suggestive of malignancy in main duct-

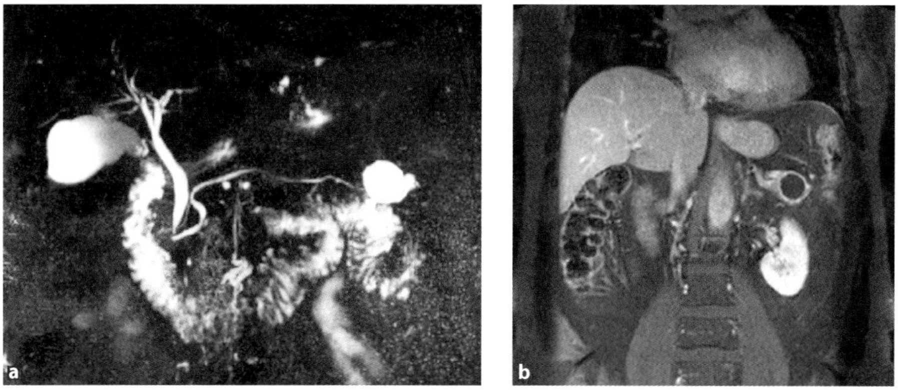

Fig. 2.5a,b MRI of a patient with a cystic neuroendocrine carcinoma in the pancreatic tail. **a** MRCP shows a normal pancreatic duct and the cystic lesion in the tail. **b** On post-contrast images, the thin enhancing rim of the lesion is visible, implicating a cystic tumor

type tumors. Among branch duct-type tumors, malignant tumors tend to be larger than benign tumors; however, this finding is variable. The presence of main pancreatic duct dilatation may be helpful in determining malignancy of branch duct-type tumors.

The treatment decision with regard to cystic neoplasms often is based on the patient's age at presentation, the lesion location, the sex and the presence or absence of symptoms, and malignant features (Kosmahl et al. 2004; Sahani et al. 2006).

In contrast to other cystic neoplasms, IPMN have a communication to the pancreatic duct but should be differentiated from pseudocysts by CT or MRI. MRI using the MRCP technique may show whether a pancreatic cystic lesion communicates with the main pancreatic duct (MPD) and demonstrate the extent of ductal involvement (Irie et al. 2000; Sugiyama et al. 1998). Due to improvements in CT technology including image post-processing such as curved reformation, the capability of CT for the evaluation of the pancreatic parenchyma and the pancreatic ducts in patients with IPMN is enhanced (Fig. 2.1).

2.4 Resectability

Resectability of pancreatic cancer usually is assessed according to presence of infiltration of adjacent tissue or vessels. In some studies, lymph node involvement and distant metastases are used as additional parameters, resulting in a strong influence of the results of the studies (Bluemke et al. 1995; Warshaw et al. 1990). CT has still shown discouraging results with lymph node assessment in pancreatic cancer. Despite advances in CT techniques, differentiation based on a morphologic parameter is not sufficient because of the small size (<1.2 cm) of many malignant lymph nodes, which is next to the commonly used cutoff size (>1 cm) used to differentiate between benign and malignant lymph nodes. (Robinson and Sheridan 2000; Taoka et al. 1999; Freeny et al. 1993).

The grading of tumor involvement of the portal and superior mesenteric veins and the celiac, hepatic, and superior mesenteric arteries based on circumferential contiguity of tumor to vessel as proposed by Lu et al. (1997) is a practicable tool for daily clinical practice (Fig. 2.6). The splenic artery has not usually been considered as critical for surgical resection. Based on a five-point scale (grade 0, no contiguity of tumor to vessel; grade 1, tumor contiguity of less than one-quarter circumference; grade 2, between one-quarter and one-half circumference; grade 3, between one-half and three-quarters circumference; and grade 4, greater than three-quarters circumferential involvement or any vessel constriction), Lu et al. obtained a sensitivity of 84%

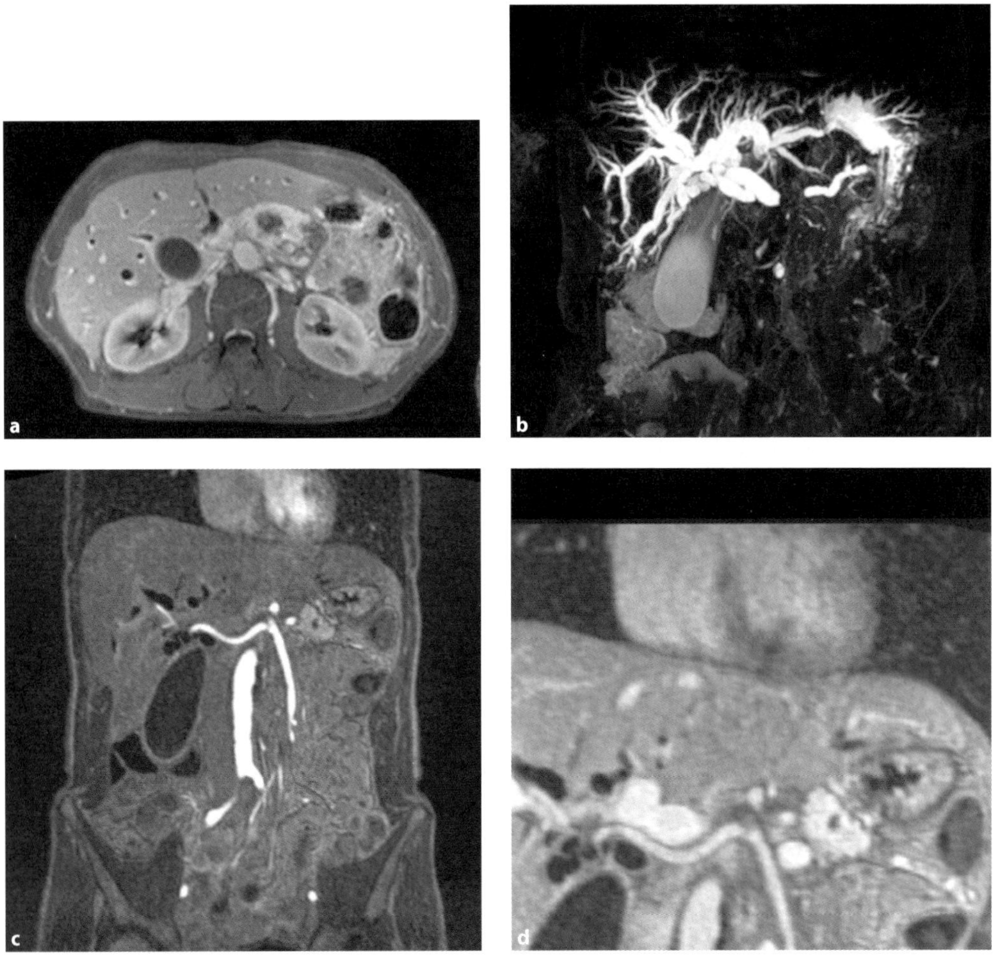

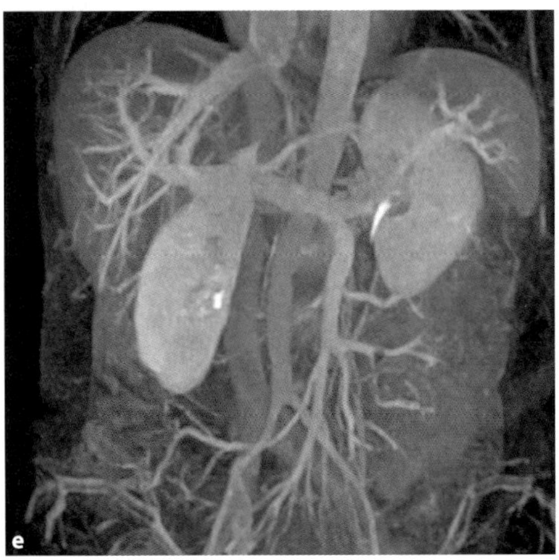

Fig. 2.6a–e All-in-one MRI in a patient with irresectable adenocarcinoma of the pancreas. **a** Contrast-enhanced T1 weighted images with fat suppression demonstrates the necrotic center of the tumor located in the pancreatic corpus but fails in the determination of the extension of the tumor. **b** MRCP shows the typical double duct sign, indicating that the tumor involves the pancreatic head. **c** Arterial MR angiography (single slice) shows aberrant origin of the hepatic artery from the superior mesenteric artery (SMA). The shifting of the SMA indicates as well a large tumor of the head. **d** Augmented view of arterial MR angiography: note the small hypodense structure over the liver artery and between celiac trunk and SMA, which was confirmed as a malignant infiltration intraoperatively. **e** Portal venous MR angiography (3D reconstruction) shows only a minor reduction of the vessel caliber around the confluens region

and a specificity of 98% for unresectability when a threshold between group 2 and group 3 was chosen. With regard to the sensitivity, specificity, and accuracy in the detection of vascular infiltration, Furukawa et al. (1998) had similar results (83.0%, 100.0%, and 89.0%). However, this score only provides a statistical probability whether a patient is resectable or not and may not substitute for surgical exploration in many cases today (Varadhachary et al. 2006).

When compared with MRI, CT still faces the problem of low contrast between the lesion and the surrounding tissue. Although some publications demonstrate that combined arterial and venous phase CT scanning will detect even small lesions, the probability of detection is reduced.

For MRI, the positive and negative predictive values for cancer nonresectability of unenhanced and contrast-enhanced MR were 90% and 83%, respectively, and the accuracy, sensitivity, and specificity were reported to be 85%, 69%, and 95%, respectively (Lopez Hänninen et al. 2002). Malignant encasement of the vessels may be optimally visualized using contrast-enhanced dynamic images.

2.5 Conclusions

In conclusion, a combination of several phases, or at least an arterial or pancreatic parenchymal phase and a portal venous phase, is essential for an optimal multiphasic CT protocol for the comprehensive evaluation of pancreatic adenocarcinomas. The addition of multiplanar and curved reformations may increase the sensitivity of CT and improves its agreement with surgical findings. Beyond abdominal MR imaging, techniques such as magnetic resonance cholangiopancreaticography (MRCP) and MR angiography should be integrated in the imaging protocol whenever possible.

Cross-sectional imaging of the pancreas enables a reliable detection rate of pancreatic tumors and is useful for the differentiation between benign and malignant lesions. Vascular infiltration as a main predictor of resectability may be visualized or excluded in most of the cases. While the differentiation of lymph node involvement is still an unsolved diagnostic challenge in imaging of pancreatic cancer, distant metastases in the liver and other organs may be detected accurately by both imaging methods.

References

Baum U, Lell M, Nomayr A (1999) Multiplanar spiral CT in the diagnosis of pancreatic tumors [in German]. Radiologe 39:958–964

Bluemke DA, Cameron JL, Hruban RH, et al. (1995) Potentially resectable pancreatic adenocarcinoma: spiral CT assessment with surgical and pathologic correlation. Radiology 197:381–385

Catalano C, Laghi A, Fraioli F (2003) Pancreatic carcinoma: the role of high-resolution multislice spiral CT in the diagnosis and assessment of resectability. Eur Radiol 13:149–156

Freeny PC (1999) Pancreatic imaging: new modalities. Gastroenterol Clin North Am 28:723–744

Freeny PC, Traverso LW, Ryan JA (1993) Diagnosis and staging of pancreatic adenocarcinoma with dynamic computed tomography. Am J Surg 165:600–606

Fuhrman GM, Charnsangavej C, Abbruzzese JL (1994) Thin-section contrast-enhanced computed tomography accurately predicts the resectability of malignant pancreatic neoplasms. Am J Surg 167:104–111

Fulcher AS, Turner M (1999) MR pancreatography: a useful tool for evaluating pancreatic disorders. Radiographics 19:5–24

Fulcher AS, Turner MA, Capps GW, Zfass AM, Baker KM (1998) Half-Fourier RARE MRCP in 300 subjects. Radiology 207:21–32

Furukawa H, Kosuge T, Mukai K (1998) Helical computed tomography in the diagnosis of portal vein invasion by pancreatic head carcinoma: usefulness for selecting surgical procedures and predicting the outcome. Arch Surg 133:61–65

Gehl HB, Urhahn R, Bohndorf K, Klever P, Hauptmann S, Lodemann KP, Matern S, Schumpelick V, Gunther RW, et al. (1993) Mn-DPDP in MR imaging of pancreatic adenocarcinoma: initial clinical experience. Radiology 186:795–798

Graf O, Boland GW, Warshaw AL, Fernandez-del-Castillo C, Hahn PF, Mueller PR (1997) Arterial versus portal venous helical CT for revealing pancreatic adenocarcinoma: conspicuity of tumor and critical vascular anatomy. AJR Am J Roentgenol 169:119–123

Ichikawa T, Erturk SM, Sou H (2006) MDCT of pancreatic adenocarcinoma: optimal imaging phases and multiplanar reformatted imaging. AJR Am J Roentgenol 187:1513–1520
Irie H, Honda H, Aibe H, et al. (2000) MR cholangiopancreatographic differentiation of benign and malignant intraductal mucin-producing tumors of the pancreas. AJR Am J Roentgenol 174:1403–1408
Kettritz U, Schlund JF, Wilbur K, Eisenberg LB, Semelka RC (1996) Comparison of gadolinium chelates with manganese-DPDP for liver lesion detection and characterization: preliminary results. Magn Reson Imaging 14:1185–1190
Kosmahl M, Pauser U, Peters K, Sipos B, Luttges J, Kremer B, Kloppel G (2004) Cystic neoplasms of the pancreas and tumor-like lesions with cystic features: a review of 418 cases and a classification proposal. Virchows Arch 445:168–178
Lopez Hänninen E, Amthauer H, Hosten N (2002) Prospective evaluation of pancreatic tumours: accuracy of MR imaging with MR cholangiopancreatography and MR angiography. Radiology 224:34–41
Lu DS, Reber HA, Krasny RM, Kadell BM, Sayre J (1997) Local staging of pancreatic cancer: criteria for unresectability of major vessels as revealed by pancreatic-phase, thin-section helical CT. AJR Am J Roentgenol 168:1439–1443
Malka D, Hammel P, Maire F, et al. (2002) Risk of pancreatic adenocarcinoma in chronic pancreatitis. Gut 51:849–852
Martin DR, Semelka RC (2000) MR imaging of pancreatic masses. Magn Reson Imaging Clin N Am 8:787–812
Morakkabati-Spitz N, Willinek WA, von Falkenhausen M (2002) Is a dynamic MRI examination of the pancreas still necessary? Rofo Fortschr Geb Rontgenstr Neuen Bildgeb Verfahr 174:433–436
Petersein J, Reisinger W, Hamm B (2002) Diagnostic value of secretin injections in dynamic MR pancreatography. Rofo Fortschr Geb Rontgenstr Neuen Bildgeb Verfahr 174:437–443
Richter GM, Simon C, Hoffmann V (1996) Hydrospiral CT of the pancreas in thin section technique [in German]. Radiologe 36:397–405
Robinson PJ, Sheridan MB (2000) Pancreatitis: computed tomography and magnetic resonance imaging. Eur Radiol 10:401–408
Romijn MG, Stoker J, van Eijck CH (2000) MRI with mangafodipir trisodium in the detection and staging of pancreatic cancer. J Magn Reson Imaging 12:261–268
Sahani DV, Kadavigere R, Blake M, Fernandez-Del Castillo C, Lauwers GY, Hahn PF (2006) Intraductal papillary mucinous neoplasm of pancreas: multidetector row CT with 2D curved reformations—correlation with MRCP. Radiology 238:560–569
Schima W, Ba-Ssalamah A (1999) Radiologic staging of liver and pancreatic malignancies [in German]. Radiologe 39:568–577
Sugiyama M, Atomi Y, Hachiya J (1998) Intraductal papillary tumors of the pancreas: evaluation with magnetic resonance cholangiopancreatography. Am J Gastroenterol 93:156–159
Taoka H, Hauptmann E, Traverso LW, Barnett MJ, Sarr MG, Reber HA (1999) How accurate is helical computed tomography for clinical staging of pancreatic cancer? Am J Surg 177:428–432
Varadhachary G, Tamm E, Abbruzzese J (2006) Borderline resectable pancreatic cancer: definitions, management, and role of preoperative therapy. Ann Surg Oncol 13:1035–1046
Warshaw AL, Gu ZY, Wittenberg J, Waltman AC (1990) Preoperative staging and assessment of resectability of pancreatic cancer. Arch Surg 125:230–233

3 Nuclear Medical Methods for the Diagnosis of Pancreatic Cancer: Positron Emission Tomography

H. Amthauer, J. Ruf

Recent Results in Cancer Research, Vol. 177

Abstract

The functional imaging approach of nuclear medicine offers important information for the characterization of a tumor's pathobiology. In oncology, positron emission tomography (PET) especially has had great impact on the staging of tumor patients and the assessment of therapy. Both the development of new, tumor-specific, tracers and the introduction of by software- and hardware-driven image fusion emphasize the potential of this modality for an all-embracing diagnostic modality.

3.1 Introduction

More than 90% of malignant pancreatic tumors are constituted by ductal adenocarcinomas, which are characterized by their poor prognosis (mean survival 13–15 months in case of locally confined disease; 3–6 months in case of systemic spread) (Gold and Goldin 1998; Pakzad et al. 2006). Currently no screening test for the early detection of pancreatic carcinoma exists. Although some cancers are detected coincidentally, more are detected at an advanced stage due to the initial lack of clinical symptoms.

As cure by surgery is only possible at the early stages, there is a need for timely detection, preferably by noninvasive diagnostic modalities (Higashi et al. 2003).

Apart from accurate detection, imaging modalities must also meet the following demands: differentiation from inflammatory pancreatic disease, assessment of metastatic spread, therapy control, and the detection of recurrence. Conventional imaging work-up usually consists of endoscopy with X-ray examination (endoscopic retrograde cholangiopancreatography, ERCP), (endo-)sonography, computed tomography (CT), magnetic resonance imaging (MRI), or a combination of them that offers anatomical information at the high spatial resolution necessary for the assessment of the primary structures and possible infiltration of neighboring structures.

These methods can be subdivided into invasive procedures such as endoscopy or endosonography that also allow interventions (e.g., Stent-placement) or biopsies (Ponchon and Pilleul 2002; Harewood and Wiersema 2002) and noninvasive imaging modalities, for which spiral CT is considered the standard imaging modality with a sensitivity between 69% and 92% and a specificity of 74%–100% for the detection of pancreatic carcinoma (Freeny 2001). While the introduction of multislice CT (MSCT) greatly improved the accuracy of CT (Catalano et al. 2003), MRI has also experienced technical improvements in recent years. This is especially true for the performance of additional MRCP and MR angiography in one imaging session (so-called "one-stop-shop"), which leads to sensitivities of up to 95% and specificities up to 82% for carcinoma detection (Lopez Hänninen et al. 2002; Ishiguchi et al. 2001).

Apart from the initial diagnosis of pancreatic carcinoma, imaging modalities are faced with the problem of differentiating tumor from chronic pancreatitis. Although morphologic imaging allows a sufficiently reliable detection of pancreatic lesions, a specific characterization, crucial for the differentiation of benign from malignant disease is often impossible. Moreover, both MRI and CT are limited in the accurate assessment of prognostic factors such as resectability or exclusion of distant metastases (Hanbidge 2002).

Both difficulties are the result of the fact that imaging modalities based on the visualization of anatomic details do not pay sufficient attention to an important aspect of tumor biology, the pathobiochemical changes associated with malignant transformation.

In contrast, the assessment of cellular characteristics such as metabolism and receptor expression is the domain of nuclear medicine. Thus, even in structures with similar morphology, the functional imaging approach can differentiate viable tumor tissue from e.g., fibrosis due to a difference in tracer uptake. Another advantage of the usually systemically administered tracers is that whole-body examinations are routinely performed, while most conventional imaging modalities are often limited to a specific region. As the pathophysiologic changes on the cellular level occur ahead of the anatomical changes on the macroscopic level, functional imaging can also provide important information concerning the assessment of therapy and prognosis.

3.2 Introduction to Nuclear Medicine Imaging

Conventional scintigraphy is usually based on the acquisition of emitted gamma-quants summed in anterior and posterior projection (planar scintigraphy). In order to increase spatial resolution and to gain information on three-dimensional tracer distribution, single photon emission tomography (SPECT) of the region in question can be performed and visualized in axial, coronal, or sagittal slicing. Somatostatin receptor scintigraphy in pancreatic tumors with neuroendocrine differentiation is a good example of a well-established tumor scintigraphy that benefits greatly from SPECT and especially hybrid SPECT/CT imaging (de Herder et al. 2005; Amthauer et al. 2005). Moreover, a bone scan may be performed if osseous metastases are suspected. More experimental approaches, still limited to studies, aim at the direct visualization and therapy of pancreatic adenocarcinoma by labeling antibodies with diagnostic and therapeutic nuclides respectively (Cardillo et al. 2004).

Positron emission tomography (PET) offers an even higher spatial resolution than SPECT and, in contrast to SPECT, allows three-dimensional visualization of the whole body. Moreover, the correction of photons for scatter and attenuation allows a determination of the concentration of the tracer in the target region of interest (ROI) or target volume of interest (VOI). This semiquantification is usually expressed as the so-called "standardized uptake value" (SUV), which reflects tracer uptake in relation to the activity administered (corrected for decay) and the body weight or mass of the patient. The resulting SUVs can then be used for intra- and interindividual comparisons.

While the traditional synthesis of functional scintigraphy and morphologic imaging as a side-by-side analysis has already greatly improved the information output of either examination, the pinnacle of this combined imaging approach is seen in the visualization of the information from both examinations in one image. For a clinical routine, software-based retrospective image fusion of separately acquired sets of data (CT, MRT, SPECT, PET) is feasible and has been validated in several studies (Amthauer et al. 2004, 2005; Ruf et al. 2006; Lemke et al. 2004). Meanwhile, both hybrid SPECT/CT and PET/CT systems are available that allow an almost simultaneous acquisition of imaging data, resulting in inherently fused images.

3.3 Positron Emission Tomography

F18-fluorodeoxyglucose positron emission tomography (FDG-PET) is increasingly becoming an important diagnostic pillar in oncology. Concerning pancreatic carcinoma, it has shown its value in the initial detection, the differentiation from pancreatitis, and the preoperative exclusion of distant metastases. In contrast to conventional imaging modalities, FDG-PET also allows a reliable detection of disease recurrence. Moreover, the assessment of glucose metabolism permits assumptions on response to therapy and prognosis. Finally, not only due to the use of hybrid PET/CT devices but also the development of more tumor-specific tracers, another breakthrough in the field of functional imaging is promising.

3.3.1 Methodic Fundamentals for the Use of FDG-PET in Pancreatic Carcinoma

3.3.1.1 Physical Aspects

In PET, both the physical prerequisites as well as the biochemical and radiochemical properties of the PET tracer have to be taken into account. The generation of a measurable signal depends on the one hand on the relation between systemic spatial resolution and tumor size and on the other hand on the relation between tracer uptake and tumor metabolism.

In essence, spatial resolution is determined by the positron energy of the nuclide utilized (effective positron range), the diameter of the PET scanner (non-colinearity), and the detector itself (material and size of a single detector-element). In the case of the most commonly used PET nuclide, fluor-18, current clinical scanners achieve a spatial resolution of approximately 4 mm. In principle, smaller structures can be detected provided that the tracer accumulation is sufficient to overcome the resulting partial volume effect (Cherry et al. 2003).

3.3.1.2 Mechanisms of Cellular Glucose Uptake

The use of radioactive glucose for tumor imaging is based on the observations of Otto Warburg et al. (1924) who noted an increased glycolysis in malignant cells. In the case of FDG, labeling is performed by replacing the hydroxyl group at the second carbon atom with the positron emitter F18. Although FDG also experiences cellular uptake via glucose transporters and consecutive phosphorylation, in contrast to regular glucose it is not subject to the further path of glycolysis. The result is an intracellular accumulation of the tracer, the so-called "metabolic trapping." As this accumulation is proportional to the glucose intake of the target tissue, metabolically active tumor tissue can be visualized. However, it has to be noted that, depending on the tumor entity, varying degrees of enzymatic activity and transport molecules exist, ultimately influencing cellular glucose accumulation (Arora et al. 1992; Smith 1999; Smith 2000). Concerning pancreatic cancer cells, an increased expression of transmembranous transport proteins such as GLUT-1 or the increased enzymatic activity of hexokinase have been identified as influential factors (Reske et al. 1997; Higashi et al. 1998, 2002; Pessin and Bell 1992).

As the PET signal is generated by the activity accumulated within a voxel of 4 mm edge length, it must be noted that the above-mentioned partial volume effects not only affect structures smaller than 4 mm, but also that the visualization of larger structures is basically the result of the respective partial volume effects of neighboring voxels. This fact emphasizes that apart from the glucose avidity of a single cell, cellularity, i.e., the cellular content per volume unit, is of great importance for tumor imaging. As pancreatic carcinoma is often accompanied by desmoplastic reactions, the bad ratio of cellular content and extracellular matrix may cause a limited sensitivity of PET (Higashi et al. 1998). One study reported several cases of tumors as large as 6 cm that did not show an elevated glucose metabolism (Higashi et al. 2003). The low cellularity as a cause of nondetection is especially plausible for the scirrhous type of adenocarcinoma, but conflicting reports exist with regards to cystic tumors (Kasperk et al. 2001; Berger et al. 2004; Sperti et al. 2005)

3.3.1.3 Clinical Factors

Hyperglycemia prior to the FDG examination has been reported to negatively affect tracer uptake (Diederichs et al. 1998). Although the actual impact of hyperglycemia is still the subject of debate, a diabetic state has to be expected in a large number of pancreatic cancer patients, either caused by the tumor itself or due to preexisting chronic pancreatitis. The results of our own analysis of 174 patients with pancreatic masses showed no statistically significant difference between the patient group with and without diabetes.

Other potential factors affecting uptake might be acute phases in patients with chronic pancreatitis or inflammatory reactions after interventional procedures, e.g., stent-insertion or dilation. The reason for this possibility lies in the increased FDG uptake of activated leukocytes (mainly monocytes), which suggests the tracers' value in inflammatory imaging. However, it also signifies that FDG is not tumor-specific, and the differentiation between benign inflammation and pancreatic carcinoma is difficult (Diederichs et al. 2000), not to mention the fact that more than 24% of the FDG uptake in cancer is due to the accompanying inflammatory reactions (Kubota et al. 1994).

According to our own data, endoscopic examinations (i.e., ERC/ERCP or ultrasound) and especially manipulations do have an influence on FDG uptake and thus specificity. Specificity of FDG-PET was with 76.9% higher in those patients that had no ERC/ERCP prior to the PET scan when compared to those that did (64%). Up to the present, no valid data on this issue or recommendations concerning a "safety interval" between intervention and PET scan exist.

3.3.1.4 Scanning Parameter for FDG-PET

A PET examination roughly consists of the intravenous tracer injection, an uptake phase for tracer distribution, and the actual scan. Especially the length of the uptake phase is currently under debate. Although the guideline of the European Association of Nuclear Medicine describes an uptake phase of approximately 60 min as sufficient (Bombardieri et al. 2003), there is a tendency for longer uptake phases (up to 2–3 h) in more recent publications, as the glucose uptake in malignomas usually increases with uptake time, thus allowing for a better specificity (Nakamoto et al. 2000).

Unfortunately, this is not true for all patients. Higashi and coworkers (2003) examined 68 patients with suspected pancreatic cancer by measuring glucose uptake 1 and 2 h after tracer injection and found 13 patients who did show a decrease in FDG uptake in the late scan, whereas 3 patients even had no noticeable uptake at all. Therefore we also adapted our scanning protocol according to their recommendations: static whole-body examination 1 h after tracer injection.

1. If positive, end of examination.
2. If negative or unambiguous, a second scan of the pancreatic region is performed 2 h after tracer injection.

3.3.1.5 Semiquantification by Standard Uptake Values

In PET imaging, the tracer uptake in a target region is measured as the standard uptake value (SUV) and reflects the radioactivity concentration within the target tissue divided by the whole body activity concentration (including tracer excretion). The tissue activity concentration (corrected for decay) is defined by an ROI or VOI (measured in Becquerel per gram, milliliter, or cm^2) whereas the whole-body activity concentration is defined as injected activity (in Becquerels) divided by the patient's respective body surface area, weight, or volume (Thie 2004). Most studies usually refer to the maximal SUV, SUVmax, that represents the maximal pixel or voxel activity of the target ROI or VOI, respectively.

3.3.1.6 Visual Versus Semiquantitative Analysis

In the middle of the 1990s, the first studies on use of semiquantification by SUV for a more objective differentiation of pancreatic carcinoma from pancreatitis were published (Inokuma et al. 1995; Koyama et al. 2001; Zimny et al. 1997; Nakata et al. 2001). However, in comparison to these one-time measurements a more reliable differentiation appears achievable by dynamic protocols that pay tribute to tracer kinetics (Voth et al. 2003; Higashi et al. 2002).

In our patient collective, an SUV of 2–13 for benign pancreatic lesions (mean: 3.6) and 2–43 for malignant lesions (mean: 4.9) was measured. Consecutive receiver operating characteristic (ROC) analysis revealed a cut-off value of 3.7 for the differentiation of benign from malignant lesions. The large overlap in SUVs for benign and malignant disease indicates the need for a critical approach to SUV utilization. Factors such as blood glucose level, body size, the length of the uptake phase, the shape and size of ROI or VOI, reconstruction parameters, and attenuation correction have to be heeded (Thie 2004). This also implies that SUV thresholds determined at one institution cannot simply be transferred to other institutions unless parameters are kept the same (Keyes 1995; Nitzsche et al. 2002).

3.4 Detection of Pancreatic Carcinoma and Differentiation from Pancreatitis

A summary of published FDG-PET studies on pancreatic cancer published form 1997 to 2005 resulted in a sensitivity of 71%–100% and a specificity of 60%–100% (Table 3.1).

Although our own results showed a high sensitivity (96%) for the detection of pancreatic carcinoma when FDG-PET was analyzed visually, we could not reproduce the high specificities reported in the literature. Using visual analysis, specificity was 35%, whereas the use of the ROC-derived SUV threshold of 3.7 only raised specificity to 68%. Therefore, the value of FDG-PET for the differentiation of pancreatitis and pancreatic carcinoma has to be regarded with care as semiquantitative imaging does not sufficiently improve specificity and the data on delayed, dual-phase, or kinetic imaging are scarce or controversial.

Despite this skepticism, the high variability in sensitivity and specificity reported must also be analyzed with regards to the patient collective, tumor size/stage, and preexistent imaging information. As a consequence, the true potential of FDG-PET can only be assessed when an

Table 3.1 Results of studies published on the use of FDG-PET in the diagnosis of pancreatic cancer

Author	Journal	Year	Pat. (*n*)	Average SUV in pancreatic cancer	FDG-PET			Computed tomography		
					Sensitivity %	Specificity %	Accuracy %	Sensitivity %	Specificity %	Accuracy %
Zimny	*Eur J Nucl Med*	1997	106	6.4+3.6	85	84	85	-	-	-
Keogan	*Am J of Roentg*	1998	37	-	88	83	-	75	83	-
Higashi	*J Nucl Med*	1998	34	4.3+1.3	93	67	88	-	-	-
Debelke	*J Nucl Med*	1999	65	5.1+2.6	92	85	91	-	-	-
Imdahl	*Br J Surg*	1999	48	7.3+2.9	96	100	-	81	89	-
Nakamoto	*Cancer*	2000	47	5.0+2.3	96	75	87	-	-	-
Diederichs	*Pancreas*	2000	159	-	-	-	86	-	-	82
Sendlar	*World J Surg*	2000	42	-	71	64	69	74	46	68
Kasperk	*World J Surg*	2001	124	-	84	66	-	82	61	-
Kalady	*Ann Surg Oncol*	2002	54	-	88	92	-	65	87	-
Koyama	*AnnNucl Med*	2002	86	3.5+1.7	82	81	81	91	62	84
Papos	*Clin Nucl Med*	2002	22	-	100	88	91	100	50	64
Higashi	*Ann Nucl Med*	2003	53	-	65	93	81	-	-	-
Lytras	*Dig Surg*	2005	112	-	73	60	64	89	65	62
Lemke	*J Nucl Med*	2004	104		84	61	-	77	64	-
Nishiyama	*Nucl Med*	2005	86	5.75±2.69	89[a]	71[a]	83[a]	-	-	-
	Comm			7.37±4.07	93[b]	71[b]	85[b]	-	-	-

SUV, standardized uptake value

[a,b] Patients studied in dual-phase technique (scanned 1 h[a] and 2 h[b]) after tracer injection

appropriate diagnostic algorithm on the basis of pretest likelihood is developed. A first analysis by Heinrich and coworkers (2005) showed that in case of a positive CT scan prior to PET imaging, FDG-PET achieved a sensitivity of 92% and a specificity of 68% for the detection of pancreatic malignoma. In case of a negative CT scan, FDG-PET achieved a sensitivity of 73% while specificity increased to 86%. In contrast, patients with unambiguous findings in CT showed detection of cancer by FDG-PET with a sensitivity of 100% and a specificity of 68% (Fig. 3.1). Although preliminary, Heinrich and coworkers' results confirm the need for staging algorithms that pay tribute to the strengths and weaknesses of either method.

3.5 Staging of Pancreatic Carcinoma by FDG-PET

3.5.1 T Stage

The determination of the T stage is limited by the spatial resolution of PET having poor anatomical orientation. Although the introduction of PET/

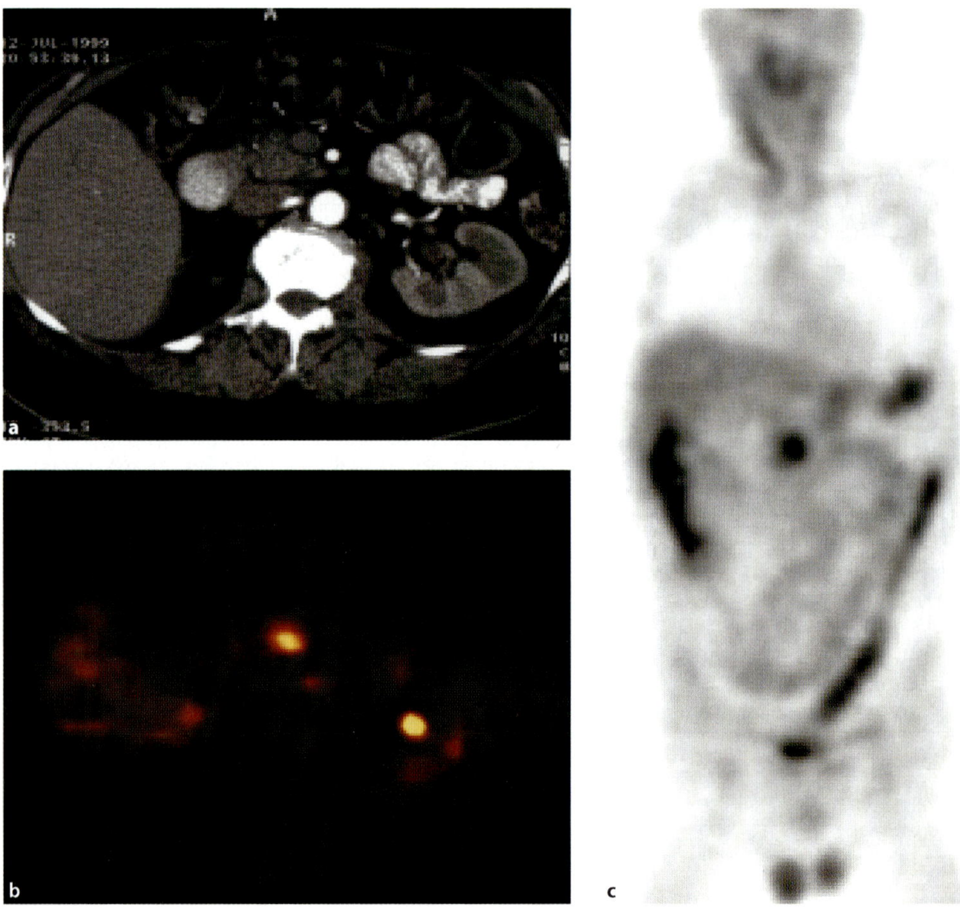

Fig. 3.1a–c A 54-year-old male patient with an inconclusive mass in the pancreatic head in MSCT **a** FDG-PET shows a significantly increased tracer uptake in the pancreatic head (SUVmax 5.1). The whole-body scan showed no evidence for locoregional (**b**) or distant metastases (**c**). Histology after surgery revealed an adenocarcinoma of pancreatic head [pT2N0(0/9)]

CT improves the topographical focus assignment in pancreatic cancer, it is doubtful that the determination of, e.g., infiltration will surpass that of multislice CT or MRI alone, as the true spatial extent of a tumor is difficult to assess by metabolic imaging and the "size" of the focus is largely dependent on the window/threshold chosen (Ruf et al. 2006).

3.5.2 N Stage

The detection and assessment of lymph node metastases is limited in both FDG-PET and conventional imaging.

In our own analysis of 53 patients, FDG-PET achieved a sensitivity of 63% and a specificity of 93%, a result comparable to the data in the literature, which reports a sensitivity of 41%–71% and a specificity of 63%–100% (Higashi et al. 2003; Pakzad et al. 2006). The low sensitivity is partially explained by partial volume effects in small lymphatic lesions that cause a lesser signal than the primary. Moreover, the focus of a peripancreatic lymph node may appear "merged" with that of the pancreatic primary, making the classification as separated lesions difficult unless morphological information is at hand.

3.5.3 M Stage

As the exclusion of distant metastases is crucial for the performance of curative surgery, FDG-PET has a decisive advantage due to the whole-body technique (Fig. 3.2).

Most frequently metastases to the lung, the bone marrow, and especially the liver are encountered. Fröhlich and coworkers (1999) reported in a preoperative study on 168 patients a sensitivity of 68% for the detection liver metastases. Their subanalysis revealed the difficulty of FDG-PET for the detection of small lesions (<1 cm; sensitivity 43%), whereas larger lesions were detected in 97% of all cases. Our own results confirm this observation with a sensitivity of 43% and 97% for metastases smaller and larger than 1 cm respectively. The reasons for the low sensitivity in small lesions are probably partial volume effects again, which especially in hepatic metastases may hinder diagnosis due to the physiological FDG uptake of hepatic tissue. Moreover, false positives based on cholangitic reactions in case of cholestasis may also occur.

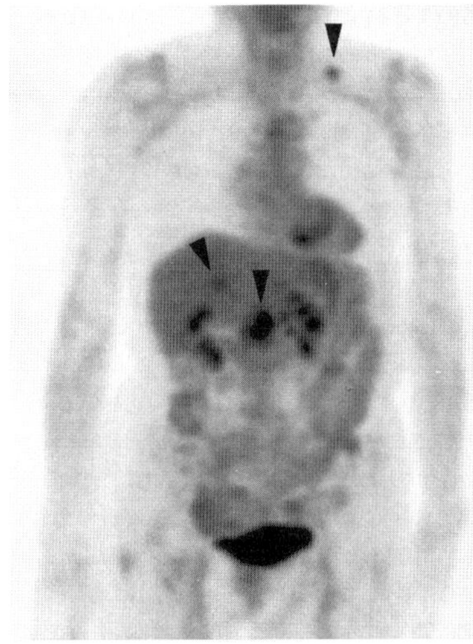

Fig. 3.2 A 63-year-old female patient with tumor-suspicious lesion in the pancreatic head. Whole-body FDG-PET detected not only the primary tumor, but also hepatic metastases and a supraclavicular lymph node metastasis (Virchow's gland)

Despite these limitations, an impact of up to 40% on the decision of the therapeutic strategy has been reported (Higashi et al. 2003; Delbeke et al. 1999).

3.6 Assessment of Prognosis

In addition to established prognostic factors for pancreatic carcinoma such as tumor stage or the height of the CA 19-9 tumor marker level, the information gained on tumor biology by metabolic FDG-PET imaging appears to deliver further information for the assessment of survival. Detailed information of the prognostic relevance of FDG-PET and the assessment of response to therapy are given in Chap. 12.

3.7 Tracers Beyond FDG

As mentioned earlier, FDG is the most common but not the only PET tracer available. For example, in the case of pancreatic tumors with neuroendocrine differentiation, somatostatin receptor PET, in analogy to somatostatin receptor scintigraphy, has become a powerful tool for the assessment of disease extent (Kowalski et al. 2003). Although the initial attempts to visualize the adenocarcinoma of the pancreas by C11-acetate (synthesis of membrane components) (Rasmussen et al. 2004) or F18-FET (amino acid metabolism) (Pauleit et al. 2005) did not prove superior to FDG, the multitude of possible combinations of ligands and positron emitting nuclides indicate the potential of PET for the assessment of tumor pathobiology, as it comes closest to the ideal of true molecular imaging. However, although PET imaging does allow for an accurate depiction, e.g., gene transfection both in vitro and in vivo (Peñuelas et al. 2005; Gambhir et al. 1998), its usefulness will be linked to the clinical realization of such therapy concepts.

3.8 Image Fusion and PET/CT

Tracer research is not the only rapidly growing field in PET imaging. With the introduction of improved hardware (e.g., new detector crystals) and software allowing for a new generation of tomographs with a higher sensitivity and better spatial resolution, the recent breakthrough of nuclear medicine imaging is the integration of functional images gained by PET and morphological images gained by CT or MRI into one image as opposed to classical side-by-side analysis (Table 3.2). This so-called image fusion was initially based on software techniques, which retrospectively generate a single data set of the separately acquired volume data of PET and CT/MRI, ready for fused visualization. Most works in this field concerning abdominal imaging have concentrated on algorithms based on "mutual information," software programs that perform a voxel-by-voxel comparison of both volume data sets in order to generate a congruent overlay of both examinations. Our group as well evaluated the image fusion of CT and FDG-PET in 102 patients with suspected pancreatic cancer with the help of such an algorithm. In 96.2% of all patients, image fusion was technically successful and the data generated were evaluable. The overall detection rate for pancreatic cancer in the fused PET/CT images was 89.1%, making it superior to the single interpretation of either CT (76.6%) or FDG-PET (84.4%) (Lemke et al. 2004). Another study compared PET/MR-fused images to the standard side-by-side analysis in

Table 3.2 Results of studies published on image fusion or the use of integrated PET-CT for the diagnosis of pancreatic cancer

Author	Journal	Year	Pat. (*n*)	Average SUV	Modality	Sensitivity	Specificity
Lemke	*J Nucl Med*	2004	104 (100)	-	PET	84	61
					CT	77	64
					Fusion	89	64
Heinrich	*Ann of Surg*	2005	59	-	PET	-	-
					CT	-	-
					PET/CT	89	69
Ruf	*Pancreatology*	2006	32	5.10 ± 1.66	PET[a]	93	41
					MRI[a]	100	76
					Fusion*	100	76

[a] Concerning pancreatic findings (although the specificity of FDG-PET was not improved by image fusion, the topographical assignment of PET foci was greatly facilitated)

32 patients, which resulted in an improved topographical assignment and interpretation of PET foci in 28% of all foci. On the downside, however, it must be noted that due to multiple metastases in those patients, the actual impact of improved focus assignment on therapy was limited (Ruf et al. 2006).

This tendency for integrated imaging took a big step at the end of the 1990s, when the first PET/CT scanners were developed. The acquisition of both data sets is performed in one imaging session, which allows for a direct overlay of both data sets using the respective coordinate system based on the position of the examination table. As a consequence of the almost simultaneous data acquisition, the technical success rate of image fusion is very high, as motion and/or positioning artifacts encountered in fusion of separately acquired sets of data can be greatly reduced. Moreover, the attenuation correction of the PET-emission scan is now performed with the rapidly acquired CT-data instead of the conventional, more time-consuming transmission by external Ge68-rod sources. This implies more patient-friendly examination times (approx. 40 instead of 80 min).

The integration of PET and modern multislice CT combines the advantages of both examinations and already has great influence especially in the field of oncology (Beyer et al. 2000; Townsend 2001).

Up to the present, only one study concerning the use of integrated PET/CT for the detection of pancreatic cancer has been published (Heinrich et al. 2005). In their examination of 59 patients with suspected pancreatic cancer, the group also addressed the impact of PET/CT on patient management and its cost-efficiency. Despite the fact that the CT component was only performed in a low-dose technique without contrast enhancement, curative surgery was abandoned in 16% of all patients as PET/CT detected previously unknown metastases. In analogy to the calculations of a preoperative PET trial for lung cancer patients (van Tinteren et al. 2002), the examination itself was even cost-effective (saving US $1.066 per patient) due to the avoidance of noncurative surgery.

On the basis of these preliminary results, the use of a true diagnostic contrast-enhanced PET/CT in pancreatic cancer patients for the selection of patients that will profit from surgery is promising.

3.9 Summary

PET has become an indispensable tool for imaging in oncology. Although the tracer FDG by itself has some limitations for the differentiation of pancreatitis from pancreatic carcinoma, its metabolic information in combination with the anatomical data from MRI or CT either by image fusion or hybrid-devices allows an extensive and complete assessment of the tumor. Apart from mere tumor visualization, the great potential of PET lies on the assessment of metabolic characteristics of the tumor, which in turn could provide useful information for a tailor-made tumor therapy.

References

Amthauer H, Ruf J, Bohmig M, Lopez-Hanninen E, Rohlfing T, Wernecke KD, Plockinger U, Gutberlet M, Lemke AJ, Steinmuller T, Wiedenmann B, Felix R (2004) Diagnosis of neuroendocrine tumours by retrospective image fusion: is there a benefit? Eur J Nucl Med Mol Imaging 31:342–348

Amthauer H, Denecke T, Rohlfing T, Ruf J, Bohmig M, Gutberlet M, Plockinger U, Felix R, Lemke AJ (2005) Value of image fusion using single photon emission computed tomography with integrated low dose computed tomography in comparison with a retrospective voxel-based method in neuroendocrine tumours. Eur Radiol 15:1456–1462

Arora KK, Parry DM, Pedersen PL (1992) Hexokinase receptors: preferential enzyme binding in normal cells to nonmitochondrial sites and in transformed cells to mitochondrial sites. J Bioenerg Biomembr 24:47–53

Berger KL, Nicholson SA, Dehdashti F, Siegel BA (2004) FDG PET evaluation of mucinous neoplasms: correlation of FDG uptake with histopathologic features. AJR Am J Roentgenol 174:1005–1008

Beyer T, Townsend DW, Brun T, Kinahan PE, Charron M, Roddy R, Jerin J, Young J, Byars L, Nutt R (2000) A combined PET/CT scanner for clinical oncology. J Nucl Med 41:1369–1379

Bombardieri E, Aktolun C, Baum RP, Bishof-Delaloye A, Buscombe J, Chatal JF, Maffioli L, Moncayo R, Mortelmans L, Reske SN (2003) FDG-PET: procedure guidelines for tumour imaging. Eur J Nucl Med Mol Imaging 30:BP115–BP124

Cardillo TM, Karacay H, Goldenberg DM, Yeldell D, Chang CH, Modrak DE, Sharkey RM, Gold DV (2004) Improved targeting of pancreatic cancer: experimental studies of a new bispecific antibody, pretargeting enhancement system for immunoscintigraphy. Clin Cancer Res 10:3552–3561

Catalano C, Laghi A, Fraioli F, Pediconi F, Napoli A, Danti M, Reitano I, Passariello R (2003) Pancreatic carcinoma: the role of high-resolution multislice spiral CT in the diagnosis and assessment of resectability. Eur Radiol 13:149–156

Cherry SR, Sorenson SA, Phelps M (2003) Positron emission tomography, physics in nuclear medicine, 3rd edn. Saunders, Philadelphia

de Herder WW, Kwekkeboom DJ, Valkema R, Feelders RA, van Aken MO, Lamberts SW, van der Lely AJ, Krenning EP (2005) Neuroendocrine tumors and somatostatin: imaging techniques. J Endocrinol Invest 28:132–136

Delbeke D, Rose DM, Chapman WC, Pinson CW, Wright JK, Beauchamp RD, Shyr Y, Leach SD (1999) Optimal interpretation of FDG PET in the diagnosis, staging and management of pancreatic carcinoma. J Nucl Med 40:1784–1791

Diederichs CG, Staib L, Glatting G, Beger HG, Reske SN (1998) FDG PET: elevated plasma glucose reduces both uptake and detection rate of pancreatic malignancies. J Nucl Med 39:1030–1033

Diederichs CG, Staib L, Vogel J, Glasbrenner B, Glatting G, Brambs HJ, Beger HG, Reske SN (2000) Values and limitations of 18F-fluorodeoxyglucose-positron-emission tomography with preoperative evaluation of patients with pancreatic masses. Pancreas 20:109–116

Freeny PC (2001) Pancreatic carcinoma: imaging update 2001. Dig Dis 19:37–46

Fröhlich A, Diederichs CG, Staib L, Vogel J, Beger HG, Reske SN (1999) Detection of liver metastases from pancreatic cancer using FDG PET. J Nucl Med 40:250–255

Gambhir SS, Barrio JR, Wu L, Iyer M, Namavari M, Satyamurthy N, Bauer E, Parrish C, MacLaren DC, Borghei AR, Green LA, Sharfstein S, Berk AJ, Cherry SR, Phelps ME, Herschman HR (1998) Imaging of adenoviral-directed herpes simplex virus type 1 thymidine kinase reporter gene expression in mice with radiolabeled ganciclovir. J Nucl Med 39:2003–2011

Gold EB, Goldin SB (1998) Epidemiology of and risk factors for pancreatic cancer. Surg Oncol Clin N Am 7:67–91

Hanbidge AE (2002) Cancer of the pancreas: the best image for early detection—CT, MRI, PET or US? Can J Gastroenterol 16:101–105

Harewood GC, Wiersema MJ (2002) Endosonography-guided fine needle aspiration biopsy in the evaluation of pancreatic masses. Am J Gastroenterol 97:1386–1391

Heinrich S, Goerres GW, Schafer M, Sagmeister M, Bauerfeind P, Pestalozzi BC, Hany TF, von Schulthess GK, Clavien PA (2005) Positron emission tomography/computed tomography influences on the management of resectable pancreatic cancer and its cost-effectiveness. Ann Surg 242:235–243

Higashi T, Tamaki N, Torizuka T, Nakamoto Y, Sakahara H, Kimura T, Honda T, Inokuma T, Katsushima S, Ohshio G, Imamura M, Konishi J (1998) FDG uptake, GLUT-1 glucose transporter and cellularity in human pancreatic tumors. J Nucl Med 39:1727–1735

Higashi T, Saga T, Nakamoto Y, Ishimori T, Mamede MH, Wada M, Doi R, Hosotani R, Imamura M, Konishi J (2002) Relationship between retention index in dual-phase (18)F-FDG PET, and hexokinase-II and glucose transporter-1 expression in pancreatic cancer. J Nucl Med 43:173–180

Higashi T, Saga T, Nakamoto Y, Ishimori T, Fujimoto K, Doi R, Imamura M, Konishi J (2003) Diagnosis of pancreatic cancer using fluorine-18 fluorodeoxyglucose positron emission tomography (FDG PET)—usefulness and limitations in "clinical reality". Ann Nucl Med 17:261–279

Imdahl A, Nitzsche E, Krautmann F, Hogerle S, Boos S, Einert A, Sontheimer J, Farthmann EH (1999) Evaluation of positron emission tomography with 2-[18F]fluoro-2-deoxy-D-glucose for the differentiation of chronic pancreatitis and pancreatic cancer. Br J Surg 86:194–199

Inokuma T, Tamaki N, Torizuka T, Magata Y, Fujii M, Yonekura Y, Kajiyama T, Ohshio G, Imamura M, Konishi J (1995) Evaluation of pancreatic tumors with positron emission tomography and F-18 fluorodeoxyglucose: comparison with CT and US. Radiology 195:345–352

Ishiguchi T, Ota T, Naganawa S, Fukatsu H, Itoh S, Ishigaki T (2001) CT and MR imaging of pancreatic cancer. Hepatogastroenterology 48:923–927

Kasperk RK, Riesener KP, Wilms K, Schumpelick V (2001) Limited value of positron emission tomography in treatment of pancreatic cancer: surgeon's view. World J Surg 25:1134–1139

Keyes JW Jr (1995) SUV: standard uptake or silly useless value? J Nucl Med 36:1836–1839
Kowalski J, Henze M, Schuhmacher J, Macke HR, Hofmann M, Haberkorn U (2003) Evaluation of positron emission tomography imaging using [68 Ga]-DOTA-D Phe(1)-Tyr(3)-octreotide in comparison to [111In]-DTPAOC SPECT. First results in patients with neuroendocrine tumors. Mol Imaging Biol 5:42–48
Koyama K, Okamura T, Kawabe J, Nakata B, Chung KH, Ochi H, Yamada R (2001) Diagnostic usefulness of FDG PET for pancreatic mass lesions. Ann Nucl Med 15:217–224
Kubota R, Kubota K, Yamada S, Tada M, Ido T, Tamahashi N (1994) Microautoradiographic study for the differentiation of intratumoral macrophages, granulation tissues and cancer cells by the dynamics of fluorine-18-fluorodeoxyglucose uptake. J Nucl Med 35:104–112
Lemke AJ, Niehues SM, Hosten N, Amthauer H, Boehmig M, Stroszczynski C, Rohlfing T, Rosewicz S, Felix R (2004) Retrospective digital image fusion of multidetector CT and 18F-FDG PET: clinical value in pancreatic lesions—a prospective study with 104 patients. J Nucl Med 45:1279–1286
Lopez Hanninen E, Amthauer H, Hosten N, Ricke J, Bohmig M, Langrehr J, Hintze R, Neuhaus P, Wiedenmann B, Rosewicz S, Felix R (2002) Prospective evaluation of pancreatic tumors: accuracy of MR imaging with MR cholangiopancreatography and MR angiography. Radiology 224:34–41
Nakamoto Y, Higashi T, Sakahara H, Tamaki N, Kogire M, Doi R, Hosotani R, Imamura M, Konishi J (2000) Delayed (18)F-fluoro-2-deoxy-d-glucose positron emission tomography scan for differentiation between malignant and benign lesions in the pancreas. Cancer 89:2547–2554
Nakata B, Nishimura S, Ishikawa T, Ohira M, Nishino H, Kawabe J, Ochi H, Hirakawa K (2001) Prognostic predictive value of 18F-fluorodeoxyglucose positron emission tomography for patients with pancreatic cancer. Int J Oncol 19:53–58
Nitzsche EU, Hoegerle S, Mix M, Brink I, Otte A, Moser E, Imdahl A (2002) Non-invasive differentiation of pancreatic lesions: is analysis of FDG kinetics superior to semiquantitative uptake value analysis? Eur J Nucl Med Mol Imaging 29:237–242
Pakzad F, Groves AM, Ell PJ (2006) The role of positron emission tomography in the management of pancreatic cancer. Semin Nucl Med 36:248–256
Pauleit D, Stoffels G, Schaden W, Hamacher K, Bauer D, Tellmann L, Herzog H, Broer S, Coenen HH, Langen KJ (2005) PET with O-(2-18F-fluoroethyl)-l-tyrosine in peripheral tumors: first clinical results. J Nucl Med 46:411–416
Peñuelas I, Haberkorn U, Yaghoubi S, Gambhir SS (2005) Gene therapy imaging in patients for oncological applications. Eur J Nucl Med Mol Imaging 32 [Suppl 2]:S384–S403
Pessin JE, Bell GI (1992) Mammalian facilitative glucose transporter family: structure and molecular regulation. Annu Rev Physiol 54:911–930
Ponchon T, Pilleul F (2002) Diagnostic ERCP. Endoscopy 34:29–42
Rasmussen I, Sorensen J, Langstrom B, Haglund U (2004) Is positron emission tomography using 18F-fluorodeoxyglucose and 11C-acetate valuable in diagnosing indeterminate pancreatic masses? Scand J Surg 93:191–197
Reske SN, Grillenberger KG, Glatting G, Port M, Hildebrandt M, Gansauge F, Beger HG (1997) Overexpression of glucose transporter 1 and increased FDG uptake in pancreatic carcinoma. J Nucl Med 38:1344–1348
Ruf J, Lopez Hänninen E, Böhmig M, Koch I, Denecke T, Plotkin M, Langrehr J, Wiedenmann B, Felix R, Amthauer H (2006) Impact of FDG-PET/MRI image fusion on the detection of pancreatic cancer. Pancreatology 6:512–519
Smith TA (1999) Facilitative glucose transporter expression in human cancer tissue. Br J Biomed Sci 56:285–292
Smith TA (2000) Mammalian hexokinases and their abnormal expression in cancer. Br J Biomed Sci 57:170–178
Sperti C, Pasquali C, Decet G, Chierichetti F, Liessi G, Pedrazzoli S (2005) F-18-fluorodeoxyglucose positron emission tomography in differentiating malignant from benign pancreatic cysts: a prospective study. J Gastrointest Surg 9:22–28
Thie JA (2004) Understanding the standardized uptake value, its methods, and implications for usage. J Nucl Med 45:1431–1434
Townsend DW (2001) A combined PET/CT scanner: the choices. J Nucl Med 42:533–534
van Tinteren H, Hoekstra OS, Smit EF, van den Bergh JH, Schreurs AJ, Stallaert RA, van Velthoven PC, Comans EF, Diepenhorst FW, Verboom P, van Mourik JC, Postmus PE, Boers M, Teule GJ (2002) Effectiveness of positron emission tomography in the preoperative assessment of patients with suspected non-small-cell lung cancer: the PLUS multicentre randomised trial. Lancet 359:1388–1393

Voth M, Opfermann T, Gottschild D (2003) The value of fluorodeoxyglucose positron emission tomography (FDG-PET) in differentiation of pancreatic lesions [in German]. Zentralbl Chir 128:375–378

Warburg O, Posener K, Negelein E (1924) Über den Stoffwechsel der Carcinomzelle. Biochem Zeitschrift 152:309–335

Zimny M, Bares R, Fass J, Adam G, Cremerius U, Dohmen B, Klever P, Sabri O, Schumpelick V, Buell U (1997) Fluorine-18 fluorodeoxyglucose positron emission tomography in the differential diagnosis of pancreatic carcinoma: a report of 106 cases. Eur J Nucl Med 24:678–682

Part II Therapy and Monitoring of Disease

4 Surgical Techniques for Resectable Pancreatic Cancer

M. Bahra, U. Neumann

Recent Results in Cancer Research, Vol. 177

Abstract

Pancreatic cancer is a highly aggressive cancer with a rising incidence in most European countries. Due to both the aggressive biology of the disease and the late diagnosis in many cases, pancreatic duct carcinoma is still a disease with a poor prognosis. Today, surgical resection of localized tumor remains the only potentially curative option available for these patients. Advances in surgical techniques and perioperative care has improved significantly in the last 20 years, causing an extension of indications for surgical intervention. However, despite new diagnostic techniques, the surgical exploration still plays the key role for the finally assessment of resectability. For evaluation of local resectability, laparoscopy alone cannot generally be recommended today and explorative laparotomy is required. Contraindications for pancreatic resection are liver metastasis, peritoneal metastasis, and tumor infiltration of visceral arteries. The surgical management of pancreatic cancer consists of two phases: first, assessment of tumor resectability and second, if resectability is given, the pancreaticoduodenectomy with consecutive reconstruction. Standard surgical strategies are the classic pancreaticoduodenectomy including a distal gastrectomy and the pylorus-preserving pancreaticoduodenectomy (PPPD) preserving antral and pyloric function, respectively. Both surgical procedures are equally effective for the treatment of pancreatic carcinoma. Delicate lymphadenectomy during pancreaticoduodenectomy is important for radical oncological enforcement. An extended lymphadenectomy showed no benefit in several trials. Despite the encouraging advances in surgical treatment, actuarial 5-year survival rates after pancreatic resection are only at about 20%.

4.1 Introduction

The only curative approach for patients with pancreatic cancer is a radical resection of the tumor. The two standard resection procedures of choice are the resection of the pancreatic head and the left-sided pancreatic resection. In case of a local advanced pancreatic carcinoma, a total pancreatectomy may be advisable in selected cases. During the last 30 years technical developments in pancreatic surgery significantly decreased the perioperative morbidity and mortality. Since pancreatic resections have become more accepted as a safe surgical procedure, two surgical approaches for patients with pancreatic head tumors are established today. The standard "Kausch-Whipple" pancreaticoduodenectomy and the pylorus-preserving pancreaticoduodenectomy [11, 23, 45]. However, although the resection rate has increased and mortality decreased, the prognosis for patients with pancreatic cancer is still poor [15].

4.2 Assessment of Resectability

The preoperative clarification of resectability should only be performed via laparotomy. Radiological (CT/MRI) signs of involvement of the superior mesenteric-portal venous confluence are no contraindication for surgical exploration. Laparoscopic evaluations can only exclude peritoneal carcinomatosis or liver metastasis, and therefore only provide incomplete information about the local resectability [14].

During the operation, the peritoneal cavity and its contents have to be carefully examined. Lesions suspicious of metastasis should be assessed histologically. Assessment of local expansion including vascular tumor involvement requires careful mobilization from the surrounding structures. Involvement of superior mesenteric artery (SMA), celiac trunk, or hepatic arteries precludes resection with curative intent, whereas invasion of the portal vein does not.

Preoperative or intraoperative biopsies are not obligatory to confirm the diagnosis of malignancy. If preoperative findings, the clinical picture, and surgical findings are consistent, resection should proceed.

4.3 Contraindications for Pancreatic Resection

Due to the locally advanced nature of the disease and the presence of early metastases in the majority of patients, for only 20% of patients is curative resection feasible at the time of diagnosis [12]. However, if possible a radical resection of the tumor should be performed. In this context, not only the question of technical feasibility is important, but more important should be the question of whether or not the patient will recover from the procedure. A definitive contraindication for a pancreaticoduodenectomy is the presence of local or distant metastases including peritoneal carcinomatosis. Metabolic disease is known as a significant predictor of short expected survival [3]. Further contraindications for radical surgery are tumor invasion of the mesenteric root or invasion of visceral arteries (SMA, celiac axis or hepatic artery). Nowadays, cancer invasion of the superior mesenteric-portal venous confluence (SMPCV) is no longer a contraindication for radical pancreaticoduodenectomy [27]. It has to be mentioned that patients with concomitant severe disease should not be operated due to the significant increased mortality risk.

Because of declining surgical mortality rates after pancreatic resection, the role of palliative resections have been discussed in recent years. Especially the question of whether a palliative pancreaticoduodenectomy should be offered to patients with hepatic metastases is still unanswered (see also Chap. 13). Some data suggest that at least a selected group of patients may benefit from palliative resections [25].

4.4 Surgical Technique

The "Kausch-Whipple" procedure is nowadays no longer regarded as the standard procedure. In recent years, pylorus-preserving pancreatoduodenectomy (PPPD) was established as the standard resection procedure for periampullary malignancies. In contrast to the Whipple operation, which includes a 2/3 gastrectomy, the PPPD necessitates the preservation of the whole stomach, including the pylorus. The duodenum is usually cut about 2 cm distal from the pyloric ring.

After transverse laparotomy and Kocher maneuver (the mobilization of the duodenum), resectability in case of malignant disease has to be ascertained, and pancreatic head resection should be performed in a standard fashion, including dissection of the distal bile duct and *en bloc* dissection of the lymph nodes in the hepatoduodenal ligament and along the celiac trunk and superior mesenteric artery. After resection of the pancreatic head with the adjacent duodenum, the first jejunal loop has to be dissected and brought up through the mesocolon in a retrocolic fashion, after which an end-to-side pancreatojejunostomy has to be performed, then a choledochojejunostomy, and finally a duodenojejunostomy.

In the past, several reports attempted to compare the standard Whipple to the pylorus-preserving procedure, also emphasizing that the operating time for PPPD is shorter [24]. Some authors have reported a higher rate of postoperative delayed gastric emptying after PPPD [49]. A prospective randomized multicenter study that compared the pylorus-preserving pancreaticoduodenectomy and standard Whipple operation with regard to duration of surgery, blood loss, hospital stay, delayed gastric emptying, and survival showed no significant differences in median blood loss and duration of operation. This study showed only a marginal difference in postoperative weight loss after the standard Whipple procedure. The overall long-term and disease-free survival was comparable for both procedures [43]. To date, the choice between both surgical procedures, standard Whipple procedure or pylorus-preserving pancreaticoduodenectomy, cannot be made on evidence-based data. However, PPPD is the preferred approach for patients with pancreatic head carcinoma today. Most important, the pylorus-preserving pancreaticoduodenectomy is a safe and radical operation that does not affect prognosis [40].

The standard procedure for surgical treatment of carcinomas of the pancreatic body or pancreatic tail is a pancreatic left resection. Due to a late onset of clinical signs such as jaundice or pain, left-sided pancreatic tumors are characterized mostly by an advanced stage at diagnosis.

After transverse laparotomy, the pancreatic left resection should be performed, based on (1) the principles of surgical oncology as a no-touch-technique and (2) standard *en bloc* dissection of the peripancreatic lymph nodes, including splenectomy. Depending on the dimension of the tumor, the resection margin has to be extended to reach the pancreatic head to enable tumor-free resection margins (subtotal, left-sided pancreatectomy). The pancreatic remnant should be provided by an end-to-side pancreatojejunostomy to avoid pancreatic fistula.

One attempt to improve the prognosis of pancreatic cancer was to perform more aggressive surgical approaches such as a total pancreatectomy [32]. Theoretical advantages for this procedure are that total pancreatectomy prevents the risk of pancreatic fistulas and provides a radical eradication of the tumor [20]. Furthermore, the risk of positive resection margins in the pancreatic remnant seemed to be eliminated. However, the experiences of the last 20 years has shown that postoperative complications are more frequent after total pancreatectomy compared to partial pancreaticoduodenectomy. One problem is severe diabetes mellitus, which is often difficult to manage. Baumel et al. reported on difficulties in glucoregulation in up to 25% of patients after total pancreatectomy [3]. Nowadays a total pancreatectomy is no longer an option for carcinomas of the pancreatic head. However, in individual cases, e.g., in case of multicentric carcinomas, an indication for total pancreatectomy may be given.

4.5 Pancreaticoenteric Anastomosis

The operative resection of pancreatic cancer includes cautious handling of the pancreatic remnant. For that, the texture and size of the remnant has to be taken into surgical consideration [46]. To prevent fatal complications such as, e.g., a leakage from the pancreaticojejunal anastomosis, different anastomotic techniques have been

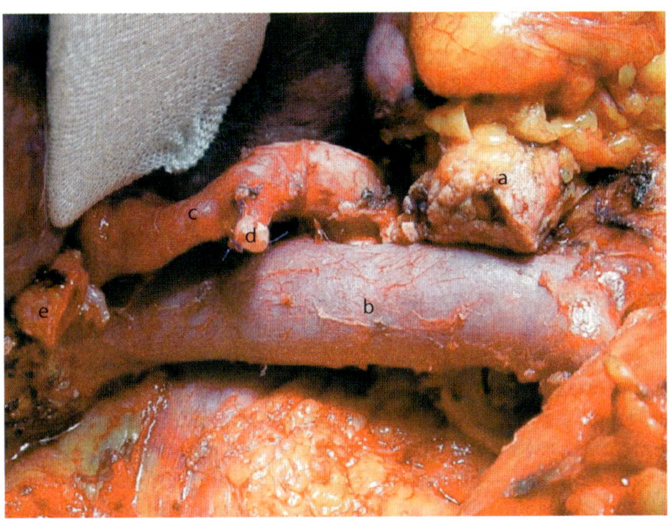

Fig. 4.1 Situs after pylorus-preserving pancreatoduodenectomy (PPPD). *a*, Pancreatic remnant; *b*, portal vein; *c*, hepatic artery; *d*, gastroduodenal artery; *e*, common bile duct

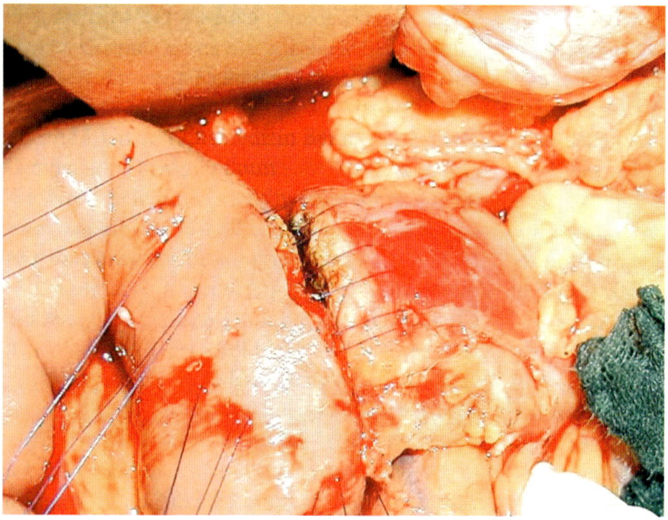

Fig. 4.2 Mattress technique for pancreatojejunostomy. After placing an incision the same size as the pancreatic cut surface in the jejunal loop and positioning U-stitches starting at the jejunal back wall, the stitches go from back to front, straight through the pancreatic remnant. With this technique, the pancreatic remnant is completely enclosed by the jejunal loop. The suture has to go straight through the pancreatic remnant

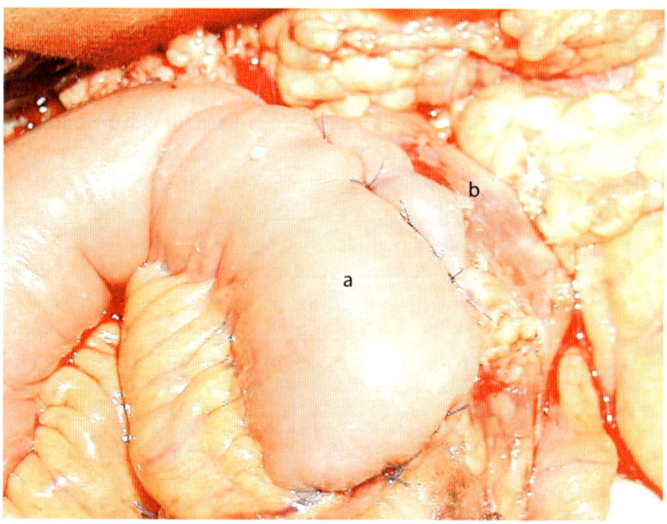

Fig. 4.3 Mattress technique for pancreaticojejunal anastomosis. A tube that drains the pancreatic juice externally is inserted to reduce the risk of anastomosis leakage. *a*, Jejunal loop; *b*, pancreatic remnant

published during recent years (Figs. 4.1, 4.2, and 4.3). To date, however, it is still not possible to decide which anastomotic technique is the best. A standard anastomotic technique is the duct-to-mucosa pancreaticojejunostomy described by Cattell and modified by Braasch [6, 7]. After removal of an area of serosa matching the cut surface of the pancreas, the back wall has to be sutured with a running suture (4-0 PDS), the bowel wall incised, and a duct-to-mucosa anastomosis performed with single stitches (5-0 Monocryl). After completion of the back wall, the front wall of the duct-to-mucosa anastomosis must also be applied with 5-0 Monocryl single stitches. Subsequently, the anterior wall of the anastomosis to the bowel has to be completed with a 4-0 PDS running suture.

A further technique is the so-called mattress technique. An incision, the same size as the pancreatic cut surface, has to be placed in the jejunal loop. Then U-stitches (4-0 PDS), starting at the jejunal back wall, from back to front, have to be positioned straight through the pancreatic remnant about 1 cm distal from the cut surface and then through the front wall of the jejunal loop. With this technique the pancreatic remnant is completely enclosed by the jejunal loop. A prospective, randomized trail comparing both techniques has shown that both techniques yield similar incidences of complications. The mattress technique seems, therefore, to be more suitable for training schedules in pancreatic surgery [26].

4.6 Pancreatogastrostomy

The pancreaticoenteric anastomosis is known as the "Achilles heel" of pancreatic surgery. Due to this perception, several approaches have been attempted to improve the safety of this anastomosis. One strategy was the introduction of a pancreatogastrostomy as an alternative reconstruction technique after pancreatic head resection [30]. Three different principles to achieve pancreatogastrostomy are in use today: the implantation of the pancreatic remnant into the stomach, the implantation of only the pancreatic duct into the stomach, and an anastomosis between the pancreatic duct and the gastric mucosa. However, the first is by far the most often performed procedure. A view through the literature shows that the surgical results after pancreatogastrostomy are similar to those yielded with pancreaticojejunostomy [2, 21, 29]. It is known that long-term pancreatic secretion into the stomach causes alkaline juice, which affects the gastric mucosa. To date, however, there is no substantial data showing a correlation between an increased risk of peptic ulcers and pancreatogastric anastomosis. Interestingly, a study by Hyodo et al. showed that pancreatogastrostomy appears to decrease the grade of *Helicobacter pylori* infection, and tends to ameliorate the severity of gastritis after pancreatogastrostomy [19]. Taken together, to date there is no convincing data that the pancreatic fluid is harmful to the stomach.

4.7 Lymphadenectomy

Affection of lymph nodes is reported to be found in more than 70% of patients after resection [4]. A radical lymphadenectomy along the hepatoduodenal ligament, celiac trunk, and superior mesenteric artery should be performed routinely as standard technique. However, to improve long-term survival in patients with pancreatic cancer, more radical surgical procedures had been proposed. One of these approaches is the extended lymph node dissection, which includes resection of bilateral paraaortal lymphatic tissue from the diaphragm down to the inferior mesenteric artery and laterally to the hilum of the right kidney [37]. Several recent studies indicated a variability in results regarding the influence of an extended lymph node clearance (Table 4.1). In a prospective randomized trail, Nimura et al. compared 51 patients after standard lymphadenectomy and 50 patients after extended lymph node dissection. No differences were found in overall survival, survival for pN0/pN1, tumor recurrence, body weight, quality of life, and bowel movements [35]. Connor et al. demonstrated that metastatic involvement of lymph node 8a (located at the common hepatic artery) is an independent prognostic factor after pylorus-preserving resection [8]. Two further randomized studies of extended lymph node dissection reported a similar overall morbidity, although the study from Baltimore reported on an increased rate of

Table 4.1 Results of standard lymph node dissection versus extended lymph node dissection for pancreatic cancer

Author	Standard dissection				Extended dissection			
	Patients (*n*)	Lymph nodes (*n*)	Morbidity (%)	1-year survival (%)	Patients (*n*)	Lymph nodes (*n*)	Morbidity (%)	1-year survival (%)
Pedrazoli [36]	40	13	5	50	41	20	15	22
Yeo [47]	56	16	34	71	58	27	40	80
Henne-Bruns [17]	26	14	0	42	46	24	0	42

delayed gastric emptying [36, 47]. Henne-Bruns et al. showed no differences in survival comparing standard and extended lymph node dissection, and concluded that further improvement of the survival rate cannot be achieved by extended retroperitoneal lymphadenectomy [17]. In conclusion, there is no evidence as yet that an extended lymph node dissection positively influences survival.

4.8 Portal Vein Resection

Tumor invasion of the portal or superior mesenteric vein has always been a controversial issue in pancreatic surgery. In only a small percentage of patients suffering from pancreatic cancer, the surgical goal of tumor-free resection margins is limited by venous tumor invasion. For these patients a radical surgical approach, including the resection of portal vein or superior mesenteric vein, is the only chance of achieving an R0-situation. In 1951, Moore et al. were the first to describe a resection of the superior mesenteric vein for pancreatic cancer [31]. In 1973, Fortner performed the successful *en bloc* removal for carcinoma of the pancreas combined with the resection and reconstruction of the portal vein, the so-called "regional pancreatectomy" [13].

Several of the technical procedures are: tangential resection and venous patch-plastic, segmental resection with splenic vein ligation, and primary anastomosis or splenic vein ligation and graft interposition. Further procedures may be the segmental resection with splenic vein preservation either with primary anastomosis or again with graft interposition. In the literature the surgical technique for resection and reconstruction is well established as a safe procedure [9, 39]. Due to this fact, cancer invasion of the mesenteric-portal venous axis should not be considered a contraindication for radical pancreaticoduodenectomy any more.

Pathological assessments of resected veins confirmed cancerous venous invasion in 20%–70% of resected specimens [5, 42]. These data indicate that a significant percentage of patients with suspected venous tumor invasion only show an inflammatory adherence. Some authors reported on small patient cohorts undergoing portal vein resection combined with arterial resection [33, 38, 44]. However, combined resections of the portal vein and visceral arteries have not yet been established as a standard technique, and therefore such procedures are only indicated in highly selected patients and should be performed as part of clinical study protocols only.

4.9 Preoperative Stenting

The significance of preoperative biliary stenting (Table 4.2) in jaundiced patients prior to pancreaticoduodenectomy has been under discussion for many years. It is well known that severe jaundice can cause multi-organ dysfunction and defects in immune function [18]. A long-term biliary tract obstruction can lead to biliary tract sepsis and septic shock. Furthermore, a correlation between obstructive jaundice and operative morbidity and mortality could be demonstrated [1]. However, studies in the more recent past showed that short-term preoperative biliary decompression does not improve surgical results after pancreatic head resection [34]. Several

Table 4.2 Preoperative biliary stenting in jaundiced patients prior pancreaticoduodenectomy. Mortality and complications

Author/group	Patients		Mortality (%)		Findings
	Total	Stent	No stent	Stent	
Povosky et al. [53]	240	126	1.8	7.9	Increased mortality/morbidity
Sohn et al. [54]	567	408	2.5	1.7	Increased wound infections
Martignoni et al. [51]	257	99	1.9	0.6	No complications
Hodul et al. [50]	300	172	1.1	0.6	Increased wound infections
Pister et al. [52]	265	172	1	0.5	Increased wound infections

retrospective and prospective reviews have failed to show a significant reduction of length of hospital stay or morbidity after preoperative biliary drainage [22, 41]. There are some indicators that preoperative stenting increases the rate of wound infections and can contaminate bile after instrumentation of the bile duct [41]. In conclusion, preoperative stenting is not indicated generally today in jaundiced patients due to pancreatic head tumor formation, and therefore it should only be used selectively.

4.10 Octreotide

The octapeptide analog of somatostatin, octreotide, has been proposed to reduce the incidence of pancreatic fistulas after pancreatic resections. While octreotide is already successfully in use for the prevention of pancreatitis and pancreatic fistulas after pancreatic transplantation [10], the role of somatostatin as prophylaxis against pancreatic anastomosis leakage is still under debate. Several randomized studies on the role of somatostatin have been published in recent years. All of the studies failed to show a significant difference in postoperative mortality. On the one hand, studies published between 1992 and 1995 showed fewer complications in patients receiving octreotide; on the other hand, in a series published between 1997 and 2002, less or no differences were seen. Only one study showed a decreased rate of postoperative pancreatic fistulas in patients after octreotide treatment [16]. Li-Ling and colleagues published a systematic review analyzing whether the use of octreotide is effective in the prevention of postoperative pancreatic complications. The analysis suggested that in centers with a high fistula rate octreotide administration reduces the rate of major complications [28]. In summary, octreotide appears to decrease the overall morbidity and the incidence of pancreatic fistulas after pancreatic resections, but not mortality. Due to this fact, octreotide may be indicated especially in patients with nonfibrotic pancreatic glands or in patients with nondilated ducts undergoing pancreatic resection.

4.11 Summary

Pancreatic cancer is the fifth leading cause of cancer mortality, with a rising incidence in most European countries. Due to both the aggressive biology of the disease and the late diagnosis in many cases, ductal pancreatic carcinoma is still a disease with a poor prognosis. Today, surgical resection of localized tumor remains the only potentially curative option available for these patients. Advances in surgical technique and perioperative care has improved significantly during last 20 years, causing an extension of indications for surgical intervention. Resections in elderly patients or removal of advanced tumors including portal vein resections are nowadays feasible with low perioperative mortality rates. Although the spectrum of indication has increased, operative mortality rates today for pancreaticoduodenectomy should not exceed 5% at centers with a high caseload. Despite new diagnostic techniques, however, surgical exploration still plays the key role for final assessment of resectability. In this context, the role of diagnostic laparoscopy in patients with pancreatic malignancies is controversial. For detection of liver or peritoneal metastasis laparoscopy before laparotomy may be reasonable. For evaluation of *local* resectability, laparoscopy alone can generally not be recommended nowadays, and explorative laparotomy should be performed.

Contraindications for pancreatic resection are liver metastasis, peritoneal metastasis, and tumor infiltration of visceral arteries. The two phases of surgical management of pancreatic cancer are: assessment of tumor resectability and, if resectability is given, the pancreaticoduodenectomy with consecutive reconstruction. Standard surgical strategies are the classic pancreaticoduodenectomy including a distal gastrectomy or PPPD, preserving antral and pyloric function respectively. Both surgical procedures are equally effective for the treatment of pancreatic carcinoma. Delicate lymphadenectomy during pancreaticoduodenectomy is important for radical oncological enforcement. In several trials, extended lymphadenectomy showed no significant benefits and is still under discussion. Despite the encouraging advances in surgical treatment, actuarial 5-year survival rates after pancreatic resection are only at about 20% [48].

References

1. Armstrong CP, Dixon JM, Taylor TV, Davies GC (1984) Surgical experience of deeply jaundiced patients with bile duct obstruction. Br J Surg 71:234–238
2. Arnaud JP, Bergamaschi R, Casa C, Serra-Maudet V (1993) Pancreatogastrostomy following pancreatoduodenectomy: a safe drainage procedure. Int Surg 78:352–353
3. Baumel H, Huguier M, Manderscheid JC, Fabre JM, Houry S, Fagot H (1994) Results of resection for cancer of the exocrine pancreas: a study from the French Association of Surgery. Br J Surg 81:102–107
4. Birk D (2000) Localisation of lymph node metastasis in pancreatic cancer. A rationale for extended resection [abstr]? Pancreas 21:41
5. Bold RJ, Charnsangavej C, Cleary KR, et al. (1999) Major vascular resection as part of pancreaticoduodenectomy for cancer: radiologic, intraoperative, and pathologic analysis. J Gastrointest Surg 3:233
6. Braasch JW, Gagner M (1991) Pylorus-preserving pancreatoduodenectomy—technical aspects. Langenbecks Arch Chir 376:50
7. Cattell RB (1943) Resection of the pancreas: discussion of special problems. Surg Clin North Am 23:753–766
8. Connor S (2002) Metastatic involvement of lymph node 8a is an independent prognostic factor in pancreatic cancer. Pancreas 27:368–420
9. Cusack JC Jr, Fuhrman GM, Lee JE, Evans DB (1994) Managing unsuspected tumor invasion of the superior mesenteric-portal venous confluence during pancreaticoduodenectomy. Am J Surg 168:352
10. Daloze P, Beauregard H, St Louis G, Corman J, Smeesters C, Aris-Jilwain N, Comtois R, Rasio E (1989) Clinical pancreas transplantation: a learning curve of its management. Transplant Proc 21:2858–2861
11. Di Carlo V (1998) Surgical treatment: Kausch-Whipple pancreatoduodenectomy with or without pylorus preserving. In: Beger H, Warshaw AL, Buchler M (eds) The pancreas. Blackwell Science, Oxford, p 1028
12. Flanders TY, Foulkes WD (1996) Pancreatic adenocarcinoma: epidemiology and genetics. J Med Genet 33:889–898
13. Fortner JG (1973) Regional resection and pancreatic carcinoma. Surgery 73:799
14. Friess H, Kleeff J, Silva JC, Sadowski C, Baer HU, Büchler MW (1998) The role of diagnostic laparoscopy in pancreatic and periampullary malignancies. J Am Coll Surg 186:675–682
15. Geer RJ, Brennan MF (1993) Prognostic indicators for survival after resection of pancreatic adenocarcinoma. Am J Surg 165:68
16. Goulillat C CJ, Baulieux J (2001) Randomized controlled multicenter trail of somatostain infusion after pancreaticoduodenectomy. Br J Surg 88:1456
17. Henne-Bruns D, Vogel I, Luttges J, Kloppel G, Kremer B (1998) Ductal adenocarcinoma of the pancreas head: survival after regional versus extended lymphadenectomy. Hepatogastroenterology 45:855
18. Hunt DR, Allison ME, Prentice CR, Blumgart LH (1982) Endotoxemia, disturbance of coagulation, and obstructive jaundice. Am J Surg 144:325
19. Hyodo M, Nagai H, Tsukahara M, Sato K (2000) Peptic diseases and Helicobacter pylori infection after pancreatogastrostomy. Hepatogastroenterology 47:1753
20. Ihse I, Anderson H, Andren S (1996) Total pancreatectomy for cancer of the pancreas: is it appropriate? World J Surg 20:288
21. Ihse I, Axelson J, Hansson L (1999) Pancreaticogastrostomy after subtotal pancreatectomy for cancer. Dig Surg 16:389
22. Jagannath P, Dhir V, Shrikhande S, Shah RC, Mullerpatan P, Mohandas KM (2005) Effect of preoperative biliary stenting on immediate outcome after pancreaticoduodenectomy. Br J Surg 92:356
23. Kausch O (1912) Das Karzinom der Papilla duodeni und seine radikal Entfernung. Beitr Klin Chir 78:439–486
24. Klinkenbijl JH, van der Schelling GP, Hop WC, van Pel R, Bruining HA, Jeekel J (1992) The advantages of pylorus-preserving pancreatoduodenectomy in malignant disease of the pancreas and periampullary region. Ann Surg 216:142–145
25. Kuhlmann K (2002) Pancreaticoduodenectomy for palliative treatment of pancreatic cancer. Pancreatology 2:336
26. Langrehr JM, Bahra M, Jacob D, Glanemann M, Neuhaus P (2005) Prospective randomized comparison between a new mattress technique and Cattell (duct-to-mucosa) pancreaticojejunostomy for pancreatic resection. World J Surg 29:1111

27. Launois B, Stasik C, Bardaxoglou E, et al. (1999) Who benefits from portal vein resection during pancreaticoduodenectomy for pancreatic cancer? World J Surg 23:926
28. Li-Ling J, Irving M (2001) Somatostatin and octreotide in the prevention of postoperative pancreatic complications and the treatment of enterocutaneous pancreatic fistulas: systematic review of randomized controlled trials. Br J Cancer 88:190
29. Mason GR (1999) Pancreatogastrostomy as reconstruction for pancreatoduodenectomy: review. World J Surg 23:221
30. Mason GR, Freeark RJ (1995) Current experience with pancreatogastrostomy. Am J Surg 169:217
31. Moore GE (1951) Radical pancreatoduodenectomy with resection and re-anastomosis of the superior mesenteric vein. Surgery 30:350
32. Moossa AR, Scott MH, Lavelle-Jones M (1984) The place of total and extended total pancreatectomy in pancreatic cancer. World J Surg 8:895
33. Nakano H, Bachellier P, Weber JC, et al. (2002) Arterial and vena caval resections combined with pancreaticoduodenectomy in highly selected patients with periampullary malignancies. Hepatogastroenterology 49:258
34. Nakeeb A, Pitt HA (1995) The role of preoperative biliary decompression in obstructive jaundice. Hepatogastroenterology 42:332
35. Nimura Y (2005) Standard versus extended lymphadenectomy. Prospective Randomized Trail. EHPBA, 6th Congress (abstract)
36. Pedrazzoli S, DiCarlo V, Dionigi R, et al. (1998) Standard versus extended lymphadenectomy associated with pancreatoduodenectomy in the surgical treatment of adenocarcinoma of the head of the pancreas: a multicenter, prospective, randomized study. Lymphadenectomy Study Group. Ann Surg 228:508
37. Schafer M, Mullhaupt B, Clavien PA (2002) Evidence-based pancreatic head resection for pancreatic cancer and chronic pancreatitis. Ann Surg 236:137
38. Settmacher U, Langrehr JM, Husmann I, et al. (2004) [Reconstruction of visceral arteries with homografts in excision of the pancreas]. Chirurg 75:1199
39. Shiraishi M, Nagahama M, Miyaguni T, Shimoji H, Kusano T, Mute Y (1998) Two-step portal bypass to reconstruct an invaded superior mesenteric vein in pancreatic cancer. Hepatogastroenterology 45:882
40. Shoenberg MH (2000) Pylorus-preserving partial duodenectomy for ductal pancreatic carcinoma—a prospective clinical trial. Dig Surg 100 (abstract)
41. Sohn TA (2000) Do preoperative biliary stents increase postpancreaticoduodenectomy complications? J Gastrointest Surg 4:258–267
42. Tashiro S, Uchino R, Hiraoka T, et al. (1991) Surgical indication and significance of portal vein resection in biliary and pancreatic cancer. Surgery 109:481–487
43. Tran KT, Smeenk HG, van Eijck CH, et al. (2004) Pylorus preserving pancreaticoduodenectomy versus standard Whipple procedure: a prospective, randomized, multicenter analysis of 170 patients with pancreatic and periampullary tumors. Ann Surg 240:738
44. Tseng JF, Raut CP, Lee JE, et al. (2004) Pancreaticoduodenectomy with vascular resection: margin status and survival duration. J Gastrointest Surg 8:935
45. Yeo CJ, Cameron JL, Maher MM, et al. (1995) A prospective randomized trial of pancreaticogastrostomy versus pancreaticojejunostomy after pancreaticoduodenectomy. Ann Surg 222:580
46. Yeo CJ, Cameron JL, Lillemoe KD, et al. (2002) Pancreaticoduodenectomy with or without distal gastrectomy and extended retroperitoneal lymphadenectomy for periampullary adenocarcinoma, part 2: randomized controlled trial evaluating survival, morbidity, and mortality. Ann Surg 236:355
47. Yeo CJ, Cameron JL, Sohn TA, et al. (1997) Six hundred fifty consecutive pancreaticoduodenectomies in the 1990 s: pathology, complications, and outcomes. Ann Surg 226:248
48. Zerbi A, Balzano G, Patuzzo R, Calori G, Braga M, Di Carlo V (1995) Comparison between pylorus-preserving and Whipple pancreatoduodenectomy. Br J Surg 82:975
49. Hodul P, Creech S, Pickleman J, Aranha GV (2003) The effect of preoperative biliary stenting on postoperative complications after pancreaticoduodenectomy. Am J Surg 186:420–425Whipple A (1942) Present day surgery of the pancreas. N Engl J Med 226:515
50. Martignoni ME, Wagner M, Krähenbühl L, Redaelli CA, Friess H, Büchler MW (2001) Effect of preoperative biliary drainage on surgical outcome after pancreatoduodenectomy. Am J Surg 181:52–59

51. Pisters PW, Hudec WA, Hess KR, Lee JE, Vauthey JN, Lahoti S, Raijman I, Evans DB (2001) Effect of preoperative biliary decompression on pancreaticoduodenectomy-associated morbidity in 300 consecutive patients. Ann Surg 234:47–55
52. Povoski SP, Karpeh MS, Conlon KC, Blumgart LH, Brennan MF (1999) Association of preoperative biliary drainage with postoperative outcome following pancreaticoduodenectomy. Ann Surg 230:131–142
53. Sohn TA, Yeo CJ, Cameron JL, Pitt HA, Lillemoe KD (2000) Do preoperative biliary stents increase postpancreaticoduodenectomy complications? J Gastrointest Surg 4:258–267

5 Postoperative Staging of Pancreatic Cancer

C. Röcken, M. P. A. Ebert

Recent Results in Cancer Research, Vol. 177

Abstract

Pancreatic cancer is a devastating disease with a 5-year survival rate of 3%–5%. The mortality of pancreatic cancer is almost identical with its incidence. The vast majority are pancreatic ductal adenocarcinomas. It is typically a tumour of the elderly. The main risk factor is smoking. Clinical and histopathological studies have identified pancreatic cancer precursor lesions. These include pancreatic intraepithelial neoplasia (PanIN), intraductal papillary mucinous neoplasia (IPMN) and mucinous cystic neoplasm (MCN). To improve patient prognosis, surgical interventions have become more aggressive, including pancreaticoduodenectomy and more or less radical lymphadenectomy. Following surgery, it is the surgical pathologist who provides valuable information regarding the exact tumour localization, histological tumour type, grading, completeness of resection, nodal status and the presence of precursor lesions. Although many tissue-based prognostic biomarkers have been characterized and can be studied by immunohistochemistry or molecular biological techniques, their impact on patient management and treatment is still limited. More recently proteomic profiling has raised hopes for early cancer detection, thereby improving the prognosis of pancreatic cancer patients.

5.1 Pancreatic Cancer

Epithelial tumours of the pancreas arise from or share similarities with the duct epithelium, acinar cells or endocrine cells (Table 5.1). The vast majority of pancreatic cancers are pancreatic ductal adenocarcinomas (PDAC), which account for 85%–90% of pancreatic tumours (Table 5.1). The incidence ranges from 3.1 to 20.8/100,000 per year for men and from 2.0 to 11.0/100,000 per year for women. Within the last 40 years the incidence of PDAC has tripled. It is typically a tumour of the elderly. Of PDAC patients, 80% are in their seventh to ninth decade of life. PDAC occurs rarely in patients younger than 40 years. The median survival of PDAC is less than 6 months and the 5-year survival rate is 3%–5%. The mortality of PDAC is almost identical with its incidence (Hamilton and Aalton 2000).

The main risk factor for PDAC is smoking. It is estimated that 25% of pancreatic cancers are related to smoking. Smokers have a twofold increased risk of pancreatic cancer compared with non-smokers. Less well defined risk factors are dietary factors, chronic pancreatitis, and diabetes mellitus. While numerous inherited germline mutations are associated with pancreatic cancer, only 10% or less of pancreatic cancers are caused by an inherited disorder. The commonest inherited genetic disorder is caused by mutations in the BRCA2 (breast cancer type 2 susceptibility protein) gene which, in addition to causing breast and ovarian tumours, can increase the frequency of pancreatic cancer. Epigenetic alterations also contribute to pancreatic cancer biology and pathogenesis (Hezel et al. 2006; Karhu et al. 2006; Maitra et al. 2006; Sato and Goggins 2006).

PDAC mainly affects the head (60%–70%) and less commonly the body and tail of the pancreas. PDAC are firm and poorly defined tumours. The cut surface is yellow to grey-white. The mean size is 2.5–3.5 cm in diameter (range 1.5–5.0 cm). Tumours of the head are usually smaller than tumours occurring in the body and tail (Hamilton and Aalton 2000).

Table 5.1 WHO classification of tumours of the exocrine pancreas (Hamilton and Aalton 2000)

Benign	
Serous cystadenoma	8441/0
Mucinous cystadenoma	8470/0
Intraductal papillary-mucinous adenoma	8453/0
Mature teratoma	9080/0
Borderline (uncertain malignant potential)	
Mucinous cystic neoplasm with moderate dysplasia	8470/1
Intraductal papillary-mucinous neoplasm with moderate dysplasia	8453/1
Solid-pseudopapillary neoplasm	8452/1
Malignant	
Ductal adenocarcinoma	8500/3
Mucinous non-cystic carcinoma	8480/3
Signet ring cell carcinoma	8490/3
Adenosquamous carcinoma	8560/3
Undifferentiated (anaplastic) carcinoma	8020/3
Undifferentiated carcinoma with osteoclast-like giant cells	8035/3
Mixed ductal-endocrine carcinoma	8154/3
Serous cystadenocarcinoma	8441/3
Mucinous cystadenocarcinoma	8470/3
- Non-invasive	8470/2
- Invasive	8470/3
Intraductal papillary-mucinous carcinoma	8453/3
- Non-invasive	8453/2
- Invasive	8453/3
Acinar cell carcinoma	8550/3
Acinar cell cystadenocarcinoma	8551/3
Mixed acinar-endocrine carcinoma	8154/3
Pancreatoblastoma	8971/3
Solid-pseudopapillary carcinoma	8452/3

5.2 Precursor Lesions

Clinical and histopathological studies have identified pancreatic cancer precursor lesions, i.e. pancreatic intraepithelial neoplasia (PanIN), intraductal papillary mucinous neoplasia (IPMN) and mucinous cystic neoplasm (MCN). PDAC probably develops from PanINs and IPMNs. The four categories of PanIN, i.e. PanIN-1A, PanIN-1B, PanIN-2 and PanIN-3, and the three categories of IPMN, i.e. IPMN adenoma, IPMN borderline and intraductal papillary mucinous carcinoma, constitute a spectrum of cytological and histological alterations of the pancreatic duct epithelium which is characterized by increased atypias and an accumulation of genetic alterations that finally lead to invasive cancer (Hruban et al. 2001, 2004). MCN is a distinct lesion which typically occurs in women and is almost always located in the tail or body of the pancreas and may progress to mucinous cystadenocarcinoma (Klimstra 2005).

5.3 Surgical Pathology Report for Pancreatic Cancer

Different surgical procedures are in use for the surgical treatment of pancreatic cancer. Among these, pancreaticoduodenectomy with or without pylorus preservation has become the standard surgical procedure for resectable pancreatic cancers of the head (Alderson et al. 2005). To improve patient prognosis, surgical interventions have become more aggressive, including more or less radical lymphadenectomy (Yeo et al. 2002). Following surgery, it is the surgical pathologist who provides valuable information regarding the exact tumour localization, histological tumour type, grading, completeness of resection, nodal status and the presence of precursor lesions. Ideally, the surgical pathology report will enclose all these clinically useful and relevant data, including tumour node metastasis (TNM) staging according to Unio Internationale Contra Cancrum (UICC) (Table 5.2). Several proposals and recommendations have been published describing requirements for the examination and reporting of pancreaticoduodenectomy specimens, forming the basis for an adequate post-operative staging and assessment of patient prognosis (Albores-Saaverda et al. 1998; Compton and Henson 1997; Lüttges et al. 1999).

Table 5.2 TNM classification of tumours of the exocrine pancreas

Primary tumour (T)			
Tx	Primary tumour cannot be assessed		
Tis	Carcinoma in situ		
T1	Tumour limited to the pancreas, 2 cm or less in greatest dimension		
T2	Tumour limited to the pancreas, more than 2 cm in greatest dimension		
T3	Tumour extends beyond pancreas, but without involvement of coeliac axis or superior mesenteric artery		
T4	Tumour involves coeliac axis or superior mesenteric artery		
Regional lymph nodes (N)			
NX	Regional lymph nodes cannot be assessed		
N0	No regional lymph node metastasis		
N1	Regional lymph node metastasis		
N1a	Metastasis in a single regional lymph node		
N1b	Metastasis in multiple regional lymph nodes		
Distant metastasis (M)			
MX	Distant metastasis cannot be assessed		
M0	No distant metastasis		
M1	Distant metastasis		
Stage grouping			
Stage 0	Tis	N0	M0
Stage IA	T1	N0	M0
Stage IB	T2	N0	M0
Stage IIA	T3	N0	M0
Stage IIB	T1, T2, T3	N1	M0
Stage III	T4	Any N	M0
Stage IV	Any T	Any N	M1

5.4 Macroscopic Examination

Duodenopancreatectomy specimens should be examined in a fresh unfixed state. The bile duct and the main pancreatic duct should be probed and the whole specimen should be cut horizontally along the probes (Lüttges et al. 1999). Fresh unfixed samples from tumour and non-lesional tissue for subsequent molecular biological investigations or research purposes should only be obtained by a trained surgical pathologist. The pancreatic carcinoma's site of origin must be identified exactly. Pancreatic cancer is a neoplasm localized in the head of the pancreas. The ampullary carcinoma has its centre in the region of the ampulla. It should be specified whether the ampullary carcinoma predominantly involves the ampulla, the intraduodenal portion of the common bile duct or the pancreatic duct. The peri-ampullary carcinoma is usually an advanced tumour that eludes any definition of its precise site of origin. Finally, the terminal bile duct carcinoma may also extend into the head of the pancreas and stems from the lower third of the bile duct. Ampullary carcinomas usually have a significantly better prognosis than pancreatic cancer. However, most tumours present in the advanced stages, often preventing specification of the exact anatomical origin.

Cystic tumours should be assessed with regard to the relationship with the main pancreatic duct, presence or absence of a pseudocapsule, whether the cystic lesion is uni- or multilocular, the character of the cystic content (serous, mucinous, bloody) and the internal surface (smooth, papillary projections), and the presence or absence of mural nodules.

Macroscopic examination should also specify the local tumour extension, i.e. tumour size at least in two dimensions, the distances from the closest margin and towards the ampulla, the dorsal resection margin, and the resection margins of the pancreatic and common bile ducts. The retroperitoneal resection margin is prognostically important and should be thoroughly sampled and labelled. In case of suspected tumour infiltration of the portal vein or superior mesenteric artery, these should be detached separately from the specimen, serially sectioned and submitted in their entirety to histology. Both vascular ends and the dorsal perivascular tissue are of high prognostic significance (Lüttges et al. 1998, 1999).

Any lymph node attached to the resection specimen should be recorded with regard to its localization and submitted to histology.

5.5 Microscopic Examination

Adequate post-operative staging of pancreatic tumours requires a thorough histological examination and classification according to WHO criteria (Table 5.1). The histological type has a significant impact on patient prognosis. Although the majority of pancreatic tumours are PDACs, other less common varieties have to be ruled out, including endocrine tumours, acinar cell carcinomas and metastases. Histological tumour typing of cystic tumours has to separate MCN and IPMN, which have a much better prognosis than cystically degenerated PDACs. While a minority of patients with PDAC survive for at least 5 years, unexpected long-term survival should raise suspicion about whether a correct diagnosis was reached by histological examination (Carpelan-Holmstrom et al. 2005). Thus, proper recognition of variants of PDAC and other malignant tumours of the pancreas requires specialist pathological expertise (Alderson et al. 2005).

Grading of PDAC is essential and an independent prognostic factor. The WHO criteria entail the combined assessment of glandular differentiation, mucin production, nuclear atypia, and mitotic activity, in which each of these four

Table 5.3 Different schemes of histological grading of pancreatic ductal carcinomas

WHO-grading system [Hamilton and Aalton 2000]				
Tumour grade (score range)	Glandular differentiation (score)	Mucin production (score)	Mitosis per 10 HPFs (score)	Nuclear features (score)
Grade 1 (1–1.6)	Well-differentiated (1)	Intensive (1)	≤5 (1)	Little polymorphism, polar arrangement (1)
Grade 2 (1.7–2.3)	Moderately differentiated duct-like structures and tubular glands (2)	Irregular (2)	6–10 (2)	Moderate polymorphism (2)
Grade 3 (2.3–3.0)	Poorly differentiated glands, mucoepidermoid and pleomorphic structures (3)	Abortive (3)	≥10 (3)	Marked polymorphism and increased size (3)

Table 5.4 Different schemes of histological grading of pancreatic ductal carcinomas

Grading system according to Adsay et al. [2005]			
Patterns[a]		Score	Grade
1+1, 1+2, 2+1	At least some fully formed glands (P1) and no non-glandular component (P3)	Scores ≤ 3	Grade 1
1+3, 2+2, 3+1	Non-grade 1 or non-grade 3	Score = 4	Grade 2
2+3, 3+2, 3+3	At least some non-glandular areas (P3) and no fully formed glandular elements (no P1)	Score ≥ 5	Grade 3

[a] Pattern 1: well-formed tubular units with complete, easily discernable borders; Pattern 2: incomplete, ill-defined borders, fusion of glands or irregular multi-lumina formation (cribriform architecture); Pattern 3: non-glandular patterns including cord-like areas, individual cell infiltration, nested or solid (sheet-like) growth patterns

categories is evaluated separately from 1 to 3, in the highest grade areas of the tumour and a score is obtained by summation of the results and its division by 4 (Tables 5.3 and 5.4). Grade 1 tumours have a score of less than 1.7; grade 2, 1.7 to 2.3; and grade 3, greater than or equal to 2.3 (Hamilton and Aalton 2000; Lüttges et al. 2000). This system has proved to be prognostically relevant. Patient prognosis significantly correlates with WHO tumour grading (Lüttges et al. 2000). However, it is a cumbersome and complicated grading system, which also relies on counting mitotic figures in high-grade areas and requires observer experience.

Recently a new grading system was proposed that is similar to the Gleason's scoring system used for prostate cancer (Adsay et al. 2005). The Gleason's system divides the histoarchitecture of prostate adenocarcinomas into five patterns. Since the morphology of PDAC and prostate carcinoma share certain similarities, this grading system can be transferred to pancreatic cancer. However, since Gleason patterns 1 and 2 are practically non-existent in PDAC, this leaves only three different patterns attributable to PDAC. PDAC pattern 1 is characterized by well-formed tubular units with complete, easily discernable borders. Pattern 2 shows incomplete, ill-defined borders, fusion of glands or irregular multi-lumina formation (cribriform architecture). Pattern 3 has non-glandular patterns including cord-like areas, individual cell infiltration, nested or solid (sheet-like) growth patterns. Finally, a score is obtained by the summation of the predominant and the secondary patterns, which is then translated into an overall grade 1 (score ≤ 3), grade 2 (score $= 4$) and grade 3 (score ≥ 5). Interestingly, this modified grading system has a moderately good reproducibility (kappa value of 0.43) and can be easily applied even by surgical pathologists with limited exposure to PDACs (Adsay et al. 2005). Furthermore, it seems to more accurately predict tumour biology and patient prognosis than the WHO grading system (Adsay et al. 2005).

However, both systems have clearly demonstrated that grading of PDAC matters and predicts patient prognosis. Future confirmatory studies are required to prove which of these different grading systems is more practicable and reliable or whether they can be used in a complementary way.

5.6 Prognostic Factors

Apart from grading, many studies, comprising more than 3,000 patients collectively, provide strong evidence that tumour size, lymphatic invasion, presence of lymph node and distant metastases, UICC tumour stage, resection margins, and infiltration of large vessels and veins correlate significantly with patient prognosis (Benassai et al. 2000; Brennan et al. 2004; Gebhardt et al. 2000; Kuhlmann et al. 2004; Lim et al. 2003; Lüttges et al. 2000; Millikan et al. 1999; Moon et al. 2006; Sohn et al. 2000; Takai et al. 2003; Tseng et al. 2004; Wenger et al. 2000). Table 5.5 gives a selection of studies which investigated independent prognostic factors of pancreatic cancer. Thus, post-operative staging necessitates a surgical pathology report that provides all this information.

However, following surgical resection, the vast majority of pancreatic cancers return, even those with R0 status and supposedly tumour-free lymph nodes. This observation has raised concern that the routine surgical examination is not sensitive enough and fails to detect minimal residual disease. Sensitivity can be increased by immunohistochemistry and molecular assays (Niedergethmann et al. 2002; Ridwelski et al. 2001). Niedergethmann et al. (2002) showed in a prospective study that immunohistochemical detection of tumour cells in paraaortic lymph nodes and PCR-based assays with respect to mutated K-*ras* in codon 12 are superior to conventional histological examination. Tumour cells were found by conventional histology in 3 out of 69 patients with PDAC, by immunohistochemistry in 5 and, using molecular assays, K-*ras* mutations identical to those of the primary tumour were found in 12 paraaortic lymph nodes. All of the latter patients had recurrence after surgery and a significant poorer survival than those without detection of mutated K-*ras* in paraaortic lymph nodes. This study supports the contention that recurrence may be related to incomplete resection of e.g. lymph node metastases.

Table 5.5 Independent prognostic factors of pancreatic cancer resected by pancreaticoduodenectomy in multivariate survival analyses

Reference	No. of patients	Study period	Resection margin		Tumour grade		Tumour size			Positive lymph nodes	Adjuvant therapy
			Negative (R0)	Positive	G1/G2	G3	>1 cm	>2 cm	< 3 cm		
			Hazard ratio [95% CI]								
Benassai et al. 2000	75	1974–1995		2.29 [1.91–2.67]		1.14 [0.86–1.42]			0.73 [0.45–1.01]	1.17 [0.86–1.48]	N.d.
Kuhlmann et al. 2004	160	1992–2002		1.57 [1.10–2.23]		1.31 [1.13–1.52]	1.25 [1.06–1.48]			1.58 [1.08–2.31]	-
Lim et al. 2003	296	1991–1996	N.d.			1.67 [1.12–2.50]		1.57 [1.10–2.26]		1.36 [1.05–1.75]	N.d.
Lüttges et al. 2000	70	1990–1997		5.4 [2.51–11.7]		2.7 [1.06–7.09]	N.d.			N.s.	N.d.
Moon et al. 2006	94	1995–2002	0.23 [0.12–0.42]		0.37 [0.19–0.72]				0.46 [0.27–0.78]	N.s.	0.61 [0.37–0.99]
Sohn et al. 2000	616	1984–1999	0.64 [0.50–0.82]		0.71 [0.56–0.90]				0.72 [0.57–0.90]	N.s[a]	0.50 [0.39–0.64]
Takai et al. 2003	167	1992–2000	N.s.[a]		N.s.				2.22[a] [1.25–3.95]	1.78 [1.04–3.06]	N.s.
Tseng et al. 2004	291	1990–2002	N.s.		N.d.		N.s.			1.5 [1.10–2.05]	N.s.

[a] Significant only on univariate analysis; tumour size>3 cm

5.7 Ancillary Techniques

Considerable research has focussed on identifying molecular events in pancreatic carcinogenesis, and their correlation with clinicopathological variables of pancreatic tumours and survival that can be used as an adjunct to predict patient prognosis (for a review, see (Garcea et al. 2005)). Using immunohistochemistry, the expression of oncogenes (K-*ras*, *cyclin D1*), tumour suppressor genes (*p53*, *p16*, *p21*, *SMAD4/DPC4*, *p27*), proteins involved in apoptosis (Bcl-2, Bax, Survivin), growth factors (TGFβ, EGF, FGFs) and growth factor receptors (EGFR-1 to -4, bFGFR), proteases (MMPs, uPA, cathepsin B, heparanse) cell–cell adhesion molecules (E-cadherin, α-catenin, β-catenin, γ-catenin), and angiogenic biomarkers (VEGF, VEGFR, PDGF, TSP-1) has been investigated (Garcea et al. 2005). The expression of several of these markers was shown to correlate significantly with patient prognosis and survival. However, their impact on patient management and treatment is still limited.

5.8 Proteomics

More recently, the investigation of the pancreatic cancer proteome has gained considerable attention. After the first two drafts of the complete human genome were published in 2001 (Lander et al. 2001; Venter et al. 2001) it was evident that there is not even half of the number of chromosomal genes that had been expected originally: both groups identified 30,000–35,000 genes instead of the expected 100,000 (Lander et al. 2001; Venter et al. 2001). The "true" number of genes is surpassed by an estimated number of proteins of several millions (Anderson et al. 2004; Anderson and Anderson 2002; Pieper et al. 2003). The genome is basically the same in every cell type and is relatively static. Mutations, chromosomal instability and epigenetic modifications do not contribute significantly to physiological cell and tissue homeostasis. The latter is accomplished by the proteome. Apart from a low gene to gene-product ratio, several studies have indicated that mRNA expression levels do not necessarily correlate with protein expression or disease progression, whereas profiles of proteins and their various isoforms are able to more accurately identify disease states, such as cancer (Wulfkuhle et al. 2003). Cancer may be genetically based, but on the functional level, it is a proteomic disease: tumour progression, invasion and metastasis depend on the functional activity of proteins, such as growth factors and proteases. Additionally, the vast majority of drug targets, including those for cancer, are proteins (Wulfkuhle et al. 2003). Furthermore, transcriptomics cannot predict the activation of key signalling molecules in important protein networks. These developments and considerations have brought the proteome back into focus (for a review see Röcken et al. 2004).

Four different sources have been searched for novel protein-based biomarkers for pancreatic cancer, i.e. serum (Bhattacharyya et al. 2004; Koopmann et al. 2004; Xia et al. 2005; Yu et al. 2005a,b), pancreatic juice (Gronborg et al. 2004; Rosty et al. 2002), pancreatic tissue (Chen et al. 2005; Shekouh et al. 2003) and culture supernatants of pancreatic cell lines (Gronborg et al. 2005). Few groups searched for biomarkers using samples from pancreatic cancer and corresponding non-neoplastic tissues (Chen et al. 2005; Shekouh et al. 2003). However, sampling of pancreatic tissue depends on adequate sampling. Tissue homogenates of undissected non-neoplastic pancreatic tissue enclose ductal and acinar cells, various neuroendocrine cells and mesenchymal cells, among others. Normal ductal epithelial cells, from which the cancer is believed to arise, represent as little as 5% of the normal pancreas. The differences between the proteomes of undissected pancreatic tissue and ductal epithelium, enriched by laser capture microdissection, was elegantly demonstrated by Shekouh et al. (2003). Thus, using undissected non-neoplastic pancreatic tissue can generate highly misleading results (Röcken and Ebert 2006).

In recent years many elaborate studies have shown that proteomics is suitable to search for novel biomarkers for pancreatic cancer. The number of differentially expressed or secreted proteins in pancreatic cancer is overwhelming. However, a meticulous analysis of their suitability in a large series of pancreatic cancer patients and an equal number of adequate controls is missing so far. To date, none of the biomarkers has reached a clinical stage.

5.9 Conclusion

Post-operative staging of pancreatic cancer necessitates a thorough surgical pathological examination of the pancreaticoduodenectomy specimen, since it harbours information that has been shown to correlate with patient prognosis and survival, i.e. tumour size, histological tumour type, tumour grade, lymphatic invasion, presence of lymph node and distant metastases, UICC tumour stage, resection margins, and infiltration of large vessels and veins. Ancillary techniques such as immunohistochemistry and molecular analysis can be used to detect micrometastases and predict patient prognosis more accurately. However, post-operative staging can only influence post-operative management of cancer patients. It does not have any impact on the major culprit of pancreatic cancer, i.e. its recognition in advanced stages. In the future, proteomic analysis of patient serum or pancreatic juice may have the potential to improve early diagnosis of pancreatic cancer patients (Ebert et al. 2006).

References

Adsay NV, Basturk O, Bonnett M, et al. (2005) A proposal for a new and more practical grading scheme for pancreatic ductal adenocarcinoma. Am J Surg Pathol 29:724–733

Albores-Saaverda J, Hefess C, Hruban RH, et al. (1998) Recommendations for the reporting of pancreatic specimens containing malignant tumours. Association of Directors of Anatomic and Surgical Pathology. Hum Pathol 29:893–895

Alderson D, Johnson CD, Neoptolomeos JP, et al. (2005) Guidelines for the management of patients with pancreatic cancer periampullary and ampullary carcinomas. Gut 54 [Suppl 5]:v1–v16

Anderson NL, Anderson NG (2002) The human plasma proteome: history, character, and diagnostic prospects. Mol Cell Proteomics 1:845–867

Anderson NL, Polanski M, Pieper R, et al. (2004) The human plasma proteome: a non-redundant list developed by combination of four separate sources. Mol Cell Proteomics 3:311–326

Benassai G, Mastrorilli M, Quarto G, et al. (2000) Factors influencing survival after resection for ductal adenocarcinoma of the head of the pancreas. J Surg Oncol 73:212–218

Bhattacharyya S, Siegel ER, Petersen GM, et al. (2004) Diagnosis of pancreatic cancer using serum proteomic profiling. Neoplasia 6:674–686

Brennan MF, Kattan MW, Klimstra D, Conlon K (2004) Prognostic nomogram for patients undergoing resection for adenocarcinoma of the pancreas. Ann Surg 240:293–298

Carpelan-Holmstrom M, Nordling S, Pukkala E, et al. (2005) Does anyone survive pancreatic ductal adenocarcinoma? A nationwide study re-evaluating the data of the Finnish Cancer Registry. Gut 54:385–387

Chen R, Yi EC, Donohoe S, Pan S, et al. (2005) Pancreatic cancer proteome: the proteins that underlie invasion, metastasis, and immunologic escape. Gastroenterology 129:1187–1197

Compton CC, Henson DE (1997) Protocol for the examination of specimens removed from patients with carcinoma of the exocrine pancreas: a basis for checklists. Cancer Committee, College of American Pathologists. Arch Pathol Lab Med 121:1129–1136

Ebert MP, Korc M, Malfertheiner P, Röcken C (2006) Advances, challenges, and limitations in serum-proteome-based cancer diagnosis. J Proteome Res 5:19–25

Garcea G, Neal CP, Pattenden CJ, et al. (2005) Molecular prognostic markers in pancreatic cancer: a systematic review. Eur J Cancer 41:2213–2236

Gebhardt C, Meyer W, Reichel M, Wunsch PH (2000) Prognostic factors in the operative treatment of ductal pancreatic carcinoma. Langenbecks Arch Surg 385:14–20

Gronborg M, Bunkenborg J, Kristiansen TZ, et al. (2004) Comprehensive proteomic analysis of human pancreatic juice. J Proteome Res 3:1042–1055

Gronborg M, Kristiansen TZ, Iwahori A, et al. (2005) Biomarker discovery from pancreatic cancer secretome using a differential proteomics approach. Mol Cell Proteomics 5:157–171

Hamilton SR, Aalton L (2000) Pathology and genetics of tumours of the digestive system. IARC Press, Lyon

Hezel AF, Kimmelman AC, Stanger BZ, et al. (2006) Genetics and biology of pancreatic ductal adenocarcinoma. Genes Dev 20:1218–1249

Hruban RH, Adsay NV, Albores-Saavedra J, et al. (2001) Pancreatic intraepithelial neoplasia: a new nomenclature and classification system for pancreatic duct lesions. Am J Surg Pathol 25:579–586

Hruban RH, Takaori K, Klimstra DS, et al. (2004) An illustrated consensus on the classification of pancreatic intraepithelial neoplasia and intraductal papillary mucinous neoplasms. Am J Surg Pathol 28:977–987

Karhu R, Mahlamaki E, Kallioniemi A (2006) Pancreatic adenocarcinoma—genetic portrait from chromosomes to microarrays. Genes Chromosomes Cancer 45:721–730

Klimstra DS (2005) Cystic, mucin-producing neoplasms of the pancreas: the distinguishing features of mucinous cystic neoplasms and intraductal papillary mucinous neoplasms. Semin Diagn Pathol 22:318–329

Koopmann J, Zhang Z, White N, et al. (2004) Serum diagnosis of pancreatic adenocarcinoma using surface-enhanced laser desorption and ionization mass spectrometry. Clin Cancer Res 10:860–868

Kuhlmann KF, de Castro SM, Wesseling JG, et al. (2004) Surgical treatment of pancreatic adenocarcinoma; actual survival and prognostic factors in 343 patients. Eur J Cancer 40:549–558

Lander ES, Linton LM, Birren B, et al. (2001) Initial sequencing and analysis of the human genome. Nature 409:860–921

Lim JE, Chien MW, Earle CC (2003) Prognostic factors following curative resection for pancreatic adenocarcinoma: a population-based, linked database analysis of 396 patients. Ann Surg 237:74–85

Lüttges J, Vogel I, Menke M, et al. (1998) The retroperitoneal resection margin and vessel involvement are important factors determining survival after pancreaticoduodenectomy for ductal adenocarcinoma of the head of the pancreas. Virchows Arch 433:237–242

Lüttges J, Zamboni G, Klöppel G (1999) Recommendation for the examination of pancreaticoduodenectomy specimens removed from patients with carcinoma of the exocrine pancreas. A proposal for a standardized pathological staging of pancreaticoduodenectomy specimens including a checklist. Dig Surg 16:291–296

Lüttges J, Schemm S, Vogel I, et al. (2000) The grade of pancreatic ductal carcinoma is an independent prognostic factor and is superior to the immunohistochemical assessment of proliferation. J Pathol 191:154–161

Maitra A, Kern SE, Hruban RH (2006) Molecular pathogenesis of pancreatic cancer. Best Pract Res Clin Gastroenterol 20:211–226

Millikan KW, Deziel DJ, Silverstein JC, et al. (1999) Prognostic factors associated with resectable adenocarcinoma of the head of the pancreas. Am Surg 65:618–623

Moon HJ, An JY, Heo JS, et al. (2006) Predicting survival after surgical resection for pancreatic ductal adenocarcinoma. Pancreas 32:37–43

Niedergethmann M, Rexin M, Hildenbrand R, et al. (2002) Prognostic implications of routine, immunohistochemical, and molecular staging in resectable pancreatic adenocarcinoma. Am J Surg Pathol 26:1578–1587

Pieper R, Gatlin CL, Makusky AJ, et al. (2003) The human serum proteome: display of nearly 3700 chromatographically separated protein spots on two-dimensional electrophoresis gels and identification of 325 distinct proteins. Proteomics 3:1345–1364

Ridwelski K, Meyer F, Fahlke J, et al. (2001) Value of cytokeratin and Ca 19-9 antigen in immunohistological detection of disseminated tumour cells in lymph nodes in pancreas carcinoma. Chirurg 72:920–926

Röcken C, Ebert MP (2006) Pancreatic cancer proteome. Gastroenterology 130:1017–1018

Röcken C, Ebert MP, Roessner A (2004) Proteomics in pathology, research and practice. Pathol Res Pract 200:69–82

Rosty C, Christa L, Kuzdzal S, et al. (2002) Identification of hepatocarcinoma-intestine-pancreas/pancreatitis-associated protein I as a biomarker for pancreatic ductal adenocarcinoma by protein biochip technology. Cancer Res 62:1868–1875

Sato N, Goggins M (2006) The role of epigenetic alterations in pancreatic cancer. J Hepatobiliary Pancreat Surg 13:286–295

Shekouh AR, Thompson CC, Prime W, et al. (2003) Application of laser capture microdissection combined with two-dimensional electrophoresis for the discovery of differentially regulated proteins in pancreatic ductal adenocarcinoma. Proteomics 3:1988–2001

Sohn TA, Yeo CJ, Cameron JL, et al. (2000) Resected adenocarcinoma of the pancreas-616 patients: results, outcomes, and prognostic indicators. J Gastrointest Surg 4:567–579

Takai S, Satoi S, Toyokawa H, et al. (2003) Clinicopathologic evaluation after resection for ductal adenocarcinoma of the pancreas: a retrospective, single-institution experience. Pancreas 26:243–249

Tseng JF, Raut CP, Lee JE, et al. (2004) Pancreaticoduodenectomy with vascular resection: margin status and survival duration. J Gastrointest Surg 8:935–949

Venter JC, Adams MD, Myers EW, et al. (2001) The sequence of the human genome. Science 291:1304–1351

Wenger FA, Peter F, Zieren J, et al. (2000) Prognosis factors in carcinoma of the head of the pancreas. Dig Surg 17:29–35

Wulfkuhle JD, Liotta LA, Petricoin EF (2003) Proteomic applications for the early detection of cancer. Nat Rev Cancer 3:267–275

Xia Q, Kong XT, Zhang GA, et al. (2005) Proteomics-based identification of DEAD-box protein 48 as a novel autoantigen, a prospective serum marker for pancreatic cancer. Biochem Biophys Res Commun 330:526–532

Yeo CJ, Cameron JL, Lillemoe KD, et al. (2002) Pancreaticoduodenectomy with or without distal gastrectomy and extended retroperitoneal lymphadenectomy for periampullary adenocarcinoma, part 2: randomized controlled trial evaluating survival, morbidity, and mortality. Ann Surg 236:355–366

Yu KH, Rustgi AK, Blair IA (2005a) Characterization of proteins in human pancreatic cancer serum using differential gel electrophoresis and tandem mass spectrometry. J Proteome Res 4:1742–1751

Yu Y, Chen S, Wang LS, et al. (2005b) Prediction of pancreatic cancer by serum biomarkers using surface-enhanced laser desorption/ionization-based decision tree classification. Oncology 68:79–86

6 Adjuvant Therapy in Patients with Pancreatic Cancer

L. Roll

Recent Results in Cancer Research, Vol. 177

Abstract

The prognosis for patients with pancreatic cancer is still very poor. A complete (R0) surgical resection of the tumor poses the only chance of cure. At the moment only postoperative chemotherapy with gemcitabine has significantly delayed the development of recurrent disease and showed an improvement in long-term survival compared to observation alone. It is essential to develop more effective adjuvant therapy strategies with involvement of all therapeutic options to change the disappointing situation.

6.1 Prognosis

The only chance of cure for patients with pancreatic cancer is a complete (R0) surgical resection of the tumor. Unfortunately, only 10%–25% of cases are potentially resectable at the time of diagnosis. The precondition for R0 resection is the absence of distant metastasis. Especially, the dimension of infiltration of peripancreatic tissue and the big vessels, the size and localization of the primary tumor, and the concomitance of involved lymph nodes are constitutive criteria for a curative-intent resection [19, 35–37]. Nonetheless, prognosis is still poor, even for those undergoing complete (R0) resection. Therefore, the development and clinical approval of effective adjuvant therapies is necessary.

6.2 Adjuvant Chemotherapy

Pancreatic cancer is a systemic disease. It has been shown that 42%–53% of resected cases develop distant metastasis in the peritoneum, 27% of cases develop extra abdominal metastasis, and more than 60% of recurrent cancer occurs in the liver. Only 20% of cases develop a solitary local recurrence. However, these patients frequently develop distant metastases soon after [13, 17, 33]. Until recently, the available drugs for palliative chemotherapy for patients with progressive pancreatic cancer were not effective. The strategies for chemotherapies have shown a high toxicity accompanied by a questionable benefit. Until the mid-1990s, all common chemotherapy regimens included 5-fluorouracil (5-FU) solely or in combination with other drugs such as methotrexate, vincristine, cyclophosphamide, cisplatin, mitomycin C, or doxorubicin.

The first and for a long time only randomized study of adjuvant systemic chemotherapy [5-FU, mitomycin C, and doxorubicin (FAM)-protocol] showed a statistically significant improvement in overall survival (OS) for the treatment group (23 months vs 11 months) [3]. However, there was a poor improvement of long-term survival (5-year survival was 4% vs 8%) and the small number of only 61 randomized patients made this study less than convincing. As published in an earlier case-control study by Splinter [32], the chemotherapy in the postoperative period was not well tolerated by patients. Only 13 of the 30 patients in the (randomized) treatment arm received all planned therapy cycles; in fact, only 24 patients started the treatment. The oral administration of 5-FU (150 mg/m^2 daily for 1 year) and mitomycin C i.v. (6 mg/m^2 on the day of surgery) resulted in a high toxicity, including one case of death. Actually, there is no convincing proof for the successful use of 5-FU in a palliative situation of pancreatic cancer [2] (Table 6.1).

Table 6.1 Adjuvant chemotherapy

	n	Chemotherapy regime	Median OS (months)	2-Y-S (%)	3-Y-S (%)	5-Y-S (%)
Splinter et al. 1989[a] [32]	36	Observation	-		28	-
	16	IV FAM	-		24	-
Bakkevold et al. 1993[b] [3]	31	Observation	11		30	8
	30	IV FAM	23		70	4
Lygidakis 2002[b] [20]	40	Observation		29	15	0
	45	SMA: CBCDA, MITX, MMC, 5-FU, FA		52	31	0
	43	SMA: CBCDA, MITX, MMC, 5-FU, FA+interleukin 2		65	49	18
Amano et al. 1999[b] [2]	158 (all)	Observation				18
		Oral 5-FU+MMC				11.5
Ishikawa et al. 1997 [15]	27	A. hepatica, v. portae: 5-FU	-		51	41
Beger et al. 1999 [4]	24	Truncus coeliacus: 5-FU/FA, MITX, CDDP	23			4-Y-S 54 R0-resected only
Beger et al. 1998[a] [5]	42	Observation	9.3			
	20	Truncus coeliacus: 5-FU/FA, MITX, CDDP	18.5			
Oettle et al. 2007[b] [26]	179	Gemcitabine 1 g/m^2 d1,8,15q28 for 6 months	13.4			
	175	Observation	6.9			

5-FU, 5-fluorouracil; 1-/2-/-3-/5-Y-S, 1-, 2-, 3-, or 5-year survival; CBCDA, carboplatin; CDDP, cisplatin; FA, folinic acid; FAM, 5-FU+doxorubicin+mitomycin C; MITX, mitoxantrone; MMC, mitomycin C; OS, overall survival; SMA, superior mesenteric artery

[a] Historical control

[b] Randomized study

To reduce the subjective and objective side effects of aggressive chemotherapy regimens on the one hand and to increase the effect of the locoregional control of the disease on the other hand, regional applied adjuvant chemotherapies have been investigated in the recent years (Table 6.1). In two nonrandomized studies, long-term survival could be improved by application of chemotherapeutics via truncus coeliacus, a. hepatica or v. portae in contrast to untreated historical control groups. A survival time of 4 years was achieved in half of the treated patients after R0 resection [4, 5, 15]. However, these data are not sufficient for a definite judgment.

6.3 Current Adjuvant Therapy Studies

In 1994, before gemcitabine was established as the palliative therapy standard, the randomization for the phase III study of the European Study Group for Pancreatic Cancer (ESPAC-1) for adjuvant therapy of resected pancreatic cancer had started. Within 7 years, 541 patients in total were recruited into this study [23, 24]; 285 patients were randomized according to the originally designated 2×2-factorial design. It divided the group into four study arms: observation ($n=69$), radiochemotherapy alone ($n=70$), chemotherapy alone ($n=74$), and combined chemotherapy and radiochemotherapy ($n=72$). The adjuvant chemotherapy consisted of 5-FU/folinic acid according to the Mayo scheme (folinic acid 20 mg/m^2+5-FU 425 mg/m^2 d1–5 every 4 weeks × 6 cycles); radiochemotherapy was applied according to the European standard (5-FU 500 mg/m^2 d1–3 and d15–17+20 Gy in 10 daily fractions over 2 weeks).

In the first publication of the pooled analysis, no survival difference was shown between the compared 175 patients receiving postoperative chemoradiotherapy and the 178 patients who did not receive such therapy. The median OS was 15.5 months vs 16.1 months. In contrast, a significant survival benefit for the 238 patients who received an adjuvant chemotherapy compared to the 235 patients who did not receive it. The median OS was 19.7 months vs 14 months, $p=0.0005$. This study has been criticized for its complex design and, hence, the difficulties in interpreting the results: Patients and clinicians were allowed to select which trial to enter and, according to their own preferences, to perform a "background" chemoradiation or chemotherapy independent from their treatment arm. In the pooled "intent-to-treat-analysis," nearly one-third of the patients in the "no chemotherapy" group and in the group for "chemotherapy alone" were treated with chemoradiotherapy [23, 24].

In a second publication after a median follow-up of 47 months the authors concluded that adjuvant radiation had a deleterious effect, possibly because it delayed sequential chemotherapy, while chemotherapy with 5-FU had a significant beneficial effect. Indeed, given the marginal activity of 5-FU in the palliative setting, the survival advantage obtained with adjuvant 5-FU in ESPAC-1 appears very surprising. A statistical comparison of the four original groups based on the 2 × 2 randomization was not possible due to lack of adequate power. For example, median survival among the 75 patients randomized to 5-FU chemotherapy was 21.6 months (95% CI, 14.2–22.5) compared with 16.9 months (95% CI, 12.3–24.8) for the 69 patients randomized to observation. Thus, 95% confidence intervals were large and widely overlapping. Since disease-free survival as well as 3-year OS data were not reported, a comparison with the results of our study is not possible [25]. In the simple and straightforwardly designed German- Austrian CONKO-001 study, an open, multicenter, randomized, controlled phase III trial, from July 1998 to December 2004, a total of 368 patients with gross complete (R0 or R1) resection of pancreatic cancer and no prior radiation or chemotherapy were enrolled. Gemcitabine was chosen by the authors as the adjuvant treatment because it was, and still is, considered the most active single agent in the treatment of locally advanced or metastasized pancreatic cancer [8, 27, 34]. Patients were prospectively randomized, with stratification for resection, tumor status, and nodal status, to receive either adjuvant chemotherapy with six cycles of gemcitabine 1,000 mg/m^2 day 1, 8, and 15 every 4 weeks (arm A) or observation (arm B). This year the primary endpoint analysis of this trial demonstrated that in accordance with study hypothesis, 6 months of adjuvant treatment with gemcitabine improved median disease-free survival (DFS) highly significantly in patients with completely resected pancreatic cancer by more than 6 months compared with observation alone (13.4 vs. 6.9 months, $p<0.001$). With a median follow-up of 53 months, the disease-free survival analysis was based on a total number of 294 (83%) observed relapses among 354 eligible patients; only 14 patients (7 in each arm) out of a total of 368 enrolled had to be excluded from the intent-to-treat population due to major violations of the entry criteria. The beneficial effect of adjuvant gemcitabine on DFS was evident in both subgroups for patients with R0 (13.1 vs 7.3 months; $p<0.001$) and R1 resection (15.8 vs 5.5 months; $p<0.001$). The estimated DFS at 3 and 5 years was 23.5% and 16.5% in the treatment arm, and 7.5% and 5.5% in the observation arm, respectively.

OS failed slightly to show a significant difference in the intent-to-treat analysis at the time of publication ($p=0.061$), with 27% of all patients still being alive. Median survival times were 22.1

vs 20.2 months in arm A and B, respectively. This relatively small difference in median survival may be explained by the fact that patients in the observation arm were regularly offered gemcitabine for palliation as soon as a relapse occurred. The divergence between the survival curves increased with longer follow-up, and estimated survival at 3 years was 34.0% in the treatment arm compared with 20.5% in the observation arm. At 5 years, approximately twice as many patients in the adjuvant treatment arm compared with observation are estimated to be alive (22.5 vs 11.5%). On the other hand, the qualified survival analysis was prespecified and designed to provide results that more closely reflect the "true" therapeutic potential of adjuvant gemcitabine in this setting. Therefore, in this analysis, only patients from the active arm who received at least one full cycle (three weekly doses) of gemcitabine, and patients from the control arm who did not receive any cytotoxic agents or radiation therapy prior to relapse were included. Patients from both arms were excluded from the analysis if minor violations of the entry criteria were identified. As anticipated from this selection process, the advantage in DFS and OS conferred by adjuvant gemcitabine over observation alone was greater in the qualified compared with the intent-to-treat (ITT) population and included a highly significant improvement in median OS (24.2 vs 20.5 months, $p=0.015$) [26]. Postoperative gemcitabine significantly delayed the development of recurrent disease after complete resection of pancreatic cancer compared with observation alone, and the increase in long-term survival was encouraging. Based on these results, gemcitabine, despite minimal toxicity and no compromise in quality of life, offers high promise to become the new standard treatment in the adjuvant pancreatic cancer setting.

6.4 Multimodal Adjuvant Therapy Regimes

In the phase II trials of the Gastrointestinal Tumor Study Group (GITSG) [12, 16], 51 patients were treated with weekly bolus 5-FU for 2 years after radiochemotherapy. The results of OS were superior to OS results of a nonpublicized follow-up study of the UK Pancreatic Cancer Trial Group. One reason could be the inclusion of R1 patients in the follow-up study. In both studies the side effects were moderate.

Preliminary study results from Johns Hopkins University demonstrated an advantage in DSF using treatment with a systemic chemotherapy comprising 5-FU, folinic acid, mitomycin C, and dipyridamole for 4 months after radiochemotherapy compared to a nonrandomized control group with no adjuvant treatment [9]. The side effects were much more aggressive compared to the study design of the GITSG. In the American phase III study, RTOG 9704, from July 1998 to July 2002, 538 patients were included, 381 with cancer of the pancreatic head. After stratification for resection, tumor size, and nodal status, patients were randomized either to receive pre- and post-chemoradiotherapy with 5-FU (continued infusion 250 mg/m^2 per day) or gemcitabine (1 g/m^2 weekly). In both arms the treatment was performed for 3 weeks before and then again for 3 weeks after 12 weeks of chemoradiotherapy with 50.4 Gy in daily fractions of 1.8 Gy and continued infusion of 5-FU (250 mg/m^2 per day). The ASCO 2006 preliminary results showed—exclusively for the subgroup of patients with pancreatic head cancer ($n=381$) among the eligible patients ($n=442$)—a significant improvement of the medial OS and the 3-year survival rate, with 36.9 months and 32% for the gemcitabine group vs 20.6 months and 21% for patients in the 5-FU-group ($p=0.047$). On the other hand, a significant difference in OS for the total study population, including cancer of pancreatic corpus and tail, failed [31]. The Picozzi phase II trial investigated 43 patients with a multimodal therapy regime consisting of cisplatin (30 mg/m^2), 5-FU (200 mg/m^2), interferon alpha, and simultaneous radiation (45–54 Gy in 25 daily fractions) followed by 5-FU (200 mg/m^2). After an average follow-up time of 31.9 months, 67% of patients were still alive and 1-/2-/ and 5-year survival rates of 95%, 64%, and 55% were demonstrated. However, this therapy regime was very toxic. Of the patients, 70% had to interrupt the therapy and 42% had to be hospitalized because of side effects such as nausea, vomiting, and diarrhea [29, 30] (Table 6.2). These encouraging results need to be validated in prospective multicenter

Table 6.2 Multimodal therapy

	n	Local therapy	Systemically chemotherapy	Median overall survival (months)	2-Y-S (%)	5-Y-S (%)
Kalser et al. 1985 [16]	21			20		19
GITSG 1987 [12]	30	45 Gy+bolus 5-FU	5-FU bolus (2 years)	18		17
UKPACA-1 1995	35	40 Gy+bolus 5-FU	5-FU bolus (2 years)		36	
Ozaki et al. 1990 [28]	16	IORT 30 Gy	MMC (local and systemically)		1-Y-S 88	
					3-Y-S 53	
Chakravarthy et al. 1998 [9]	28	50 Gy+bolus 5-FU/ FA+dipyridamole	-		45	
	12	50 Gy+bolus 5-FU/ FA+dipyridamole	5-FU Bolus, FA, MMC, dipyridamole		After 9 months: recurrence-free 81	
Abrams et al. 1999 [1]	23	5-FU/FA+3–27 Gy liver	5-FU ci+FA	15.9		
		50–54 Gy lymph nodes				
		50–57 Gy tumor				
Morganti et al. 1999 [22]	8	pre-op. 40 Gy+ci 5-FU+IORT	5-FU/MMC/ADR	18.5		
Picozzi et al. 2003 [29, 30]	43	45–54 Gy+CDDP/ ci 5-FU/IFN-alpha	5-FU ci 2x6 weeks		1-Y-S 95	55
					2-Y-S 64	
Friedman et al. 1999 [11]	11	45–54 Gy+ci 5-FU	Gemcitabine 4–6 months			
Demols et al. 2005 [10]	30	45 Gy+Gem 300 mg/m^2	Gemcitabine 2#	19		
RTOG 9704 2006[b] [31]	187	50.4 Gy 1.8 Gy/fx per day 5-FU ci	5-FU ci 3 weeks pre- and 12 weeks post-RCT	20.6 (pancreatic head cancer)	3-Y-S 21 (pancreatic head cancer)	
	194	50.4 Gy 1.8 Gy/fx per day 5-FU ci	Gemcitabine 3 weeks pre- and 12 weeks post-RCT	36.9 (pancreatic head cancer)	3-Y-S 32 (pancreatic head cancer)	

5-FU, 5-fluorouracil; 1-/2-/-3-/5-Y-S, 1-, 2-, 3-, or 5-year survival; ADR, doxorubicin; CDDP, cisplatin; ci, continued infusion; FA, folinic acid; fx, fraction; gemcitabine 2#, gemcitabine for two cycles (or for 2 months pre-RCT); IFN, interferon; IORT, intraoperative radiotherapy; MMC, mitomycin C; pre-op., before surgery; RCT, radiochemotherapy

[a] Randomized study

studies. Furthermore, therapy regimes have to be modified to minimize the toxic effect for patients in the adjuvant situation. Experiences with new substances such as gemcitabine as the radiosensitive agent and as systemic treatment remain to be made [14, 18].

6.5 Adjuvant Immunotherapy

Systemic treatment with monoclonal antibodies was not beneficial in the adjuvant situation. The disappointing results of four studies with antibody MAb 17-1A in the palliative therapy of pancreatic cancer led to abandonment for the present in the adjuvant situation. In a phase II study, the murine antibody MAb BW494 showed only limited activity in nonresectable pancreatic cancer cases [6]. The results of a small, randomized study with 61 eligible patients treated with MAb BW494 after resection did not reach a statisticall significance in median OS: 428 days for the treatment group and 386 days for the control group [7]. Lygidakis et al. investigated the efficacy of a combined locoregional chemotherapy and immunotherapy. In matched groups, 80 patients were enrolled to receive either no specific therapy or a regional therapy administered via a. lienalis and a. mesenterica superior. This complex therapy regime consists of combined chemotherapy with 5-FU, folinic acid, cisplatin, mitomycin C, and immunotherapy with interleukin-2 and interferon-gamma for 3 years after resection. It was shown that the median OS was significant higher for the treatment group in contrast to the untreated patients (30 months vs 16.8 months, $p<0.001$). A further investigative trial demonstrated a higher rate of complete remission of the disease with the same immunotherapy combined with a modified chemotherapy consisting of carboplatin, docetaxel, and gemcitabine after a curative intended resection [21]. A subsequent randomized phase III study with 128 patients could underline the benefit of a locoregional chemotherapy combined with immunotherapy. Patients were randomized in three groups: arm A (observation only), arm B (locoregional chemotherapy via SMA with carboplatin, mitoxantrone, mitomycin C, 5-FU, folinic acid), and arm C (locoregional chemotherapy like arm B and additional immunotherapy with interleukin-2). The analysis demonstrated significant results in the survival rates after 2 and 5 years (29% and 0% in arm A, 52% and 0% in arm B, 65% and 18% in arm C) [20]. To gain confidence in the feasibility of this complex therapy, these promising results have to be supported in further multicenter studies, including an examination of the intraoperative implantation of the catheter in the a. mesenterica superior.

References

1. Abrams RA, Grochow LB, Chakravarthy A, et al. (1999) Intensified adjuvant therapy for pancreatic and periampullary adenocarcinoma: survival results and observations regarding patterns of failure, radiotherapy dose and CA19-9 levels. Int J Radiat Oncol Biol Phys 44:1039–1046
2. Amano H, Takada T, Kato H, et al. (1999) Five-year results of a randomized study of postoperative adjuvant chemotherapy for resected pancreatic-biliary carcinomas (meeting abstract). ASCO 1999
3. Bakkevold KE, Arnesjo B, Dahl O, et al. (1993) Adjuvant combination chemotherapy (AMF) following radical resection of carcinoma of the pancreas and papilla of Vater—results of a controlled, prospective, randomised multicentre study. Eur J Cancer 29A:698–703
4. Beger HG, Gansauge F, Buchler MW, et al. (1999) Intraarterial adjuvant chemotherapy after pancreaticoduodenectomy for pancreatic cancer: significant reduction in occurrence of liver metastasis. World J Surg 23:946–949
5. Beger HG, Link KH, Gansauge F (1998) Adjuvant regional chemotherapy in advanced pancreatic cancer: results of a prospective study. Hepatogastroenterology 45:638–643
6. Buchler M, Friess H, Malfertheiner P, et al. (1990) Studies of pancreatic cancer utilizing monoclonal antibodies. Int J Pancreatol 7:151–157
7. Buchler M, Friess H, Schultheiss KH, et al. (1991) A randomized controlled trial of adjuvant immunotherapy (murine monoclonal antibody 494/32) in resectable pancreatic cancer. Cancer 68:1507–1512
8. Burris HA 3rd, Moore MJ, Andersen J, et al. (1997) Improvements in survival and clinical benefit with gemcitabine as first-line therapy for patients with advanced pancreas cancer: a randomized trial. J Clin Oncol 15:2403–2413
9. Chakravarthy A, Yeo C (1998) Preliminary result of a phase II study of adjuvant combined modality therapy for resected pancreatic and periampullary adenocarcinoma using local irradiation, 5-FU, leucovorin, dipyridamole and mitomycin-C (meeting abstract). ASCO 1998

10. Demols A, Peeters M, Polus M, et al. (2005) Adjuvant gemcitabine and concurrent continuous radiation (45 Gy) for resected pancreatic head carcinoma: a multicenter Belgian phase II study. Int J Radiat Oncol Biol Phys 62:1351–1356
11. Friedman N, Brenner MJ, Linder JA, Bosley JA, Burdick RK, Didolkar MS (1999) Adjuvant radiation and continuous 5-FU followed by gemcitabine as adjuvant treatment for resected pancreatic cancer (meeting abstract). ASCO 1999
12. Gastrointestinal Tumor Study Group (1987) Further evidence of effective adjuvant combined radiation and chemotherapy following curative resection of pancreatic cancer. Cancer 59:2006–2010
13. Griffin JF, Smalley SR, Jewell W, et al. (1990) Patterns of failure after curative resection of pancreatic carcinoma. Cancer 1990 66:56–61
14. Hoffman JP, Lipsitz S, Pisansky T, et al. (1998) Phase II trial of preoperative radiation therapy and chemotherapy for patients with localized, resectable adenocarcinoma of the pancreas: an Eastern Cooperative Oncology Group study. J Clin Oncol 1998 16:317–323
15. Ishikawa O, Ohigashi H, Imaoka S, et al. (1997) Regional chemotherapy to prevent hepatic metastasis after resection of pancreatic cancer. Hepatogastroenterology 1997 44:1541–1546
16. Kalser MH, Ellenberg SS (1985) Pancreatic cancer. Adjuvant combined radiation and chemotherapy following curative resection. Arch Surg 120:899–903
17. Kayahara M, Nagakawa T, Ueno K, et al. (1993) An evaluation of radical resection for pancreatic cancer based on the mode of recurrence as determined by autopsy and diagnostic imaging. Cancer 1993 72:2118–2123
18. Kudrimoti M, Regine W, John W, et al. (1999) Concurrent infusional gemcitabine and radiation in the treatment of advanced unresectable GI malignancy: a phase I/II study (meeting abstract). ASCO 1999
19. Lillemoe KD, Pitt HA (1996) Palliation. Surgical and otherwise. Cancer 78:605–614
20. Lygidakis NJ, Sgourakis G, Georgia D, et al. (2002) Regional targeting chemoimmunotherapy in patients undergoing pancreatic resection in an advanced stage of their disease: a prospective randomized study. Ann Surg 2002 236:806–813
21. Lygidakis NJ, Stringaris K (1996) Adjuvant therapy following pancreatic resection for pancreatic duct carcinoma: a prospective randomized study. Hepatogastroenterology 43:671–680
22. Morganti AG, Trodella L, Valentini V, et al. (1999) Preoperative radiochemotherapy in pancreatic cancer: preliminary results. Tumori 1999 85: S27–32
23. Neoptolemos JP, Dunn JA, Stocken DD, et al. (2001) Adjuvant chemoradiotherapy and chemotherapy in resectable pancreatic cancer: a randomised controlled trial. Lancet 2001 358:1576–1585
24. Neoptolemos JP, Stocken DD, Dunn JA, et al. (2001) Influence of resection margins on survival for patients with pancreatic cancer treated by adjuvant chemoradiation and/or chemotherapy in the ESPAC-1 randomized controlled trial. Ann Surg 2001 234:758–768
25. Neoptolemos JP, Stocken DD, Friess H, et al. (2004) A randomized trial of chemoradiotherapy and chemotherapy after resection of pancreatic cancer. N Engl J Med 350:1200–1210
26. Oettle H, Post S, Neuhaus P, et al. (2007) Adjuvant chemotherapy with gemcitabine vs observation in patients undergoing curative-intent resection of pancreatic cancer: a randomized controlled trial. JAMA 297:267–277
27. Oettle H, Riess H (2002) Gemcitabine in combination with 5-fluorouracil with or without folinic acid in the treatment of pancreatic cancer. Cancer 95:912–922
28. Ozaki H, Kinoshita T, Kosuge T, et al. (1990) Effectiveness of multimodality treatment for resectable pancreatic cancer. Int J Pancreatol 1990 7:195–200
29. Picozzi V (2003) Adjuvant therapy for resected pancreas cancer (PC) using alpha-interferon (IFN)-based chemoradiation: completion of a phase II trial. ASCO 2003
30. Picozzi VJ, Kozarek RA, Traverso LW (2003) Interferon-based adjuvant chemoradiation therapy after pancreaticoduodenectomy for pancreatic adenocarcinoma. Am J Surg 185:476–480
31. Regine WF, Winter KW, Abrams R, et al. (2006) RTOG 9704, a phase III study of adjuvant pre and post chemoradiation (CRT) 5-FU vs. gemcitabine (G) for resected pancreatic adenocarcinoma. ASCO Annual Meeting Proceedings Part I. J Clin Oncol 24:18S
32. Splinter TA, Obertop H, Kok TC, et al. (1989) Adjuvant chemotherapy after resection of adenocarcinoma of the periampullary region and the head of the pancreas. A non-randomized pilot study. J Cancer Res Clin Oncol 115:200–202

33. Staley CA, Lee JE, Cleary KR, et al. (1996) Preoperative chemoradiation, pancreaticoduodenectomy, and intraoperative radiation therapy for adenocarcinoma of the pancreatic head. Am J Surg 171:118–124
34. Tempero MA, Behrman S, Ben-Josef E, et al. (2005) Pancreatic adenocarcinoma: clinical practice guidelines in oncology. J Natl Compr Canc Netw 3:598–626
35. Trede M, Schwall G, Saeger HD (1990) Survival after pancreatoduodenectomy. 118 consecutive resections without an operative mortality. Ann Surg 211:447–458
36. Watanapa P, Williamson RC (1992) Surgical palliation for pancreatic cancer: developments during the past two decades. Br J Surg 79:8–20
37. Yeo CJ, Abrams RA, Grochow LB, et al. (1997) Pancreaticoduodenectomy for pancreatic adenocarcinoma: postoperative adjuvant chemoradiation improves survival. A prospective, single-institution experience. Ann Surg 225:621–633

7 First-Line Chemotherapy in Advanced Pancreatic Cancer

U. Pelzer

Recent Results in Cancer Research, Vol. 177

Abstract

This chapter focuses on first-line therapy in inoperable pancreatic cancer.

7.1 Introduction

Pancreatic cancer is currently placed seventh in global cancer mortality [1]. In the United States of America, it is the fourth leading cause of cancer-related death. Because less than 10% of cases hold the potential of curative resections, systemic chemotherapy is the major treatment option. Patients with metastatic disease have a median untreated survival of 3–6 months. Due to tumor-related symptoms, such as pain, weight loss, nausea, and vomiting, quality of life (QoL) is impaired significantly.

Gemcitabine was the first drug that demonstrated a benefit in survival (4.4 versus 5.6 months), as well as an improvement in disease-related symptoms in a randomized study [2]. Single-agent chemotherapy with gemcitabine is to date considered the standard of care for patients with advanced pancreatic cancer [3] and it serves as reference in recently published trials. Nevertheless, results for gemcitabine monotherapy are poor and urgently deserve further improvement.

Recently, results for gemcitabine have been challenged by the combination of gemcitabine and erlotinib. One randomized trial demonstrated a significant increase in median survival (6.4 versus 5.9 months; $p=0.03$) for the combination of gemcitabine and erlotinib [4]. Whether this difference is clinically meaningful is a matter of discussion.

7.2 First-Line Chemotherapy

7.2.1 Locally Advanced Disease

Systemic therapy has been accepted as a standard in locally advanced disease. Overall there is no significant benefit for patient treated with chemoradiation [5].

Chemoradiation may have a role as a consolidation treatment for patients who do not have progressive disease during chemotherapy. This approach improved survival from 12 to 15 months in a retrospective analysis of data from phase II/III trials on stage III disease in the Groupe d'Etude et de Recherche en Cancréologie Onco-Radiothérapic (GERCOR) experience [6]. Otherwise we have to note that this overall survival can also be reached with systemic chemotherapeutic treatment without the side effects of radiation. Therefore, chemoradiation may have a marginal impact, only in the individual treatment of patients with local advanced pancreatic cancer.

Last year preliminary results of an important randomized study were published comparing chemoradiation and chemotherapy for patients with locally advanced disease [7]. This trial seems to answer the final question about the impact of chemoradiation on this disease. A median overall survival of 8 months (after 16 months of observation) for patients with chemoradiation (cisplatin/5-FU/radiation) followed by gemcitabine versus 14.5 months for patients with gemcitabine standard therapy is a significant indicator for the use of gemcitabine standard therapy for this patient group.

There are also many other experimental treatment options such as chemoembolism/selected arterial perfusion and many others. None of them seems to be generally recommended for those patients, but the options often serve as a way to individualize treatment design.

7.2.2 Metastatic Disease

Until a decade ago, nihilistic behavior in the treatment of those patients prevailed. In the foreground was the main question about the general use of systemic chemotherapy at all [8, 9]. Two trials comparing chemotherapy with best supportive care suggested that chemotherapy may improve survival time and the quality of life [10, 11]. Further improvement was obtained by using of gemcitabine [2]. In spite of the lack of confirmatory trials and the use of a nonvalidated primary endpoint (clinical benefit), gemcitabine became a standard of care in advanced pancreatic cancer. Gemcitabine achieves an objective response rate of 4%–26%, a median progression-free survival of 2.0–3.8 months, and a 1-year overall survival of 17%–28% [12–19]. The therapeutic activity of gemcitabine administered as a fixed dose rate infusion instead of the standard 30-min infusion did not significantly improve the outcome of patients with advanced pancreatic cancer [12]. The addition of a second cytotoxic agent or other drugs to gemcitabine also did not improve treatment efficacy over single-agent gemcitabine [12–18, 20]. A metaanalysis surmised that the addition of 5-fluorouracil (5-FU), cisplatin, or a platinum compound to gemcitabine may improve 1-year overall survival by 4% [21]. Completed randomized trials comparing standard therapy gemcitabine and combination treatment such as gemcitabine/5-FU, gemcitabine/cisplatin or gemcitabine/capecitabine suggested a survival improvement for patients with good conditions [21]. The authors advise a combination therapy for those patients to get a maximum response. But these results are based only on subgroup analyses. A recent large randomized trial (CONKO 004) will prospectively examine this point of interest [22].

After a cohort of unsuccessful trials, two gemcitabine-based doublets yielded a statistically significant outcome improvement over a single agent in phase III trials [4, 23]. However, the results of the gemcitabine/capecitabine combination could not be confirmed in another phase III trial [24]. Altogether, the advantage obtained by gemcitabine/capecitabine and by a gemcitabine/erlotinib combination in overall survival was of marginal clinical significance, consisting of an absolute 7% improvement at 1 year (from 17%–19% with gemcitabine alone to 24%–26% with combined therapy) [4, 23]. Overall, from a clinical perspective, these trials confirmed the lack of a significant impact of double-agent combination therapy on the clinical course of pancreatic cancer.

7.3 Summary

Recapitulating the trials done to date, we have to notice that there is only a weak argument for combination therapy. In line with clinical considerations we have to recognize that the inclusion of new drugs into the therapy of advanced pancreatic cancer does not result in a milestone for the outcome in this poorly served patient group.

Gemcitabine remains the standard drug in the therapy of pancreatic cancer, and only in a selected patient pool is the use of intensive therapy (combination with capecitabine or cisplatin) reasonable. The combination treatment of gemcitabine with erlotinib is useful for patients who display the cutaneous side effects of erlotinib within 6–8 weeks of treatment start, indicating the effective impact of this treatment schedule.

References

1. Parkin DM, Bray F, Ferlay J, Pisani P (2001) Estimating the world cancer burden: Globocan 2000. Int J Cancer 94:153–156
2. Burris HA, Moore MJ, Andersen J, Green MR, Rothenberg ML, Modiano MR, Cripps MC, Portenoy RK, Storniolo AM, Tarassoff P, Nelson R, Dorr FA, Stephens CD, Von Hoff DD (1997.) Improvements in survival and clinical benefit with gemcitabine as first-line therapy for patients with advanced pancreas cancer: a randomized trial. J Clin Oncol 15:2403–2413

3. Van Cutsem E, Aerts R, Haustermans K, Topal B, Van Steenbergen W, Verslype C (2004) Systemic treatment of pancreatic cancer. Eur J Gastroenterol Hepatol 16:265–274
4. Moore MJ, Goldstein D, Hamm J, Kotecha J, Gallinger S, Au HJ, et al. (2005) Erlotinib improves survival when added to gemcitabine in patients with advanced pancreatic cancer. A phase III trial of the National Cancer Institute of Canada Clinical Trials Group [NCIC-CTG]. ASCO Gastrointestinal Cancers Symposium abstr 77
5. Kondo S, Ueno H, Okusaka T, Ikeda M, Morizane C, Najima M (2006) Gemcitabine monotherapy versus chemoradiotherapy using 5-FU in patients with locally advanced pancreatic cancer. 2006 Gastrointestinal Cancers Symposium, ASCO Abstr 137
6. Huguet F, André T, Hammel P, et al. (2006) Chemoradiotherapy (CRT) after chemotherapy (CT) improves survival for locally-advanced (LA) pancreatic cancer patients: retrospective analysis of 181 patients enrolled in prospective phases II and III GERCOR studies. J Clin Oncol 23:4095
7. Chauffert B, Mornex F, Bonnetain F, Triboulet JP, Bouche O, Rougier P, Bosset JF, Aparicio T, Masskouri F, Bedenne L (2006) Phase III trial comparing initial chemoradiotherapy (intermittent cisplatin and infusional 5-FU) followed by gemcitabine vs. gemcitabine alone in patients with locally advanced non metastatic pancreatic cancer: a FFCD-SFRO study. ASCO Annual Meeting Proceedings Part I (June 20 Supplement) 4008. J Clin Oncol 24:18S
8. Lionetto R, Pugliese V, Bruzzi P, Rosso R (1995) No standard treatment is available for advanced pancreatic cancer. Eur J Cancer 31A:882–887
9. Taylor I (1993) Should further studies of chemotherapy be carried out in pancreatic cancer? Eur J Cancer 29:1076–1078
10. Glimelius B, Hoffman K, Sjoden PO, Jacobsson G, Sellstrom H, Enander LK, Linne T, Svensson C (1996) Chemotherapy improves survival and quality of life in advanced pancreatic and biliary cancer. Ann Oncol 7:593–600
11. Palmer KR, Kerr M, Knowles G, Cull A, Carter DC, Leonard RC (1994) Chemotherapy prolongs survival in inoperable pancreatic carcinoma. Br J Surg 81:882–885
12. Poplin E, Levy DE, Berlin J, Rothenberg L, Cella D, Mitchell E, Alberts S, Benson A 3rd (2006) Phase III trial of gemcitabine (30-minute infusion) versus gemcitabine (fixed-dose-rate infusion [FDR]) versus gemcitabine + oxaliplatin (GEMOX) in patients with advanced pancreatic cancer (E6201). J Clin Oncol 24:4004
13. Berlin JD, Catalano P, Thomas JP, Kugler JW, Haller DG, Benson AB (2002) Phase III study of gemcitabine in combination with fluorouracil versus gemcitabine alone in patients with advanced pancreatic carcinoma: Eastern Cooperative Oncology Group Trial E2297. J Clin Oncol 20:3270–3275
14. Moore MJ, Hamm J, Dancey J, et al. (2003) Comparison of gemcitabine versus the matrix metalloproteinase inhibitor BAY 12-9566 in patients with advanced or metastatic adenocarcinoma of the pancreas: a phase III trial of the National Cancer Institute of Canada Clinical Trials Group. J Clin Oncol 21:3296–3302
15. Rocha Lima CM, Green MR, Rotche R, Miller WH Jr, Jeffrey GM, Cisar LA, Morganti A, Orlando N, Gruia G, Miller LL (2004) Irinotecan plus gemcitabine results in no survival advantage compared with gemcitabine monotherapy in patients with locally advanced or metastatic pancreatic cancer despite increased tumor response rate. J Clin Oncol 22:3776–3783
16. Bramhall SR, Schulz J, Nemunaitis J, Brown PD, Baillet M, Buckels JA (2002) A double-blind placebo-controlled, randomised study comparing gemcitabine and marimastat with gemcitabine and placebo as first line therapy in patients with advanced pancreatic cancer. Br J Cancer 87:161–167
17. Bramhall SR, Rosemurgy A, Brown PD, Bowry C, Buckels JA; Marimastat Pancreatic Cancer Study Group (2001) Marimastat Pancreatic Cancer Study Group. Marimastat as first-line therapy for patients with unresectable pancreatic cancer: a randomized trial. J Clin Oncol 19:3477–3455
18. Oettle H, Richards D, Ramanathan RK, van Laethem JL, Peeters M, Fuchs M, Zimmermann A, John W, Von Hoff D, Arning M, Kindler HL (2005) A phase III trial of pemetrexed plus gemcitabine versus gemcitabine in patients with unresectable or metastatic pancreatic cancer. Ann Oncol 16:1639–1645

19. Van Cutsem E, van de Velde H, Karasek P, Oettle H, Vervenne WL, Szawlowski A, Schoffski P, Post S, Verslype C, Neumann H, Safran H, Humblet Y, Perez Ruixo J, Ma Y, Von Hoff D (2004) Phase III trial of gemcitabine plus tipifarnib compared with gemcitabine plus placebo in advanced pancreatic cancer. J Clin Oncol 22:1430–1438
20. Louvet C, Labianca R, Hammel P, et al. (2005) Gemcitabine in combination with oxaliplatin compared with gemcitabine alone in locally advanced or metastatic pancreatic cancer: results of a GERCOR and GISCAD phase III trial. J Clin Oncol 23:3509–3516
21. Banu E, Oudard S, Banu A, et al. (2005) Cumulative meta-analysis of randomized trials comparing gemcitabine-based chemotherapy versus gemcitabine alone in patients with advanced or metastatic pancreatic cancer (PC). J Clin Oncol (meeting abstracts) 23:4101
22. Pelzer U, Stieler J, Roll L, Stauch M, Opitz B, Scholten T, Hahnfeld S, Dörken B, Riess H, Oettle H (2006) A prospective, randomized trial of simultaneous pancreatic cancer treatment with enoxaparin and chemotherapy (PROSPECT—CONKO 004). ASCO Annual Meeting Proceedings Part I. J Clinic Oncol 24:18S [June 20 Suppl]:4110
23. Cunningham D, Chau I, Stocken DD, Davies C, Dunn JA, Valle J, Smith D, Steward WP, Harper P, Neoptolemos J (2005) Phase III randomised comparison of gemcitabine versus gemcitabine plus capecitabine in patients with advanced pancreatic cancer. Eur J Cancer 3 [Suppl 4]:12
24. Herrmann R, Bodoky G, Ruhstaller T, Glimelius B, Saletti P, Bajetta E, Schueller J, Bernhard J, Dietrich D, Scheithauer W (2005) Gemcitabine (G) plus capecitabine (C) versus G alone in locally advanced or metastatic pancreatic cancer. A randomized phase III study of the Swiss Group for Clinical Cancer Research (SAKK) and the Central European Cooperative Oncology Group (CECOG). J Clin Oncol 23(16S)

8 Second-Line Chemotherapy in Advanced Pancreatic Cancer

U. Pelzer

Recent Results in Cancer Research, Vol. 177

Abstract

This chapter focuses on second-line therapy in inoperable pancreatic cancer.

8.1 Introduction

Gemcitabine became the new standard in the treatment of advanced pancreatic cancer (APC) [1] in the late 1990s. Since then there have been no similar significant drug advances reported. In spite of this, the median survival for patients with advanced metastatic cancer has increased to 10–12 months in the last decade [2]. But this is not an effect due to new therapeutic drugs in first-line therapy; rather it is a benefit of the extensive use of second-line regimens for appropriate patients. However, no standard second-line treatment has yet been defined for these patients. Several phase II studies (see Table 8.1) refer to effective drugs and drug combinations in second-line therapy. Most drugs are adopted from salvage therapy regimens of advanced colorectal cancer or lung cancer. Trials are missing that compare the new approach with the standard procedure after failing first-line therapy. Only one small, randomized trial could show a significant improvement for a second-line regimen [3].

8.2 Second-Line Chemotherapy

Following the use of gemcitabine as a second-line drug [4], there has been a large variety of chemotherapy regimens that realize small advantages. The use of chemotherapy in advanced pancreatic cancer was heavily dependent on the experiences of the local oncologists. Many patients were treated with individual designs. But due to there being so many different first- and second-line patient schedules, the idea of analysis was impractical. The process of the implementation of sequential therapies into the treatment of advanced pancreatic cancer led to a development of several regimens (Table 8.1).

A small study [5] with flutamide in second-line therapy after failing the current standard, 5-fluorouracil (5-FU), in the early 1990s led to a median survival of 4.7 months in this deadly disease. But with only 14 patients in this setting and no further evaluations of this drug in pancreatic cancer, we cannot assess any impact on therapy guidelines.

Irinotecan has shown activity as a second-line therapy, and a combination of irinotecan and the thymidylate synthase inhibitor raltitrexed led to a median overall survival of 6.5 months [6]. Interestingly, the addition of irinotecan to existing first-line therapy on which patients had progressed (gemcitabine/5-FU/FA/cisplatin, G-FLIP) was associated with some benefit, and the median overall survival of patients was 10.3 months from the start of G-FLIP [7]. Another trial with 17 patients in refractory disease after a multiple combination in first-line therapy (gemcitabine/mitomycin/oxaliplatin) used the combination of irinotecan and 5-FU. A progression-free survival of 4 months was noted. A similar result was observed with a combination of irinotecan and 5-FU/folinic acid (FolFIri) in pretreated patients with a gemcitabine-containing regimen [8]. A study with paclitaxel showed second-line activity with a median survival time of 17.5 weeks from the start of therapy [9].

Table 8.1 Second-line drug combinations

Author	*N*	1st line	2nd line	Result	Source
Rothenberg	74	5-FU	Gem	MS 3.85 months	[4]
Sharma	14	5-FU	Flutamide	MS 4.7 months	[5]
Oettle	18	Gem or Gem/FU/FA	Paclitaxel	OS 12 months	[9]
Klapdor	17	Gem/Mito/Oxa	IRI/FU	PFI 4 months	[16]
Kozuch	34	Gem/FU/Cis	Gem/IRI/FU/Cis	OS 10.3 months	[7]
Pelzer	23	Gem	Oxa/FU/FA	OS 12.5 months	[2]
Ulrich-Pur[a]	38	Gem	Raltitrexed	MS 4.3 months	[6]
			IRI+raltitrexed	MS 6.5 months	
Aklilu	13	Gem+other	Arsenic trioxide	MS 4.2 months	[10]
Milella	20	Gem+other	Celecoxib/FU	MS 3.5 months	[11]
Ng	15	Gem+other	FolFIri	MS 3.5 months	[8]
Blaszkowsky	30	Gem+other	Capecitabine+erlotinib	MS 6.7 months	[15]
Oettle[a]	23	Gem	Oxa/FU/FA	MS 4 months	[3]
	23	Gem	BSC	MS 2 months	
Tsavaris	30	Gem	Oxa/FU/FA	MS 5.5 months	[12]
Demols	31	Gem	Gem/Oxa	MS 6 months	[13]
Reni	41	Gem+other	Oxa/raltitrexed	MS 5.2 months	[14]

Cis, cisplatin; FA, folinic acid; FolFIri, 5-FU/folinic acid and irinotecan; FU, fluorouracil; IRI, irinotecan; Gem, gemcitabine; MS, median survival; OS, overall survival; Oxa, oxaliplatin; PFI, progression-free survival; RR, response rate

[a] Randomized study

Arsenic trioxide (AT) after a gemcitabine-containing regimen led to a median survival of 16.6 weeks and a progression-free interval of 7 weeks in 13 patients [10]. A combination of celecoxib and 5-FU continuous venous infusion (c.v.i.) after failing a gemcitabine based regime in 20 patients with advanced pancreatic or biliary tract cancer led to a median survival of 14 weeks with a progression-free survival in second-line therapy of 8 weeks [11].

The combination of oxaliplatin/folinic acid and 5-FU after failing first-line standard therapy with gemcitabine led to an overall survival of 12.5 months in 23 patients [2]. Tsavaris et al. [12] also used the combination of oxaliplatin/5-FU/FA in patients with gemcitabine refractory disease. This small phase II study used a different weekly regimen, so more neutropenia was observed and granulocyte-stimulating factor (GSF) had to given in 17 patients. The median time to progression was 22 weeks, median survival 5.5 months. Gemcitabine and oxaliplatin in combination after failing gemcitabine monotherapy in the first line could reach an interesting median survival in the second line of 6 months. The addition of oxaliplatin may break through the first resistance of gemcitabine for any length of time [13]. Oxaliplatin and raltitrexed in 41 patients led to a similar result [14]. Erlotinib and capecitabine are drugs that have found their employment now in primary therapy. In combination after failing a gemcitabine-containing regimen in 30 patients, we noticed a promising median survival in second-line therapy of 6.7 months [15].

The results of Oettle et al. [3] compare favourably with those seen in some other second-line treatments. Remarkable is the design of their study. The authors randomized the patients who failed first-line therapy into the standard procedure with best supportive care and a chemotherapy group with the combination of oxaliplatin/5-FU and folinic acid. Sequential oxaliplatin

Table 8.2 Ongoing trials

Author	*n*	1st line	2nd line	Aim	Source
Moore	37	Gem+other	E7389	RR/OS	Clinicaltrials.gov[a]
Rocha Lima	45	Gem+other	Docetaxel/capecitabine	RR/OS	
Messersmith	65	Any	Capecitabine	RR/OS	
Astra Zeneca[a]	64	Gem	A: AZD6244	Unknown	
			B: Capecitabine		
Oettle[a]	165	Gem	A: Oxa/FU/FA	RR/OS	
			B: FU/FA		
Heinemann[b]	Unknown	Gem	Capecitabine/erlotinib	Unknown	
		Capecitabine	Gem/erlotinib	Unknown	
Ramesh	45	Any	Gefitinib/docetaxel	Unknown	
O'Reilly	30	Any	Docetaxel/flavopiridol	Unknown	

FA, folinic acid; FU, fluorouracil; Gem, gemcitabine; OS, overall survival; Oxa, oxaliplatin; RR, response rate

[a] National Institutes of Health and the National Library of Medicine [17]

[b] Randomized study

and 5-FU/FA following gemcitabine led to a median overall survival of 39.6 (range 30.4–48.8) weeks from the start of first-line treatment versus 34.4 weeks without second-line chemotherapy ($p=0.03$). A median time of 21 weeks in group A versus 10 weeks in group B shows a significant difference between these two groups regarding survival time after gemcitabine failure ($p=0.008$). The combination of oxaliplatin and 5-FU used in this study was remarkably well tolerated. As expected, haematotoxicity and neurotoxicity were common. However, in the majority of cases, toxicities were WHO grade 1 or 2.

8.3 Summary

There is no established second-line therapy for patients with refractory disease under/after a gemcitabine-containing first-line chemotherapy. Therefore, a variety of different chemotherapy combinations continue to be investigated. All patients with refractory disease should be recruited into clinical trials to address the question about the best effective regimen for those patients. Unfortunately, a far too individual landscape is to be found in practice.

The CONKO 003 trial [3] was the first randomized study that showed a significant survival benefit for a second-line treatment with chemotherapy in patients with advanced pancreatic cancer. This small trial answered the main question about the use of second-line therapy in principle. But urgent need for more effective drugs and designs is obvious, and many clinical trials are now in progress (Table 8.2).

References

1. Burris HA 3rd, Moore MJ, Andersen J, et al. (1997) Improvements in survival and clinical benefit with gemcitabine as first-line therapy for patients with advanced pancreas cancer: a randomized trial. J Clin Oncol 15:2403–2413
2. Pelzer U, Hempel C, Stieler J, et al. (2002) Oxaliplatin (OXA) in combination with high dose 5-FU (24 h)/folinic acid (FA) as salvage therapy in patients with gemzar-refractory advanced pancreatic cancer. Proc Am Soc Clin Oncol 21:A684
3. Oettle H, Pelzer U, Stieler J, et al. (2005) Oxaliplatin/folinic acid/5-fluorouracil [24 h] (OFF) plus best supportive care versus best supportive care alone (BSC) in second-line therapy of gem-

citabine-refractory advanced pancreatic cancer (CONKO 003). 2005 ASCO Annual Meeting Proceedings. J Clin Oncol [June 1 Suppl] 23:4031
4. Rothenberg ML, Moore MJ, Von Hoff DD, et al. (1996) A phase II trial of gemcitabine in patients with 5-FU-refractory pancreas cancer. Ann Oncol 7:347–353
5. Sharma JJ, Razvillas B, Stephens CD, Hilsenbeck SG, Sharma A, Rothenberg ML (1997) Phase II study of flutamide as second line chemotherapy in patients with advanced pancreatic cancer. Invest New Drugs 15:361–364
6. Ulrich-Pur H, Raderer M, Verena Kornek G, Schull B, Schmid K, Haider K, Kwasny W, Depisch D, Schneeweiss B, Lang F, Scheithauer W (2003) Irinotecan plus raltitrexed vs raltitrexed alone in patients with gemcitabine pretreated advanced pancreatic cancer. Br J Cancer 88:1180–1184
7. Kozuch P, Grossbard ML, Barzdins A, Araneo M, Robin A, Frager D, Homel P, Marino J, DeGregorio P, Bruckner HW (2001) Irinotecan combined with gemcitabine, 5-fluorouracil, leucovorin and cisplatin (G-FLIP) is an effective and noncross-resistant treatment for chemotherapy refractory metastatic pancreatic cancer. Oncologist 6:488–495
8. Ng M, Norman AR, Cunningham D, et al. (2004) Phase II trial evaluating a 2 weekly regimen of irinotecan (IR) and 5-FU/leucovorin (LV) in patients with metastatic pancreatic cancer refractory to chemotherapy. 2004 ASCO Annual Meeting Proceedings. J Clin Oncol 22A:4229
9. Oettle H, Arnold D, Esser M, Huhn D, Riess H (2000) Paclitaxel as weekly second-line therapy in patients with advanced pancreatic carcinoma. Anticancer Drugs 11:635–638
10. Aklilu M, Kindler HL, Nattam S, Brich A, Vokes EE (2004) A multicenter phase II study of arsenic trioxide (AT) in patients with advanced pancreatic cancer (PC) refractory to gemcitabine. 2004 ASCO Annual Meeting Proceedings. J Clin Oncol 22:A4114
11. Milella M, Gelibter A, Di Cosimo S, Bria E, Ruggeri EM, Carlini P, Malaguti P, Pellicciotta M, Terzoli E, Cognetti F, et al. (2004) Exploratory phase II study of celecoxib and infusional fluorouracil as second-line treatment for advanced pancreatic (PDAC) and biliary tree cancer (BTC). 2004 ASCO Annual Meeting Proceedings. J Clin Oncol 22:A4183
12. Tsavaris N, Kosmas C, Skopelitis H, Gouveris P, Kopterides P, Loukeris D, Sigala F, Zorbala-Sypsa A, Felekouras E, Papalambros E (2005) Second-line treatment with oxaliplatin, leucovorin and 5-fluorouracil in gemcitabine-pretreated advanced pancreatic cancer: a phase II study. Invest New Drugs 23:603
13. Demols A, Peeters M, Polus M, et al. (2006) Gemcitabine and oxaliplatin (GEMOX) in gemcitabine refractory advanced pancreatic adenocarcinoma: a phase II study. Br J Cancer 27:481–485
14. Reni M, Pasetto L, Aprile G, et al. (2006) Raltitrexed-eloxatin salvage chemotherapy in gemcitabine-resistant metastatic pancreatic cancer. Br J Cancer 27:785–791
15. Blaszkowsky LS, Kulke KH, Ryan DP, Clark JW, Meyerhardt J, Zhu AX, et al. (2005) A phase II study of erlotinib in combination with capecitabine in previously treated patients with metastatic pancreatic cancer. 2005 ASCO Annual Meeting Proceedings. J Clin Oncol 23:4099
16. Klapdor R, Fenner C (2000) Irinotecan (CamptoR): efficacy as third/fourth line therapy in advanced pancreatic cancer. Anticancer Res 20:5209–5212
17. National Institutes of Health and the National Library of Medicine (2007) ClinicalTrials.gov. http://www.clinicaltrials.gov. Cited 2 Aug 2007

9 Neoadjuvant and Adjuvant Strategies for Chemoradiation

A. Kaiser, V. Budach

Recent Results in Cancer Research, Vol. 177

Abstract

There is an increasing body of evidence showing that patients with resectable pancreatic cancer might benefit from adjuvant therapy. Based on phase III trials, potential options for adjuvant treatment are chemotherapy alone or a multimodal approach involving radiotherapy. Available data are heterogeneous and have been discussed controversially. Hitherto, a worldwide standard of care has not yet been established. Adequate patient selection might be the key element for a tailored adjuvant treatment. Clinical research currently focusses on gemcitabine alone or in combination, and some molecular biologic approaches with epidermal growth factor receptor monoclonal antibodies (EGFR-MoABs) and anti-angiogenic drugs. Recent advances in radiooncology offer better dose conformality and reduced morbidities. Currently, the co-operative Radiotherapy and Gastrointestinal Groups have launched a multicentric European Organization for Research and Treatment of Cancer (EORTC) trial investigating the impact of radiotherapy in combination with gemcitabine in R0-resected pancreatic head cancer.

9.1 Introduction

Only about 10%–20% of pancreatic cancer patients are deemed to be resectable and could be ideal candidates for adjuvant or neoadjuvant treatment strategies (Evans 2005; Kelly and Benjamin 1995; Sener et al. 1999). Surgery is the only possibly curative treatment option. Remarkable progress has been made in terms of clear resection margins, which could be increased from 26% to 43%. From the 1970s through the 1990s, perioperative mortality improved from 30% to 0.9%, respectively. Five-year survival rates increased from 14% in the 1970s to more than 30% in the 1990s (Yeo et al. 1995; Yeo and Cameron 1999). In the 1990s more than 65% of patients received some form of adjuvant therapy compared to less than 25% in the 1980s. This reflects a major change in the treatment paradigms from therapeutic nihilism to intensified adjuvant therapy.

Prognostic factors after surgery are performance status, extent of tumour spread and tumour size, nodal status, grading and status of resection margins (Kalser et al. 1985; Kalser and Ellenberg 1985; Neoptolemos et al. 2001, 2004; Sohn et al. 2000). Additional and well-known factors are blood loss during pancreaticoduodenectomy and time to recovery. Less common ampullary carcinoma and intrapancreatic bile duct carcinoma have a more favourable prognosis than pancreatic ductal adenocarcinoma (Magee et al. 2002). For pancreatic cancer, a prolonged median survival of about 15–20 months can be expected after R0 surgery compared to 8 to 12 months after R1 surgery (Evans et al. 1998). Even after R0 surgery, however, relapses occur regularly. Local recurrences account for the majority (80%), recurrence in the peritoneal cavity for 25%, and liver metastasis for about 50% of all cases (Wayne et al. 2002). Metastases to other regions such as lung are rare and usually occur at a late stage.

Though there is remarkable progress of pancreatic cancer treatment, survival data are still dismal. Therefore, adjuvant therapy is of major importance.

9.2 Adjuvant Chemoradiation

The Gastrointestinal Tumor Study Group (GITSG) GI-9173 data published in 1985 has proved that post-operative chemoradiation (CRT) is highly effective (Kalser and Ellenberg 1985). This randomized trial investigated surgery followed by a 40-Gy split-course radiotherapy (RT) combined with 5-fluorouracil (5-FU) versus surgery alone. The treatment arm ($n=21$) was superior to surgery alone ($n=22$), resulting in median survival of 20 months versus 12 months. These results were confirmed by the GITSG in a non-randomized controlled phase II study in 1987 (Gastrointestinal Tumor Study Group 1987). Both studies had great impact on adjuvant treatment of pancreatic cancer in the USA. This treatment regimen has become the new standard of care, and until recently it was in widespread use in the United States. A number of additional studies confirmed these results (Foo et al. 1993; Foo and Gunderson 1998; Mehta et al. 2000; Paulino 1999; Yeo et al. 1995, 1997). The combination of 5-FU with leucovorin seemed to be only marginally effective (Abrams et al. 1999). A recent study from Johns Hopkins University compared two schemes of chemoradiation with surveillance. Chemoradiation was either intensified 50–57 Gy to the pancreas and a prophylactic dose of 23–27 Gy to the liver combined with 5-FU or a standard dose of 40–45 Gy to the pancreas combined with 5-FU/leucovorin. Patients receiving adjuvant therapy had a median survival of 19.5 months compared with only 13.5 months after resection alone. More intense treatment schemes did not appear to further improve survival (Sohn et al. 2000; Yeo et al. 1997). A European Organization for Research and Treatment of Cancer (EORTC) multi-centre trial including 207 evaluable patients combined split-course RT with 5-FU and also found a statistically insignificant improved survival trend of 24.5 versus 19 months (Klinkenbijl et al. 1999). Subgroup analysis indicated a benefit for pancreatic head cancer patients with survival of 17.1 versus 12.6 months.

Some of these studies have methodological limitations. Patient accrual was either slow or the numbers of patients were statistically insufficient. Patient selection was non-uniform, thereby including patients with pancreatic cancer and those with periampullary cancer, who have a better prognosis. Mono-institutional studies suffered from selection bias. Up to 25% of the patients did not receive the planned radiochemotherapy because of withdrawal of consent, lack of post-operative recovery or rapid tumour progression. There was no stratification for tumour sites, nor was there a detailed analysis of resection margins. From the current point of view, treatment was often suboptimal, with split-course RT and a heterogeneous dose distribution, and 5-FU given as bolus instead of as continuous infusion.

A rather modern treatment scheme was applied to 52 patients by Mehta et al. (2000). RT was intensified from 45 Gy (R0) to 54–60 Gy (R1) and in a few cases intraoperative RT was added. This was combined with a continuous infusion of 5-FU. The resulting median survival was a promising 32 months and morbidities were only moderate.

9.3 Adjuvant Chemotherapy

The first randomized trial to demonstrate a positive effect of adjuvant chemotherapy without RT was published in 1993 (Bakkevold et al. 1993). Sixty-one radically resected patients were randomized either for post-operative adjuvant combination chemotherapy using 5-FU, doxorubicin and mitomycin C (AMF), or as controls (no adjuvant chemotherapy). The median survival in the treatment group was 23 months compared to 11 months in the control group. The authors concluded that adjuvant chemotherapy prolongs the incidence of recurrence during the first 2 years following radical surgery; however, an increased cure rate was not observed.

The benefits of chemoradiation have been questioned since the publication of the European Study Group for Pancreatic Cancer (ESPAC) 1 trial (Neoptolemos et al. 2001, 2004). This was the most ambitious and largest adjuvant trial in pancreatic cancer with 548 patients involved. It had a 2×2 factorial design: of 541 eligible patients, 289 were assigned to chemotherapy versus radiochemotherapy, 68 to chemoradiotherapy only versus no chemoradiotherapy with record of background chemotherapy and 188 to chemotherapy only versus no chemotherapy with record of background chemotherapy. The 289 patients of the first group were assigned to observation, chemoradiotherapy, chemotherapy, or chemoradiotherapy and chemotherapy. The treatment concepts were those of other published trials: surgery followed by 5-FU/FA bolus, surgery followed by 40 Gy split-course RT+5-FU bolus, or surgery followed by both. In summary the 2×2 factorial design showed no survival benefit with CT or CRT to observation. When all patients were pooled, a survival benefit for adjuvant CT, not for adjuvant CRT, was observed. The Kaplan-Meier analysis showed a reduced survival rate following radiochemotherapy compared to no radiochemotherapy of 29% versus 41%, respectively, after 2 years and of 10% versus 20% after 5 years, which was statistically significant.

These data actually suggest that adjuvant radiochemotherapy might even harm patients after a potentially curative resection. This trial had substantial impact on therapeutic decisions in Europe, where radiochemotherapy has virtually been abandoned and adjuvant chemotherapy has become the European standard of care.

The results of ESPAC-1, however, need to be discussed, and substantial criticisms have been raised. The trial used various randomization procedures. Because of interaction between the therapy arms, the study might be regarded as underpowered. Background chemotherapy was allowed, which was not part of the study medication. Additionally, about 40% of the patients did not receive the originally planned treatment. There was no standardized quality assurance for surgery nor for the radiochemotherapy procedures, and 30% of the RT patients received a non-uniform dose or even no radiation at all. Chemoradiation started on average 2 weeks later than chemotherapy. Neither RT nor chemotherapy was optimal according to modern standards. And last but not least, from a tumour biologic point of view, there is no rationale conceivable for a shorter relapse-free survival with chemoradiation. Insufficient treatment quality for the chemoradiation arm might also have contributed to the enhanced treatment-related toxicity (Choti 2004; Koshy et al. 2005). In summary, the published results of the ESPAC-1 trial have to be considered premature and are in no way suited to rule out adjuvant chemoradiation for pancreatic cancer.

Recently, a meta-analysis summarized individual data of 875 patients treated in five randomized controlled trials (Stocken et al. 2005). The ESPAC-1 trial contributed 550 patients. The pooled hazard ratio reduction was 25% corresponding to a significant reduction of the death risk after chemotherapy. The median survival was 19 months with, and 13.5 months without, chemotherapy, respectively. In this meta-analysis an increased risk of death with the addition of RT to chemotherapy could not be observed. The median survival was the same (15.8 months with chemoradiation and 15.2 without). Subgroup analysis revealed that chemoradiation was more effective compared with chemotherapy in patients with positive resection margins. Still, the authors concluded that the initial use of chemoradiotherapy might have delayed the effective use of chemotherapy and thereby reduced survival.

The ESPAC-3 trial has meanwhile launched to confirm the beneficial role of adjuvant chemotherapy and to differentiate between the efficacies of 5-FU and gemcitabine (Neoptolemos et al. 2003). A randomization between 5-FU/FA and gemcitabine is used; for ampullary cancer a third arm with observation only is installed. After amendment, 680 patients need to be enrolled, so final results will take some time.

Gemcitabine has come into focus recently. It is a potent radiation sensitizer of pancreatic tumour cells in vitro (Lawrence et al. 1996). It is active in pancreatic cancer and improves clinical benefit (23.8 versus 4.8%) and survival rate (5.7 versus 4.4 months) over 5-FU, which led to the Gemzar (Eli Lilly, Indianapolis) registration (Burris and Storniolo 1997; Burris et al. 1997; Rothenberg et al. 1996). Toxicity is minimal and it can be administered on an outpatient setting.

Preliminary data of the CONKO-001 study, presented at the American Society of Clinical Oncology annual meeting (ASCO) 2005, confirmed the efficacy of gemcitabine. In a randomized manner, median survival with gemcitabine was 14 months, without it, 7 months (Neuhaus et al. 2005).

9.4 Pre-operative Chemoradiotherapy

The concept of pre-operative radiochemotherapy is alluring, but its value for resectable cancer is not yet clear. Using radiochemotherapy first, a possibly systemic disease could receive a systemic treatment without the delay of post-operative recovery. Multi-modal treatment ought to start with the least toxic treatment, thus sparing surgery in patients, who currently suffer from rapid progression or metastasis. Further possible advantages have been suggested, including the prevention of intraoperative tumour spread and improved radiosensitivity, as tumour oxygenation has not been hampered by surgery and the higher probability of R0 resection (Bergenfeldt and Albertsson 2006; Crane et al. 2006b; Evans 2005).

There have been very promising data from a sequence of trials performed by the MD Anderson Cancer Centre. Only patients with a possibly resectable disease were included, surgical techniques and pathological evaluation were standardized. First, 5-FU and concomitant RT with 50.4 Gy did result in a median survival of 18 months. Toxicity, though, was severe enough to necessitate hospital admission in one-third of the patients (Evans et al. 1992). The subsequent trials did use an accelerated, so-called "rapid fractionation" programme delivered over 2 weeks, with a 30-Gy total dose and a 3-Gy single fraction dose. During surgery an additional intraoperative RT of 10–15 Gy was administered. Combining this scheme with 5-FU led to a median survival of 25 months (Pisters et al. 1998). Paclitaxel was less effective, with a median survival of 19 months (Pisters et al. 2002). Best results were achieved when combining RT with gemcitabine. Median survival was 36 months, toxicities were manageable, with a hospitalization rate of 43% (Wolff et al. 2001). These trials all suffered from a positive selection bias. Recently, results of a French phase II study have been published combining 5-FU with cisplatin and concurrent RT to 50 Gy in a pre-operative setting for potentially resectable pancreatic cancer. Among 40 evaluable patients, 15 did not undergo resection of the pancreatic tumour because of local or metastatic progression. Median survival for those patients, who completed treatment, was 11.7 months. The scheme was concluded to be feasible, but the use of more efficient drugs such as gemcitabine and optimized RT seemed justified (Mornex et al. 2006).

Numerous trials investigated pre-operative chemoradiotherapy (Bergenfeldt and Albertsson 2006) based on heterogeneous patient populations including patients with locally advanced disease. Pre-operative chemoradiation seems to offer a downstaging effect, shifting patients from locally advanced to potentially resectable stages (White et al. 1999, 2001). Median survival in those patients who were resected exceeded 16 months. When comparing 5-FU-based chemoradiation in a pre-operative and post-operative setting, actuarial survival rates at 2, 3 and 5 years were 39% versus 52%, 35% versus 40% and 28% versus 40%, respectively, in favour of adjuvant treatment. This difference did not reach statistical significance and was attributed to larger, more locally advanced tumours in the preoperative therapy group (Spitz et al. 1997). Pathological findings after pre-operative chemoradiotherapy showed fewer involved lymph nodes, more negative resection margins, similar toxicity and a non-significant median survival difference of 20 versus 25 months (Pendurthi et al. 1998).

So far, randomized controlled trials proving an overall survival benefit for neoadjuvant treatment approaches are missing.

9.5 Intraoperative Radiotherapy

A possible advantage of intraoperative radiotherapy (IORT) is the ability to deliver high doses of radiation to sites at high risk of local recurrence while organs at risk can be shielded. IORT has been used in the adjuvant and neoadjuvant situation, alone or in combination with chemotherapy (for an overview see Bergenfeldt and Albertsson 2006). IORT has been proved effective over surgery alone in pancreatic cancer with respect to local recurrence, which was reduced by half (Reni et al. 2001). This trial also found a survival benefit for selected stage I–II patients. Operative morbidity and mortality were not increased. In a subgroup analysis, a combination of IORT with

RT and chemotherapy improved survival significantly (Di Carlo et al. 1997).

IORT can act as a valuable partner in a combined modality treatment setting that includes chemoradiation. However, accelerated re-population during the interval between IORT and external RT has to be taken into account (Wilkowski et al. 2005).

9.6 Radiotherapy Treatment Planning

Many of the patients treated in the aforementioned trials had their RT based on 2D-treatment planning, which led to large dose burden on the surrounding healthy normal tissue and consequential acute and late radiation damage. The introduction of a split-course technique and a total dose not exceeding 40 Gy was mainly driven by the acute toxicities observed. 2D dose distributions in the target volume often were less than optimal, leading to cold and hot spots. In the meantime, technical progress enables 3D-treatment planning with optimized protection of normal tissue, thus offering the opportunity to treat without a split to higher total doses of 54 to 60 Gy. Still, the critical dose-limiting structures neighbouring the target volume is the small bowel, which has a tolerance dose of 45–50 Gy, depending on the single fraction dose, and the kidney, which has a tolerance dose of about 23 Gy to the whole organ. With regard to a potentially enhanced toxicity by combining with chemotherapy, no more than 30% of the kidneys should reach a dose level of 20 Gy. In contrast to these structures, the liver, as an organ with great regeneration capacities, tolerates much higher doses, up to 50 Gy in up to 1/3 of the liver volume. A rather conservative approach with regard to possible toxic damage of the liver is 12.5 Gy to 75%, 25 Gy to 50% and 37.5 Gy to 25% of liver volume (Emami et al. 1991; Wilkowski et al. 2005).

Pancreatic cancer carries a high risk, exceeding 80%, for dissemination to loco-regional lymph nodes. The lymphatic drainage from the pancreas consists of peripancreatic nodes and along the upper mesenteric artery, the a. gastroduodenalis, a. hepatica communis, a. lienalis and coeliac trunk. Involvement of nodes near the portal vein and para-aortal and para-caval nodes happens frequently (Kayahara et al. 1995, 1996, 1999).

Treatment planning should be based on a pre-operative 3D data set with intravenous contrast medium and contrast enhancement of the small bowel. The patients should be immobilized with raised arms. A clinical target volume (CTV) should be defined, which includes the primary tumour region, involved lymph nodes and any subclinical region at risk, with an additional margin of 0.5 cm. To reduce toxicity, part of the pancreatic tail, which is not involved, may be excluded. Loco-regional lymph nodes should be included, at least between the upper mesenteric artery and coeliac trunk. The planning target volume is equal to the CTV plus a safety margin to account for patient and organ movement of 1–3 cm. An extension of the target volume to include the liver for prophylactic reasons did not result in an increased survival (Yeo et al. 1997). Shrinking of the planning target volume (PTV) after 45 Gy is recommended. Dose should be prescribed according to the guidelines of the International Commission on Radiation Units, report 50 (ICRU-50), dose heterogeneity should not exceed ±5% (see EORTC 40013 (Wilkowski et al. 2005)). When sophisticated techniques such as intensity modulated RT (IMRT) or stereotactically guided RT (SRT) are involved, ICRU-50 criteria might not be fulfilled; still, dose homogeneity should be aimed for.

9.7 Advances in Radiotherapy

Stereotactically guided RT is a means to further reduce the irradiated volume by shrinking the PTV (Fig. 9.1). The technique is still emerging since set-up uncertainties caused by breathing and organ motion are of concern. A stereotactically guided boost of 25 Gy following an IMRT treatment of 45 Gy combined with 5-FU enabled dose escalation up to 70 Gy with a tolerable acute toxicity. Of 19 patients, 16 completed treatment, local control was excellent and overall survival was not influenced in these patients suffering from advanced disease (Koong et al. 2005). On the other hand, a trial from Denmark reports unacceptable toxicity, poor outcome and a ques-

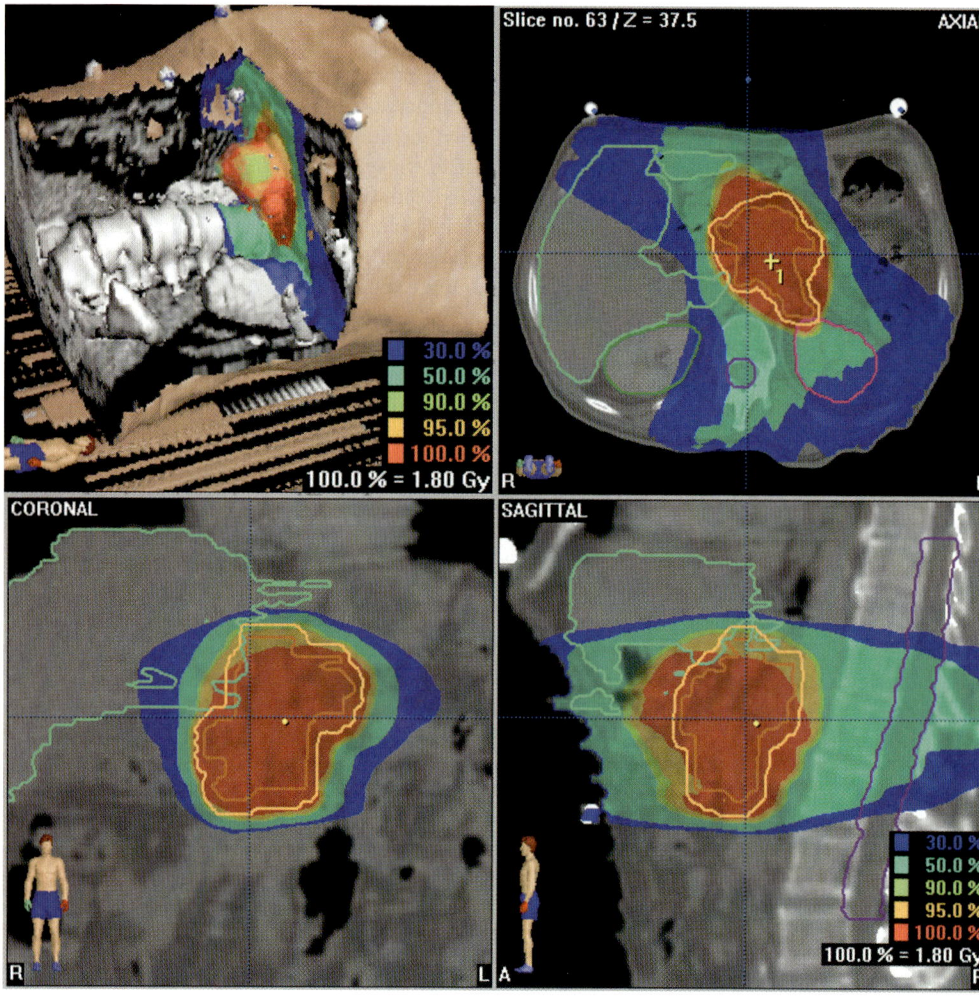

Fig. 9.1 Dose distributions of a stereotactically guided radiotherapy. (Courtesy of Dr. Wurm, Charité, Berlin)

tionable palliative effect of a fractionated stereotactically guided treatment of 15 × 3 Gy, again in locally advanced cancer (Hoyer et al. 2005).

Inverse treatment planning and IMRT allows specific dose distributions in order to either escalate the total dose given to the tumour without a further protection of surrounding organs at risk, such as the small bowel, or to better protect the organs at risk at the same total dose level (Landry et al. 2002). In general, the high dose volume is reduced, whereas the low dose volume is increased. A dosimetric analysis using different planning techniques revealed an advantage for using an integrated boost with doses of up to 64.8 Gy, which could have been given safely (Brown et al. 2006). A first phase I study combining gemcitabine 350 mg/m^2 with IMRT 33 Gy in 11 fractions had to be closed due to excessive toxicity. Even after reducing gemcitabine to 250 mg/m^2, patients suffered from dose-limiting gastrointestinal toxicity and myelosuppression (Crane et al. 2001a). A trial using IMRT as a boost following conventionally fractionated RT of 30 Gy with another 21–30 Gy, and a 3-Gy single fraction dose combined with 5-FU had a tolerable acute toxicity and some palliative effect in locally advanced cancer (Bai et al. 2003). Without dose escalation, IMRT has been found to be effective and tolerable in combination with capecitabine (Ben-Josef et al. 2004). Currently, the PARC study is investigating IMRT in combination with cetuximab and gemcitabine (Krempien et al. 2005).

9.8 Advances in Chemotherapy in the Combined Therapy Setting

Gemcitabine has been widely investigated in the adjuvant and neoadjuvant setting to replace 5-FU-based regimens. In the United States, the randomized Radiation Therapy Oncology Group (RTOG) 9704 trial tested the sequence 5-FU/FA→5-FU/RT→5-FU/FA versus gemcitabine (Gem)→5-FU/RT→Gem. The data were presented at the ASCO 2006 meeting (Regine and Abrams 1998; Saif 2006). From 1998 to 2002, 538 patients entered the trial (stage T1–T4, N0–N1); 381 had pancreatic head carcinoma, and 442 patients were eligible and analysable. Haematological toxicity was elevated in the gemcitabine arm, but manageable. For patients with pancreatic head carcinoma, median survival improved to 36.9 months compared to 20.6 months without gemcitabine. There was no improvement in survival for patients with tumours of the pancreatic body or tail. It was concluded that gemcitabine might be considered as a new standard adjuvant therapy, at least for pancreatic head carcinoma.

Data on gemcitabine combined with RT is emerging, but dose finding is still an issue. About 170 patients were treated in approx. 15 phase II trials. The gemcitabine dose was limited to 300 mg/m^2 weekly. The RT dose was 50.4 Gy for a limited target volume of less than 1,500 cm^3 (Van Laethem et al. 2003). There was a promising activity combined with moderate and manageable haematological and gastrointestinal toxicity. Median survival was 15 months, disease-free survival was 6 months; grade 3–4 haematological and non-haematological toxicity was 25%–36%. The Eastern Cooperative Oncology Group (ECOG) 4201 study evaluating gemcitabine plus RT versus gemcitabine alone was closed recently.

There were dose-finding phase I/II-studies of gemcitabine with concurrent radiation for advanced pancreatic cancer with a significant grade 3–4 toxicity of anorexia and dehydration when doses exceeded 350 mg/m^2 (McGinn and Zalupski 2003; Wolff et al. 2001). Toxicity was related to radiation dose. The infusion rate is related to the systemic efficacy (Crane et al. 2001b). Since gemcitabine as a prodrug must be phosphorylated to its active metabolites there is tissue saturation. Administration with a fixed dose rate is feasible (Tempero et al. 2003); data on combination with RT is not available.

In general, the therapeutic index seemed to be rather narrow (Crane et al. 2002). A dose of 40 mg/m^2 twice weekly concurrent to RT following an induction therapy of irinotecan/gemcitabine was feasible too (Blackstock et al. 1999, 2002) but of only moderate activity (Mishra et al. 2005). Combination of gemcitabine with cisplatin and concomitant with RT was feasible (Wilkowski et al. 2003). Other partners are under evaluation. Of special interest are non-cytotoxic partners such as trastuzumab or epidermal growth factor receptor (EGFR) antibodies. Inhibitors of the ras protein, metalloproteinases, COX inhibitors, and vascular-endothelial-growth-receptor (VEGF) inhibitors are being investigated pre-clinically or in early clinical studies (Wayne et al. 2002).

Three major randomized studies are evaluating the role of bevacizumab and cetuximab with gemcitabine and irinotecan with docetaxel (Saif 2006). The ECOG 2204 trial, activated in February 2006 is a phase II randomized study of adjuvant therapy comprising bevacizumab versus cetuximab in combination with gemcitabine, capecitabine, and RT in patients with completely resected carcinoma of the pancreas (see the ECOG homepage). Activity is of interest for a possible combined regimen with RT as the toxicity profiles are favourable. A phase I trial combining capecitabine and bevacizumab with RT in locally advanced pancreatic cancer had shown promising results, although there was ulceration and bleeding in the RT field (Crane et al. 2006).

In Europe, the EORTC is recruiting patients in the protocol 22012/40013 (Fig. 9.2; see the EORTC homepage). This is a multi-institutional trial of the gastrointestinal tract cancer group and the RT group, with the Fédération Francophone de la Cancérologie Digestive (FFCD) co-oper-

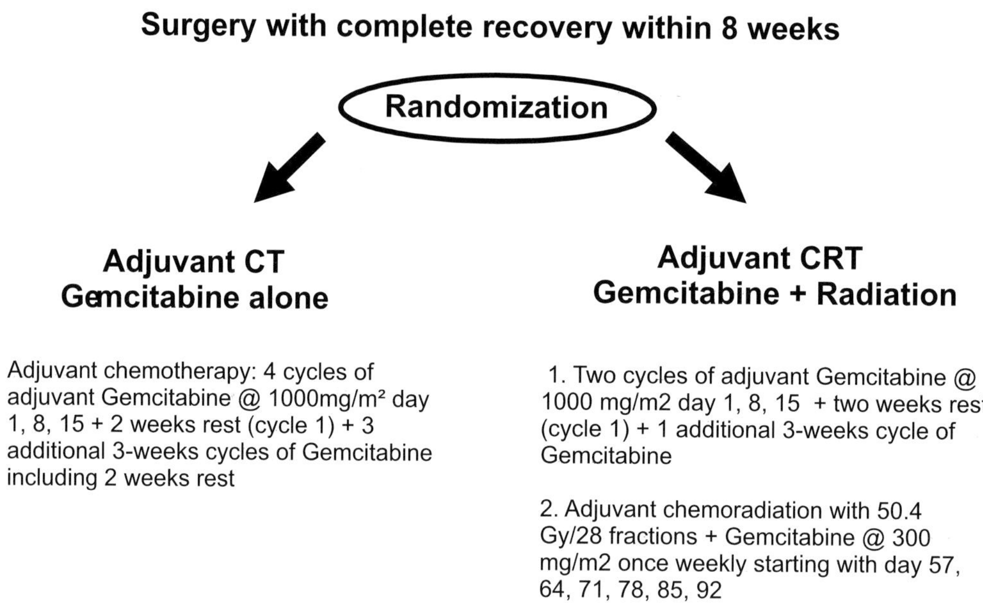

Fig. 9.2 EORTC Trial 44013 / 22012: Randomized phase II/III study comparing gemcitabine followed by gemcitabine plus concomitant radiation (50.4 Gy) versus gemcitabine alone after curative pancreaticoduodenectomy for pancreatic head cancer

ating. There is a phase II feasibility part with a planned 80 patients, followed by a phase III part with a planned 540 patients. Endpoint will be an improvement in disease-free survival by 10%. A strict patient selection will take place, as only patients with pancreatic head carcinoma after R0 pancreaticoduodenectomy will be included. Taking into account the ESPAC-1 data, an initially planned surveillance arm was dropped. After a first amendment, the standard arm now offers gemcitabine 1,000 mg/m^2 for four cycles. The experimental arm offers gemcitabine 1,000 mg/m^2 for two cycles followed by chemoradiotherapy with gemcitabine 300 mg/m^2 once weekly with concurrent 50.4 Gy RT. Eligibility criteria include R0 pancreaticoduodenectomy for pancreatic head cancer with a complete recovery within 8 weeks. So far the accrual has reached 80 patients.

In 2006, during the German Cancer Congress, the first data from the Heidelberg Phase III Trial CapRI (post-operative cisplatin, interferon alpha-2b, and 5-FU combined with external radiation treatment versus 5-FU alone for patients with resected pancreatic adenocarcinoma) was reported. In all, 52 patients were enrolled. The treatment scheme was less toxic than expected; patients could be treated on an outpatient basis. The main common toxicity criteria (CTC) grade III toxicities are leukopenia, hand-foot-syndrome, stomatitis, fatigue syndrome and hypo-calcemia. The treatment scheme was deemed to be feasible, but an experienced interdisciplinary group is needed (Knaebel et al. 2005).

A phase II study of the CAO/ARO/AIO evaluating a pre-operative radiochemotherapy for potentially resectable patients with cancer of the pancreatic head has started. Gemcitabine 300 mg/m^2 weekly is combined with cisplatin 30 mg/m^2 weekly and concurrent RT to 50.4–55.8 Gy followed by surgery versus surgery alone (see the AIO homepage, www.aio-portal.de).

9.9 Summary and Conclusion

As surgery has improved, the outcome has remained predictable by factors such as tumour size, resection margin status, N-stage, grading and blood loss at surgery.

In the United States, the adjuvant standard of care is a combined chemoradiation with 5-FU based on the GITSG study results from 1985 with a very limited number of patients. Results have been confirmed by several authors and the randomized EORTC 40891 study, which was, however, underpowered.

In Europe, most patients receive adjuvant chemotherapy only, with 5-FU or with gemcitabine based on the ESPAC-1 data, which have been criticized for considerable inherent limitations concerning statistical power and quality assurance. Gemcitabine is currently evaluated in combined modality treatment with other partners, varying doses and administration forms, and especially with concurrent RT. Still, in the United States and Europe there is a strong belief in adjuvant therapy based on a survival advantage in the major randomized studies.

Many trials investigating adjuvant therapy in pancreatic cancer are outdated or statistically questionable. This is why the recent phase III studies, ESPAC-3 and EORTC 22012/40013, deserve support.

When planning adjuvant therapy, some precautions have to be taken into consideration.

- Patients should be selected carefully.
- Chemoradiotherapy may be more effective for patients with cancer of the pancreatic head than pancreatic body and tail and for patients with positive resection margins.
- Treatment planning should be state-of-the-art to minimize treatment-related toxicity.
- RT planning should be three-dimensional, and should aim for 50-Gy doses without split.
- IMRT or IORT should be evaluated.

The concurrent chemotherapy can be 5-FU, given as continuous infusion with 200–250 mg/m^2 per day, 7 days per week during the entire treatment cycle. Possible partners are interferon-α and cisplatin, but toxicity has to be monitored carefully. Finally, gemcitabine to a dose of 300 mg/m^2 once weekly concurrent to RT is a safe and possibly more effective treatment, which is being evaluated in a randomized multi-centre trial of the EORTC.

References

Abrams RA, Grochow LB, Chakravarthy A, Sohn TA, Zahurak ML, Haulk TL, Ord S, Hruban RH, Lillemoe KD, Pitt HA, Cameron JL, Yeo CJ (1999) Intensified adjuvant therapy for pancreatic and periampullary adenocarcinoma: survival results and observations regarding patterns of failure, radiotherapy dose and CA19–9 levels. Int J Radiat Oncol Biol Phys 44:1039–1046

Bai YR, Wu GH, Guo WJ, Wu XD, Yao Y, Chen Y, Zhou RH, Lu DQ (2003) Intensity modulated radiation therapy and chemotherapy for locally advanced pancreatic cancer: results of feasibility study. World J Gastroenterol 9:2561–2564

Bakkevold KE, Arnesjø B, Dahl O, Kambestad B (1993) Adjuvant combination chemotherapy (AMF) following radical resection of carcinoma of the pancreas and papilla of Vater—results of a controlled, prospective, randomised multicentre study. Eur J Cancer 29A:698–703

Ben-Josef E, Shields AF, Vaishampayan U, Vaitkevicius V, El-Rayes BF, McDermott P, Burmeister J, Bossenberger T, Philip PA (2004) Intensity-modulated radiotherapy (IMRT) and concurrent capecitabine for pancreatic cancer. Int J Radiat Oncol Biol Phys 59:454–459

Bergenfeldt M, Albertsson M (2006) Current state of adjuvant therapy in resected pancreatic adenocarcinoma. Acta Oncol 45:124–135

Blackstock AW, Bernard SA, Richards F, Eagle KS, Case LD, Poole ME, Savage PD, Tepper JE (1999) Phase I trial of twice-weekly gemcitabine and concurrent radiation in patients with advanced pancreatic cancer. J Clin Oncol 17:2208–2212

Blackstock AW, Melin SA, Butler JM, Patton S, Pineau B, Albertson D, Howerton R, Levine E (2002) Irinotecan/gemcitabine followed by twice-weekly gemcitabine/radiation in locally advanced pancreatic cancer. Oncology 16[Suppl 5]:25–28

Brown MW, Ning H, Arora B, Albert PS, Poggi M, Camphausen K, Citrin D (2006) A dosimetric analysis of dose escalation using two intensity-modulated radiation therapy techniques in locally advanced pancreatic carcinoma. Int J Radiat Oncol Biol Phys 65:274–283

Burris HA, Moore MJ, Andersen J, Green MR, Rothenberg ML, Modiano MR, Cripps MC, Portenoy RK, Storniolo AM, Tarassoff P, Nelson R, Dorr FA, Stephens CD, Von Hoff DD (1997) Improvements in survival and clinical benefit with gemcitabine as first-line therapy for patients with advanced pancreas cancer: a randomized trial. J Clin Oncol 15:2403–2413

Burris H, Storniolo AM (1997) Assessing clinical benefit in the treatment of pancreas cancer: gemcitabine compared to 5-fluorouracil. Eur J Cancer 33 [Suppl 1]:S18–S22

Choti MA (2004) Adjuvant therapy for pancreatic cancer—the debate continues. N Engl J Med 350:1249–1251

Crane CH, Antolak JA, Rosen II, Forster KM, Evans DB, Janjan NA, Charnsangavej C, Pisters PW, Lenzi R, Papagikos MA, Wolff RA (2001a) Phase I study of concomitant gemcitabine and IMRT for patients with unresectable adenocarcinoma of the pancreatic head. Int J Gastrointest Cancer 30:123–132

Crane CH, Wolff RA, Abbruzzese JL, Evans DB, Milas L, Mason K, Charnsangavej C, Pisters PW, Lee JE, Lenzi R, Lahoti S, Vauthey JN, Janjan NA (2001b) Combining gemcitabine with radiation in pancreatic cancer: understanding important variables influencing the therapeutic index. Semin Oncol 28:25–33

Crane CH, Abbruzzese JL, Evans DB, Wolff RA, Ballo MT, Delclos M, Milas L, Mason K, Charnsangavej C, Pisters PW, Lee JE, Lenzi R, Vauthey JN, Wong AB, Phan T, Nguyen Q, Janjan NA (2002) Is the therapeutic index better with gemcitabine-based chemoradiation than with 5-fluorouracil-based chemoradiation in locally advanced pancreatic cancer? Int J Radiat Oncol Biol Phys 52:1293–1302

Crane CH, Ellis LM, Abbruzzese JL, Amos C, Xiong HQ, Ho L, Evans DB, Tamm EP, Ng C, Pisters PW, Charnsangavej C, Delclos ME, O'Reilly M, Lee JE, Wolff RA (2006a) Phase I trial evaluating the safety of bevacizumab with concurrent radiotherapy and capecitabine in locally advanced pancreatic cancer. J Clin Oncol 24:1145–1151

Crane CH, Varadhachary G, Wolff RA, Pisters PW, Evans DB (2006b) The argument for pre-operative chemoradiation for localized, radiographically resectable pancreatic cancer. Best Pract Res Clin Gastroenterol 20:365–382

Di Carlo V, Zerbi A, Balzano G, Villa E (1997) Intraoperative and postoperative radiotherapy in pancreatic cancer. Int J Pancreatol 21:53–58

Emami B, Lyman J, Brown A, Coia L, Goitein M, Munzenrider JE, Shank B, Solin LJ, Wesson M (1991) Tolerance of normal tissue to therapeutic irradiation. Int J Radiat Oncol Biol Phys 21:109–122

Evans DB (2005) Preoperative chemoradiation for pancreatic cancer. Semin Oncol 32:S25–S29

Evans DB, Rich TA, Byrd DR, Cleary KR, Connelly JH, Levin B, Charnsangavej C, Fenoglio CJ, Ames FC (1992) Preoperative chemoradiation and pancreaticoduodenectomy for adenocarcinoma of the pancreas. Arch Surg 127:1335–1339

Evans DB, Pisters PW, Lee JE, Bold RJ, Charnsangavej C, Janjan NA, Wolff RA, Abbruzzese JL (1998) Preoperative chemoradiation strategies for localized adenocarcinoma of the pancreas. J Hepatobiliary Pancreat Surg 5:242–250

Foo ML, Gunderson LL, Nagorney DM, McLlrath DC, van Heerden JA, Robinow JS, Kvols LK, Garton GR, Martenson JA, Cha SS (1993) Patterns of failure in grossly resected pancreatic ductal adenocarcinoma treated with adjuvant irradiation +/− 5 fluorouracil. Int J Radiat Oncol Biol Phys 26:483–489

Foo ML, Gunderson LL (1998) Adjuvant postoperative radiation therapy +/− 5-FU in resected carcinoma of the pancreas. Hepatogastroenterology 45:613–623

Gastrointestinal Tumor Study Group (1987) Further evidence of effective adjuvant combined radiation and chemotherapy following curative resection of pancreatic cancer. Gastrointestinal Tumor Study Group. Cancer 59:2006–2010

Hoyer M, Roed H, Sengelov L, Traberg A, Ohlhuis L, Pedersen J, Nellemann H, Kiil Berthelsen A, Eberholst F, Engelholm SA, von der Maase H (2005) Phase-II study on stereotactic radiotherapy of locally advanced pancreatic carcinoma. Radiother Oncol 76:48–53

Kalser MH, Barkin J, MacIntyre JM (1985) Pancreatic cancer. Assessment of prognosis by clinical presentation. Cancer 56:397–402

Kalser MH, Ellenberg SS (1985) Pancreatic cancer. Adjuvant combined radiation and chemotherapy following curative resection. Arch Surg 120:899–903

Kayahara M, Nagakawa T, Ueno K, Ohta T, Tsukioka Y, Miyazaki I (1995) Surgical strategy for carcinoma of the pancreas head area based on clinicopathologic analysis of nodal involvement and plexus invasion. Surgery 117:616–623

Kayahara M, Nagakawa T, Futagami F, Kitagawa H, Ohta T, Miyazaki I (1996) Lymphatic flow and neural plexus invasion associated with carcinoma of the body and tail of the pancreas. Cancer 78:2485–2491

Kayahara M, Nagakawa T, Ohta T, Kitagawa H, Ueno K, Tajima H, Elnemr A, Miwa K (1999) Analysis of paraaortic lymph node involvement in pancreatic carcinoma: a significant indication for surgery? Cancer 85:583–590

Kelly DM, Benjamin IS (1995) Pancreatic carcinoma. Ann Oncol 6:19–28

Klinkenbijl JH, Jeekel J, Sahmoud T, van Pel R, Couvreur ML, Veenhof CH, Arnaud JP, Gonzalez DG, de Wit LT, Hennipman A, Wils J (1999) Adjuvant radiotherapy and 5-fluorouracil after curative resection of cancer of the pancreas and periampullary region: phase III trial of the EORTC gastrointestinal tract cancer co-operative group. Ann Surg 230:776–782

Knaebel HP, Märten A, Schmidt J, Hoffmann K, Seiler C, Lindel K, Schmitz-Winnenthal H, Fritz S, Herrmann T, Goldschmidt H, Mansmann U, Debus J, Diehl V, Büchler MW (2005) Phase III trial of postoperative cisplatin, interferon alpha-2b, and 5-FU combined with external radiation treatment versus 5-FU alone for patients with resected pancreatic adenocarcinoma—CapRI: study protocol [ISRCTN62866759]. BMC Cancer 5:37

Koong AC, Christofferson E, Le QT, Goodman KA, Ho A, Kuo T, Ford JM, Fisher GA, Greco R, Norton J, Yang GP (2005) Phase II study to assess the efficacy of conventionally fractionated radiotherapy followed by a stereotactic radiosurgery boost in patients with locally advanced pancreatic cancer. Int J Radiat Oncol Biol Phys 63:320–323

Koshy MC, Landry JC, Cavanaugh SX, Fuller CD, Willett CG, Abrams RA, Hoffman JP, Thomas CR (2005) A challenge to the therapeutic nihilism of ESPAC-1. Int J Radiat Oncol Biol Phys 61:965–966

Krempien R, Muenter MW, Huber PE, Nill S, Friess H, Timke C, Didinger B, Buechler P, Heeger S, Herfarth KK, Abdollahi A, Buchler MW, Debus J (2005) Randomized phase II—study evaluating EGFR targeting therapy with cetuximab in combination with radiotherapy and chemotherapy for patients with locally advanced pancreatic cancer—PARC: study protocol [ISRCTN56652283]. BMC Cancer 5:131

Landry JC, Yang GY, Ting JY, Staley CA, Torres W, Esiashvili N, Davis LW (2002) Treatment of pancreatic cancer tumors with intensity-modulated radiation therapy (IMRT) using the volume at risk approach (VARA): employing dose-volume histogram (DVH) and normal tissue complication probability (NTCP) to evaluate small bowel toxicity. Med Dosim 27:121–129

Lawrence TS, Chang EY, Hahn TM, Hertel LW, Shewach DS (1996) Radiosensitization of pancreatic cancer cells by 2',2'-difluoro-2'-deoxycytidine. Int J Radiat Oncol Biol Phys 34:867–872

Magee CJ, Ghaneh P, Hartley M, Sutton R, Neoptolemos JP (2002) The role of adjuvant therapy for pancreatic cancer. Expert Opin Investig Drugs 11:87–107

McGinn CJ, Zalupski MM (2003) Radiation therapy with once-weekly gemcitabine in pancreatic cancer: current status of clinical trials. Int J Radiat Oncol Biol Phys 56:10–15

Mehta VK, Fisher GA, Ford JM, Oberhelman HA, Vierra MA, Bastidas AJ, Poen JC (2000) Adjuvant radiotherapy and concomitant 5-fluorouracil by protracted venous infusion for resected pancreatic cancer. Int J Radiat Oncol Biol Phys 48:1483–1487

Mishra G, Butler J, Ho C, Melin S, Case LD, Ennever PR, Magrinat GC, Bearden JD, Minotto DC, Howerton R, Levine E, Blackstock AW (2005) Phase II trial of induction gemcitabine/CPT-11 followed by a twice-weekly infusion of gemcitabine and concurrent external beam radiation for the treatment of locally advanced pancreatic cancer. Am J Clin Oncol 28:345–350

Mornex F, Girard N, Scoazec JY, Bossard N, Ychou M, Smith D, Seitz JF, Valette PJ, Roy P, Rouanet P, Ducreux M, Partensky C (2006) Feasibility of preoperative combined radiation therapy and chemotherapy with 5-fluorouracil and cisplatin in potentially resectable pancreatic adenocarcinoma: the French SFRO-FFCD 97-04 Phase II trial. Int J Radiat Oncol Biol Phys 65:1471–1478

Neoptolemos JP, Dunn JA, Stocken DD, Almond J, Link K, Beger H, Bassi C, Falconi M, Pederzoli P, Dervenis C, Fernandez-Cruz L, Lacaine F, Pap A, Spooner D, Kerr DJ, Friess H, et al. (2001) Adjuvant chemoradiotherapy and chemotherapy in resectable pancreatic cancer: a randomised controlled trial. Lancet 358:1576–1585

Neoptolemos JP, Cunningham D, Friess H, Bassi C, Stocken DD, Tait DM, Dunn JA, Dervenis C, Lacaine F, Hickey H, Raraty MG, Ghaneh P, Buchler MW (2003) Adjuvant therapy in pancreatic cancer: historical and current perspectives. Ann Oncol 14:675–692

Neoptolemos JP, Stocken DD, Friess H, Bassi C, Dunn JA, Hickey H, Beger H, Fernandez-Cruz L, Dervenis C, Lacaine F, Falconi M, Pederzoli P, Pap A, Spooner D, Kerr DJ, et al. (2004) A randomized trial of chemoradiotherapy and chemotherapy after resection of pancreatic cancer. N Engl J Med 350:1200–1210

Neuhaus P, Oettle H, Post S, et al. (2005) A randomised, prospective, multicenter, phase III trial of adjuvant chemotherapy with gemcitabine vs. observation in patients with resected pancreatic cancer. ASCO Annual Meeting, abstr LBA4013

Paulino AC (1999) Resected pancreatic cancer treated with adjuvant radiotherapy with or without 5-fluorouracil: treatment results and patterns of failure. Am J Clin Oncol 22:489–494

Pendurthi TK, Hoffman JP, Ross E, Johnson DE, Eisenberg BL (1998) Preoperative versus postoperative chemoradiation for patients with resected pancreatic adenocarcinoma. Am Surg 64:686–692

Pisters PW, Abbruzzese JL, Janjan NA, Cleary KR, Charnsangavej C, Goswitz MS, Rich TA, Raijman I, Wolff RA, Lenzi R, Lee JE, Evans DB (1998) Rapid-fractionation preoperative chemoradiation, pancreaticoduodenectomy, and intraoperative radiation therapy for resectable pancreatic adenocarcinoma. J Clin Oncol 16:3843–3850

Pisters PW, Wolff RA, Janjan NA, Cleary KR, Charnsangavej C, Crane CN, Lenzi R, Vauthey JN, Lee JE, Abbruzzese JL, Evans DB (2002) Preoperative paclitaxel and concurrent rapid-fractionation radiation for resectable pancreatic adenocarcinoma: toxicities, histologic response rates, and event-free outcome. J Clin Oncol 20:2537–2544

Regine WF, Abrams RA (1998) Adjuvant therapy for pancreatic cancer: back to the future. Int J Radiat Oncol Biol Phys 42:59–63

Reni M, Panucci MG, Ferreri AJ, Balzano G, Passoni P, Cattaneo GM, Cordio S, Scaglietti U, Zerbi A, Ceresoli GL, Fiorino C, Calandrino R, Staudacher C, Villa E, Di Carlo V (2001) Effect on local control and survival of electron beam intraoperative irradiation for resectable pancreatic adenocarcinoma. Int J Radiat Oncol Biol Phys 50:651–658

Rothenberg ML, Moore MJ, Cripps MC, Andersen JS, Portenoy RK, Burris HA 3rd, Green MR, Tarassoff PG, Brown TD, Casper ES, Storniolo AM, Von Hoff DD (1996) A phase II trial of gemcitabine in patients with 5-FU-refractory pancreas cancer. Ann Oncol 7:347–353

Saif MW (2006) Pancreatic cancer: highlights from the 42nd annual meeting of the American Society of Clinical Oncology, 2006. Jop 7:337–348

Sener SF, Fremgen A, Menck HR, Winchester DP (1999) Pancreatic cancer: a report of treatment and survival trends for 100,313 patients diagnosed from 1985–1995, using the National Cancer Database. J Am Coll Surg 189:1–7

Sohn TA, Yeo CJ, Cameron JL, Koniaris L, Kaushal S, Abrams RA, Sauter PK, Coleman J, Hruban RH, Lillemoe KD (2000) Resected adenocarcinoma of the pancreas-616 patients: results, outcomes, and prognostic indicators. J Gastrointest Surg 4:567–579

Spitz FR, Abbruzzese JL, Lee JE, Pisters PW, Lowy AM, Fenoglio CJ, Cleary KR, Janjan NA, Goswitz MS, Rich TA, Evans DB (1997) Preoperative and postoperative chemoradiation strategies in patients treated with pancreaticoduodenectomy for adenocarcinoma of the pancreas. J Clin Oncol 15:928–937

Stocken DD, Büchler MW, Dervenis C, Bassi C, Jeekel H, Klinkenbijl JH, Bakkevold KE, Takada T, Amano H, et al. (2005) Meta-analysis of randomised adjuvant therapy trials for pancreatic cancer. Br J Cancer 92:1372–1381

Tempero M, Plunkett W, Ruiz Van Haperen V, Hainsworth J, Hochster H, Lenzi R, Abbruzzese J (2003) Randomized phase II comparison of dose-intense gemcitabine: thirty-minute infusion and fixed dose rate infusion in patients with pancreatic adenocarcinoma. J Clin Oncol 21:3402–3408

Van Laethem JL, Demols A, Gay F, Closon MT, Collette M, Polus M, Houbiers G, Gastelblum P, Gelin M, Houtte PV, Closset J (2003) Postoperative adjuvant gemcitabine and concurrent radiation after curative resection of pancreatic head carcinoma: a phase II study. Int J Radiat Oncol Biol Phys 56:974–980

Wayne JD, Abdalla EK, Wolff RA, Crane CH, Pisters PW, Evans DB (2002) Localized adenocarcinoma of the pancreas: the rationale for preoperative chemoradiation. Oncologist 7:34–45

White R, Lee C, Anscher M, Gottfried M, Wolff R, Keogan M, Pappas T, Hurwitz H, Tyler D (1999) Preoperative chemoradiation for patients with locally advanced adenocarcinoma of the pancreas. Ann Surg Oncol 6:38–45

White RR, Hurwitz HI, Morse MA, Lee C, Anscher MS, Paulson EK, Gottfried MR, Baillie J, Branch MS, Jowell PS, McGrath KM, Clary BM, Pappas TN, Tyler DS (2001) Neoadjuvant chemoradiation for localized adenocarcinoma of the pancreas. Ann Surg Oncol 8:758–765

Wilkowski R, Thoma M, Heinemann V, Rau HG, Wagner A, Stoffregen C, Dühmke E (2003) Radiochemotherapy with gemcitabine and cisplatin in pancreatic cancer—feasible and effective [in German]. Strahlenther Onkol 179:78–86

Wilkowski R, Thoma M, Weingandt H, Dühmke E, Heinemann V (2005) Chemoradiation for ductal pancreatic carcinoma: principles of combining chemotherapy with radiation, definition of target volume and radiation dose. Jop 6:216–230

Wolff RA, Evans DB, Gravel DM, Lenzi R, Pisters PW, Lee JE, Janjan NA, Charnsangavej C, Abbruzzese JL (2001) Phase I trial of gemcitabine combined with radiation for the treatment of locally advanced pancreatic adenocarcinoma. Clin Cancer Res 7:2246–2253

Yeo CJ, Cameron JL (1999) Improving results of pancreaticoduodenectomy for pancreatic cancer. World J Surg 23:907–912

Yeo CJ, Cameron JL, Lillemoe KD, Sitzmann JV, Hruban RH, Goodman SN, Dooley WC, Coleman J, Pitt HA (1995) Pancreaticoduodenectomy for cancer of the head of the pancreas. 201 patients. Ann Surg 221:721–731

Yeo CJ, Abrams RA, Grochow LB, Sohn TA, Ord SE, Hruban RH, Zahurak ML, Dooley WC, Coleman J, Sauter PK, Pitt HA, Lillemoe KD, Cameron JL (1997) Pancreaticoduodenectomy for pancreatic adenocarcinoma: postoperative adjuvant chemoradiation improves survival. A prospective, single-institution experience. Ann Surg 225:621–633

10 Primary Advanced Unresectable Pancreatic Cancer

R. Wilkowski, M. Wolf, V. Heinemann

Recent Results in Cancer Research, Vol. 177

Abstract

Median as well as overall survival of pancreatic cancer patients in the advanced stage is extremely low despite advances in cancer therapy regarding tumor cell biology, therapy resistance, and diagnosis. In matters of chemoradiation therapy (CRT) in locally advanced pancreatic cancer, favorable positive effect has been reached with different radiotherapy proceedings such as intraoperative radiation therapy with or without external chemo-/radiation therapy or with CRT alone with regard to local tumor pain, local tumor remission, or local control of disease and overall survival. Primary (chemo-) radiation therapy only rarely leads to local remission. Intraoperative radiation therapy (IORT) merely reaches pain palliation in most cases. By administering up-to-date primary CRT, especially with gemcitabine-associated CRT, local remission in up to 50% of patients can be observed. By applying neoadjuvant CRT, better resectability and the reduction of postoperative positive lymph node metastasis has been seen in patients with resectable or possibly resectable pancreatic cancer. With primary CRT, resectability can also be achieved in patients with primary unresectable pancreatic cancer. It has been shown at the evaluation of patients' progression samples—either treated with neoadjuvant or primarily with radiotherapy (with conventional radiation technique)—that the rate of local recurrence or local progression can be reduced in comparison with historical cohorts. By contrast, the rate on distant metastases was not affected. Whereas concurrent CRT leads to favorable local tumor control, this procedure has a minor effect as to the survival in most of the studies. Because metastases occur mostly out of the irradiation field and because of partly advanced local tumor progression, the concept of combined CRT with continuing chemotherapy was developed.

Median survival of pancreatic patients in the advanced stage is approx. 3–5 months, with a 12-month survival probability of 10% despite advances in cancer therapy. On the other hand, the 5-year survival probability is 0.4%–3.0% (Bramhall et al. 1995, 1998).

The causes of such a dismal prognosis can be understood first of all in the commonly late diagnosis (Haycox et al. 1998), second in the aggressive tumor cell biology with continuing therapy resistance (Magee et al. 2001), and finally because an acceptable resection rate can be achieved only in specialized centers (Birkmeyer et al. 2002; Neoptolemos et al. 1997).

Only 10%–15% of patients can be resected after the diagnosis of pancreatic cancer. Resection is considered a potential curative therapy. However, median survival of these patients amounts to only 13–18 months, with a 5-year survival of 10%–20% (Bramhall et al. 1995; Yeo et al. 1997). The survival rate did not improve with a radical resection and extended lymphadenectomy (Pedrazzoli et al. 1998).

Furthermore, 15%–30% of primary nonmetastatic pancreatic cancer is unresectable due to extended vessel infiltration at time of diagnosis. The prognosis for these patients is very dismal due to lack of specific therapy; moreover, median overall survival is a maximum of 6–8 months (Niederhuber et al. 1995; Shinchi et al. 2002).

10.1 Chemotherapy of Advanced Pancreatic Cancer

Although more chemotherapeutic agents have been examined for the purposes of the therapy of advanced pancreatic cancer, only 5-FU, mitomycin-C (MMC) (Haycox et al. 1998) and, lately, gemcitabine (Burris et al. 1997; Moore et al. 1995; Rothenberg et al. 1996) have shown reproductible outcomes with objective results.

A 5-FU-based combined chemotherapy has shown a clear survival advantage compared to patients without treatment in randomized controlled studies (Glimelius et al. 1996; Mallinson et al. 1980; Palmer et al. 1994). However, compared to monotherapy with 5-FU, a toxicity increase without additional improvement of survival has been reported (Cullinan et al. 1990).

Gemcitabine belongs to a series of new chemotherapeutic agents tested for pancreatic cancer. It has shown superior efficacy both in monotherapy and in combined therapies (Berlin et al. 2002; Burris et al. 1997; Heinemann et al. 1999b, 2000). Nevertheless, the application of fluoropyrimidine continues to be of interest in trials where the efficacy of 5-FU after portal vein infusion (PVI) application and the development of orally applicable chemotherapeutic agents is sought (Neoptolemos et al. 2004). The National Cancer Research Institute in Britain has recently started a Gem-Cap phase III trial where gemcitabine (Gem) will be applied with capecitabine (Cap).

The survival advantage with gemcitabine is minor compared to bolus 5-FU (Burris et al. 1997). Nevertheless, it is being used in advanced pancreatic cancer increasingly as the standard therapy.

However, a significant breakthrough in the therapy of advanced pancreatic cancer with chemotherapy has not been found yet.

10.2 Chemoradiation in Locally Advanced Pancreatic Cancer

A favorable positive effect has been reached with different radiotherapy proceedings such as intraoperative radiation therapy (IORT) with or without external chemo-/radiation therapy or with chemoradiation (CRT) alone with regard to both local tumor symptomatic (local tumor pain), local tumor remission, or local control of disease and overall survival (Fossati et al. 1995; Nishimura et al. 1997; Staley et al. 1996). Therefore, chemoradiation with a total irradiation dose of 45.0–50.0 Gy (eventually up to 60.0 Gy) with conventional fractionation and a concurrent chemotherapy with 5-FU (eventually PVI during the whole therapy with 200–225 mg/m^2 per day) was recommended as the standard and most effective therapy procedure for patients in good general condition (German Cancer Association 2002).

Randomized trials reporting significant improvement of median survival after chemoradiation are listed in Table 10.1 (Moertel et al. 1981; Li et al. 2003; Shinchi et al. 2002).

For decades, 5-FU has been considered the agent of choice with regard to the chemotherapeutic agents administered concurrently or sequentially to radiation. Combined chemotherapies such as FAM (5-FU, doxorubicin, mitomycin-C) or SMF (streptozotocin, mitomycin-C, 5-FU), or the Mallinson regimen (5-FU, cyclophosphamide, methotrexate and vincristine) resulted in increased toxicity and no improvement as to survival (Bruckner et al. 1993; Cullinan et al. 1990). Even newer agents tested recently for pancreatic cancer such as paclitaxel, docetaxel, irinotecan, topotecan, and oxaliplatin could not be established as treatment (Ashamalla et al. 2003; Kamthan et al. 1997). Only after the introduction of the pyrimidine analog gemcitabine it was possible to reach an improved response rate for unresectable (Epelbaum et al. 2002; Kornek et al. 2001; Okusaka et al. 2004; Safran et al. 2002) or metastatic (Burris et al. 1997; Carmichael et al. 1996; Casper et al. 1994; Heinemann et al. 1999a; Rothenberg et al. 1996) patients in different studies. Gemcitabine has a favorable side effect profile: positive clinical benefit response, practically no hepato- or nephrotoxicity. Only hematotoxicity can be seen as a dose-limiting factor. Because of that, radiation-sensitizing effects have been experimentally proved for gemcitabine (Lawrence et al. 1996; McGinn et al. 1996; Mose et al. 1999; Shewach et al. 1994), which suggests some hope for successful administration of this agent concurrent to radiation.

Table 10.1 Randomized trials to chemoradiation in locally advanced pancreatic cancer

Author	Patients	Therapy	Med. Surv. (in months)	Remark
Moertel et al. 1969	32	35–40 Gy	6.3	Sig.
	32	35–40 Gy+5-FU→5-FU	10.4	
Moertel et al. 1981	83	40 Gy (split)+5-FU→5-FU	9.6	Sig.
	86	60 Gy (split)+5-FU→5-FU	9.2	
	25	60 Gy (split)	5.2	
GITSG 1985	24	54 Gy→SMF	10.5	Sig.
	24	SMF	8.0	
GITSG 1988	73	60 Gy (split)+5-FU	8.4	N.s.
	72	60 Gy (split)+Adri	7.5	
Klaasen et al. 1985	47	40 Gy+5-FU	8.3	N.s.
	44	5-FU	8.2	
Shinchi et al. 2002	16	EBRT 50 Gy+5-FU (PVI)	13.2	Sig.
	15	No therapy	6.4	
Li et al. 2003	16	50.4–61.2 Gy+5FU	6.7	Sig.
	18	50.4–61.2 Gy+G	14.4	
Cohen et al. 2005	104	59.4 Gy	7.1	N.s.
		59.4 Gy+5-FU/MMC	8.4	
Chauffert 2006; ASCO	59	60.0 Gy+5-FU (PVI), Cis→G (to PD)	8.4	Sig.
	60	G(1,000) (to PD)	14.3	
Wilkowski 2006; ASCO	32	50.0 Gy+5-FU (PVI)	9.0	N.s.
	33	50.0 Gy+G/C	9.6	
	31	50.0 Gy+G/C→G/C (4 cycles)	6.1	

5-FU, 5-fluorouracil; Med. Surv., median survival; N.s., not significant; Pat., number of patients; SMF, streptozotocin, mitomycin-C, 5-FU; split, split-course radiation; sq, sequential chemotherapy; sig., significant

10.3 Local Remission After Primary (Chemo-)Radiation Therapy

Radiation therapy alone or the combination of external beam radiation therapy (EBRT) with IORT leads to local remission only rarely. The administration of IORT has been explained primarily with providing the benefit of good to best pain palliation [pain control in 57% (Okamoto et al. 1994; Tuckson et al. 1988) to 100% (Manabe et al. 1988)].

Whittington et al. (1984) and Mohiuddin et al. (1988) have reported on a patient cohort where the combination of EBRT with iodine-125 seed implantation increased local control (clinical, local symptomatic) from 22% (historical patient group) to 81%.

It has been possible to observe objective remission in images only recently, since the advent of the concurrent administration of radiation sensitizing agents (chemotherapeutic agents, in the first-line 5-FU or combination therapies with 5-FU) for EBRT (Aristu et al. 2003; Luderhoff et al. 1996).

The frequency of local remission in up to 50% of patients can be observed when administering up-to-date primary chemoradiation (Ikeda et al. 2002; Li et al. 2003; Rich and Evans 1995; Spitz et al. 1997; Wolff et al. 2000).

It is possible to achieve these response rates especially with gemcitabine-associated chemoradiation therapy. Remission was seen in 50% vs 13% of the patients in a randomized comparison of gemcitabine-CRT with 5-FU-CRT. Of a total of 18 gemcitabine-CRT patients, 4 have shown total remission (Li et al. 2003).

Bruckner et al. (1998) observed downstaging in 30% of a group of unresectable patients in International Union Against Cancer (UICC) stages II and III. The therapy concept included radiation therapy (54 Gy) with 5-FU and streptozotocin and cisplatin, followed by systemic chemotherapy with 5-FU–folic acid. Local tumor regression was surprisingly positive in resected patients. Fibroses were found in the histology of five of the resected patients, but no cancer cells.

A histological response (tumor cell destruction) has been seen in more than 5 in 10 (50%) of the resected patients from a group of 34 that were examined (Joensuu et al. 2004). These patients were treated primarily with concurrent chemoradiation with gemcitabine. Of these, 3 patients (11%) had a tumor cell destruction of more than 90%.

Wilkowski et al. (2004) have shown in an analysis of 47 patients with primary unresectable carcinoma that, especially during a concurrent sequential CRT with gemcitabine and cisplatin (GC), a high rate of local remission (69% during GC-ssqCRT) can be achieved, which can be proved by imaging diagnostics. It is possible to reach complete pathological remissions: R0 resection was achieved in 13 patients. Of these, 4 patients had no histologically verified tumor.

10.4 Secondary Resection After Primary (Chemo-)Radiation Therapy

Better resectability and the reduction of postoperative positive lymph node metastasis has been seen especially in patients with resectable or possibly resectable pancreatic cancer after neoadjuvant chemoradiation.

The restaging after chemoradiation has led the enrolled cancer patients in UICC stage II and III to resection rates between 43% and 74% in Evans et al. (1992), Ishikawa (1996), Rich et al. (1985), and Hoffman et al. (1998). Patients in UICC stage IV were studied by Jeekel and Treurniet-Donker (1991), Bruckner et al. (1998), Todd et al. (1998), and Kim et al. (2002)). Accordingly, resection rates were between 3.4% and 19% after neoadjuvant multimodality therapy in UICC stage IV.

Resectability can be achieved in patients with primary unresectable pancreatic cancer with primary chemoradiation too. This has been reported first of all after concurrent chemoradiation with gemcitabine (Ammori et al. 2003; Brunner et al. 2003; Crane et al. 2002; Epelbaum et al. 2002; Pipas et al. 2001; Wilkowski et al. 2004). R0 resection has been reached only in individual cases after concurrent administration of PVI 5-FU (application during radiation). Concurrent combination chemotherapies (CDDP+5-FU+/−paclitaxel) (Aristu et al. 2003) has led to complete remission in the framework of a resection only in individual cases.

10.5 Local and Systemic Progression After Primary (Chemo-)Radiation Therapy

It can be shown at the evaluation of patients' progression samples—either treated neoadjuvant or primarily with (chemo-) radiotherapy (with conventional radiation technique)—that the rate of local recurrence or local progression can be reduced in comparison with historical cohorts; moreover, it can be expected only in 6%–27% of the patients (Ishikawa et al. 1994, 1998; Kornek et al. 2001; Luderhoff et al. 1996; Okusaka et al. 2001).

By contrast, the rate on distant metastases, especially peritoneal carcinosis and liver metastasis, was not affected. This rate was assessed in 97% of the patients as a cause for therapy failure (Okusaka et al. 2004; Poggi et al. 2002; Shinchi et al. 2002).

Time to distant metastasis was even extended in the patient groups if a systemic chemotherapy was integrated in the treatment regimen as sequential chemotherapy. Kornek et al. (2000) report a progression-free survival of 10 months after concurrent sequential chemoradiation with 5-FU/leucovorin and cisplatin. Favorable effect was achieved with local liver perfusion with 5-FU too (Ishikawa et al. 1998).

The prognosis was favorable for the group of patients undergoing resection after neoadjuvant or primary (chemo-) radiation therapy (Al-Sukhun et al. 2003). Downstaging has been found in only 2 of 16 patients in a historical comparison by Jessup (1993), who administered neoadjuvant radiotherapy with 54 Gy and continuous 5-FU infusion. Median survival was 8 months in this group. The two successfully treated and resected neoadjuvant patients had a tumor-free interval of 20 and 22 months, respectively.

Ishikawa et al. (1994) have found in a case control study that preoperative radiation therapy resulted in downstaging and consequently in oncological resection in 17 of 23 patients. These patients had a reduction in local recurrence and have not died of the consequences of them. The first manifestations of disease development in the group of Ishikawa were frequently liver metastases. These metastases have caused lethal consequences more frequently in a year compared to a historical control group.

Median time to progression (TTP) of only 4.4 months was observed by Azria et al. (2002) after sequential chemo-radiotherapy (sCRT) with 5-FU (600 mg/m^2, day 1–5, week 1 and 5) and cisplatin (100 mg/m^2, day 2, weeks 1 and 5).

Okusaka et al. reporton a median progression-free interval of 5.8 months and a therapy failure due to distant metastasis (78%) in a series of 41 primary unresectable patients treated with ssqCRT (concurrent cisplatin 5 mg/m^2 per day, sequential 5-FU). Only 21% of the patients developed a local recurrence.

A median TTP of 2.7 vs 7.1 months ($p=0.019$), a median TTLP of 2.7 vs 7.4 months ($p=0.0016$), and a median time to systemic progression (TTSP) of 3.1 vs 6.1 months (n.s.) have been observed in a randomized trial by Li et al. (2003) where 5-FU-CRT vs gemcitabine-CRT has been compared.

10.6 Overall Survival After Primary (Chemo-)Radiotherapy

In 1969, Moertel et al. were able to achieve a better median survival in locally advanced pancreatic cancer with the administration of the combination of external radiation (EBRT) and 5-FU compared to radiation alone. Hereby was the importance of radio sensitizing through concurrent chemotherapy established.

5-FU, as an integrative part in CRT, has not been substituted yet by other agents, new combinations, or regional applications. The role of PVI 5-FU application, the administration of gemcitabine as radio sensitizer, or hyperfractionation of radiation during CRT is not clear.

Significant advantage of gemcitabine-CRT (concurrent gemcitabine, weekly 600 mg/m^2 per day 6× and sequential gemcitabine) compared to 5-FU-CRT (bolus 5-FU 500 mg/m^2 per day, days 1–3 and sequential gemcitabine) has been shown only in one randomized study (Li et al. 2003). However, there have been only 18 vs 16 patients compared, and 5-FU has been applied as bolus on three subsequent days of weeks 1, 3, and 5 of radiotherapy. Median survival of 14.5 months was achieved with gemcitabine-CRT, 6.7 months with 5-FU-CRT.

However, a median survival of 13.2 months has been reported in a further randomized trial by Shinchi et al. (2002) with PVI 5-FU-CRT (200 mg/m^2 per day). Median survival was 6.4 months in case of an untreated group of patients.

We should conclude in comparing these two studies alone that gemcitabine-CRT can be seen as equivalent to PVI 5-FU-CRT. A retrospective analysis by Mehta et al. (2001) does not support this conclusion. He has compared 27 patients with either bolus 5-FU or PVI 5-FU CRT. Median survival was 6 months for both groups in this trial. However, bolus 5-FU-CRT shows no improvement as to overall survival in comparison with untreated patients.

Whereas concurrent CRT leads to favorable local tumor control, this procedure has a minor effect as to the survival in most of the studies. This is because of the development of metastases out of the irradiation field. The concept of combined CRT with continuing chemotherapy was developed as a logical consequence due to these metastases and because of partly advanced local tumor progression. The Gastrointestinal Tumour Study Group (GITSG) completed a trial in 1981 that divided the patients in three study arms as follows: 60 Gy EBRT without radio sensitizing with 5-FU, 60 Gy EBRT with radio sensitizing with 5-FU and subsequent 5-FU application, 40 Gy EBRT with radio sensitizing with 5-FU and subsequent 5-FU application. Median survival was 23, 40, and 42 weeks, respectively. That is, a high dose of chemotherapy had no additional use. Better results were reached especially with concurrent or subsequent chemotherapy.

A median survival of 8.2 months after chemotherapy alone with weekly bolus 5-FU has been reported in the phase III study of the Eastern Cooperative Oncology Group (ECOG) of a total of 91 patients with unresectable pancreatic cancer. A median survival of 8.3 months has been seen in the direct comparison within the group treated with 5-FU-CRT and subsequent chemotherapy (Klaasen et al. 1985). Significantly higher toxicity (51%) has been observed in the study arm with combination therapy compared to 5-FU therapy alone (27%).

It has been possible to show in the phase I/II study of the Radiation Therapy Oncology Group (RTOG) enrolling 81 patients that, in spite of the fact that a prophylactic liver radiation can reduce the incidence of hepatic metastasis, this procedure can affect neither the local tumor control nor the intraabdominal tumor spread, and consequently, prophylactic liver irradiation cannot be generally recommended (Komaki et al. 1992).

A median survival of 17 months was seen in recent studies after CRT combined with triple chemotherapy (5-FU, streptozocin, and cisplatin) (Terk et al. 1997). Favorable median survival of 14 months was shown in a further trial of combined chemoradiation with 5-FU, leucovorin, and cisplatin (Kornek et al. 2000).

Hypofractionation (Luderhoff et al. 1996) or hyperfractionation (Crane et al. 2001; de Lange et al. 2002) of the irradiation in the framework of chemoradiation and sequential chemotherapy has been also administered. These regimens cannot be recommended as routine therapies due to considerable toxicities.

No survival advantage was achieved for patients with combined or IORT or brachytherapy alone (Nishimura et al. 1988; Calvo et al. 1991; Fossati et al. 1995; Kasperk et al. 1995; Okamoto et al. 2004).

Although recent studies have been reporting about acceptable survival after CRT, the results are not convincing in comparison with chemotherapy alone (especially using gemcitabine) (Fisher et al. 1999; Saad et al. 2002); possibly, it would be seen as even more unfavorable for the total cohort of patients (Chauffert et al. 2006).

10.7 Effect of Radiation Dose on Progression and Overall Survival After Primary (Chemo-)Radiotherapy

The initial data about the irradiation of pancreatic cancer have shown that “very high” doses would have been considered necessary in order to treat local tumors effectively. The effect of radiation has been reported as depending on dose, and a median survival of 10 months was achieved with a total dose of 68–75 Gy in the target field (Wiegel et al. 2000). A cure after radiation alone has been assessed as barely possible. Accordingly, the further aspect of local palliation (reduction of pain symptomatic in 65%–70% of the cases) has been formulated as the treatment aim. Necessary dose escalation was reached through IORT, eventually followed by EBRT. It was not possible to show a convincing remission rate or a substantial improvement of progression-free and total survival in studies with EBRT alone (Moertel et al. 1969, 1981), with IORT (Abe et al. 1993; Goldson 1991; Nishimura et al. 1988), or with a combination of EBRT and IORT (Kawamura et al. 1992; Gilly et al. 1990), although a median survival of 12.0 months has been reported in patients in stages I and II, respectively, with the combined use of EBRT and IORT (Manabe et al. 1988; Abe et al. 1991, 1993; Okamoto et al. 1994).

Downstaging for potential resectable patients has been reported first with the administration of chemoradiation with 5-FU and the administration of a radiation dose of 45–54 Gy (Scherer 1987). However, it has been shown that with the additional administration of IORT, a median survival of 18 months can be reached only for resectable patients, and the median survival amounts to 8.0–16.5 months for unresectable patients in this case (Kojima et al. 1991; Wood et al. 1982; Shipley et al. 1984).

The concept of dose escalation with IORT has been discussed in recent studies in combination with chemoradiation as a rule (Okamoto et al. 2003). Convincing data were not shown in comparison with chemoradiation alone. Accordingly, Okamoto et al. (2003) have reported a median overall survival of 8.6 months.

Thus, it can be formulated that the "effectuating" of the therapy for locally advanced pancreatic patients can be strived for with radiation dose escalation only in cases where the "optimization" of the concurrent or sequential chemotherapy regimen can affect the systemic progression procedure of the carcinoma significantly. This is supported by the fact that local progression results after chemoradiation can be seen substantially later in the median survival than in the overall survival of the patients. That means that patients have no local relapses or local progression after chemoradiation with a local dose of 50.0 Gy, which is considered moderate regarding possible late consequences.

10.8 Primary Concurrent Chemoradiation with Gemcitabine

Since the effectiveness of gemcitabine compared to 5-FU or 5-FU-associated polychemotherapies has been proved in the treatment of pancreatic patients with metastasis (Burris et al. 1997), this agent has been examined also as a combination agent for concurrent chemoradiation in the treatment of locally advanced pancreatic cancer.

The selected therapy applications of concurrent chemotherapy with gemcitabine were and are:

- Normal gemcitabine chemotherapy dose (or combination therapy (Muler et al. 2004)) with total radiation dose- and/or volume reduction with accelerated radiation (McGinn et al. 2001; Muler et al. 2004)
- Reduced gemcitabine chemotherapy with total dose reduction with accelerated radiation (Crane et al. 2001)
- Reduced gemcitabine chemotherapy dose with hypofractionated radiation (de Lange et al. 2002)
- Escalation of gemcitabine chemotherapy dose with weekly applications up to a toxic dose with normal dose radiation (Morganti et al. 2003; Poggi et al. 2002; Safran et al. 2002)
- De-escalation of gemcitabine chemotherapy dose with weekly applications to a tolerable dose with normal dose radiation (Brunner et al. 2003)
- Reduced gemcitabine chemotherapy dose with weekly applications and a normal dose radiation (Ikeda et al. 2002; Okusaka et al. 2004)
- Reduced gemcitabine chemotherapy dose with 24-h infusion and weekly applications and normal dose radiation ((Kudrimoti et al. 1999; Mohiuddin et al. 2002) respectively)
- Reduced gemcitabine chemotherapy dose with weekly applications and "split course" radiation (Van Laethem et al. 2003)
- Reduced gemcitabine chemotherapy doses twice a week and normal dose radiation (Pipas et al. 2001; Blackstock et al. 1999, 2003)
- Reduced gemcitabine chemotherapy doses three times a week and normal dose radiation (Epelbaum et al. 2002)
- Combined chemotherapy, gemcitabine with 5-FU and normal dose radiation (Talamonti et al. 2000; Wilkowski et al. 2000)
- Combined chemotherapy, gemcitabine with cisplatin (dose reduced or normal dose) and normal dose or accelerated radiation (Martenson et al. 2003; Wilkowski et al. 2002)

Tolerable concurrent gemcitabine doses with weekly application are defined as 250 mg/m^2–300 mg/m^2 with conventional dose radiation (up to 50.4 Gy and 28 fractions) and with the involvement of regional lymph nodes in the radiation volume (TV II) (Wolff et al. 2001; Ikeda et al. 2002; Morganti et al. 2003). Gemcitabine doses could be increased to 440 mg/m^2 per day with weekly applications when there is a reduction of radiation volume (only with the involvement of macroscopic tumor = TV I) (Poggi et al. 2002).

A gemcitabine dose of 300 mg/m^2 has been applied with hypofractionated radiation (3 × 8.0 Gy) (de Lange et al. 2002).

A maximum gemcitabine dose of 300 mg/m^2 or 75 mg/m^2 per day, and weekly application for each, has been determined for the purposes of a concurrent combined chemotherapy with cisplatin or paclitaxel, respectively (Brunner et al. 2003; Safran et al. 2002).

It has also been proved to be possible to apply a dose of 40–90 mg/m^2 per day gemcitabine every 2 weeks concurrent with normal dose radiation (Blackstock et al. 1999, 2003; Yavuz et al. 2001).

Kornek et al. have examined the concurrent 24-h infusion of gemcitabine and determined an applicable dose of 130 mg/m^2 per day and weekly application.

It can be seen on the basis of the data above that neither the gemcitabine dose, the application rhythm, nor the applicable radiation dose or radiation volume could have been recommended as standard up to now.

The problem is that the different combinations of gemcitabine with radiation have led to different toxicity profiles which partly correspond to grade 3 or 4 toxicity.

Generally, a normal dose or weekly reduced gemcitabine dose, even with a reduced radiation dose or reduced volume, has led to increased gastrointestinal complications (McGinn et al. 2001; Muler et al. 2004). Hematotoxicity (leukocytopenia and/or thrombocytopenia grade 3–4 up to 66%) has been seen with high probability with the dose reduction of gemcitabine and normal dose radiation (Wolff et al. 2001; Blackstock et al. 2003; Okusaka et al. 2004). Dose-reduced combined chemotherapies with normal dose radiation have led to significant hematotoxicity too (Wilkowski et al. 2002; Brunner et al. 2003).

One possible solution for the problem has been seen in the application of gemcitabine as sequential chemotherapy alone (Li et al. 2003; Kachnic et al. 2001; Ben-Josef et al. 2004) and the concurrent application of a chemotherapy with 5-FU or capecitabine (Ben-Josef et al. 2004).

It has been shown that for the majority of patients treated concurrently with gemcitabine, a local remission could have been achieved with the possibility of secondary R0 resection in comparison with patients treated with concurrent 5-FU (Crane et al. 2002), independently from toxicity, which was assessed as moderate (Brunner et al. 2003) to intolerable (Talamonti et al. 2000). Response rates have been reported in 29%–50% of the patients (de Lange et al. 2002; Ikeda et al. 2002; Li et al. 2003), and absence of tumor after neoadjuvant treatment and secondary resection (ypT0 stages) has been observed (Brunner et al. 2003; Epelbaum et al. 2002). Thus, pathologically complete remissions are possible after gemcitabine-associated CRT.

Median TTP has been reported between 4.4 (Okusaka et al. 2004) and 7.1 months (de Lange et al. 2002; Li et al. 2003). Local therapy failure (local progression or local relapse after remission) has been observed in up to 65% (de Lange et al. 2002) and distant metastasis in 75% of the patients (de Lange et al. 2002). Median overall survival was between 8.3 (Kornek et al. 2001) and 14.5 months (Li et al. 2003).

Concurrent chemoradiation with 5-FU has been compared with gemcitabine monotheapy only in one prospective randomized study; sequential chemotherapy has been administered in both arms with gemcitabine monotherapy until progress (Li et al. 2003). Significantly better remission rates (13% vs 50%) and significantly improved median progression-free (2.7 vs 7.1 months) and median overall survival (6.7 vs 14.1 months) have been observed only in the case of a few patients (16 vs 18 patients) during gemcitabine-CRT.

10.9 Primary (Chemo-)Radiotherapy: Does It Make Sense and Is It Efficient?

Different studies (Crane et al. 2002; Li et al. 2003) point out that sequential concurrent chemoradiation, especially with gemcitabine, positively affect the progression-free and overall survival in primary unresectable pancreatic patients in comparison with concurrent chemoradiation and radiotherapy alone. Prospective randomized studies are warranted to prove the significant differences as to different combinations of concurrent and sequential chemotherapy with 5-FU +/−gemcitabine or gemcitabine+/−cisplatin.

IORT alone or in combination should not be induced because there have been negative results with possible deterioration of the prognosis.

The most important positive prognostic factor is remission after chemoradiation. Especially patients undergoing secondary R0 resection after image-proved remission show a significant improvement in progression-free and overall survival and reach can 5-year survival (24.9% of the patient cohort; R. Wilkowski, unpublished).

The therapy aim for locally advanced primary unresectable nonmetastatic pancreatic cancer is the local treatment of the disease, considering its systemic aggressiveness. A proper combination agent should be found for concurrent chemoradiation that has a high systemic effect and/or is capable of achieving this effectiveness in sequential application.

References

Abe M, Shibamoto Y, Ono K, Takahashi M (1991) Intraoperative radiation therapy for carcinoma of the stomach and pancreas. Front Radiat Ther Oncol 25:258–269

Abe M, Shibamoto Y, Nishimura Y (1993) Intraoperative radiotherapy for pancreatic cancer in Japan: multi-institutional and Kyoto University experiences. In: Schildberg FW, Willich N, Krämling HJ (eds) Intraoperative radiation therapy. Verlag Die blaue Eule, Essen, pp 278–281

Al-Sukhun S, Zalupski MM, Ben-Josef E, Vaitkevicius VK, Philip PA, Soulen R, Weaver D, Adsay V, Heilbrun LK, Levin K, Forman JD, Shields AF (2003) Chemoradiotherapy in the treatment of regional pancreatic carcinoma: a phase II study. Am J Clin Oncol 26:543–549

Ammori JB, Colletti LM, Zalupski MM, Eckhauser FE, Greenson JK, Dimick J, Lawrence TS, McGinn CJ (2003) Surgical resection following radiation therapy with concurrent gemcitabine in patients with previously unresectable adenocarcinoma of the pancreas. J Gastrointest Surg 7:766–772

Aristu J, Canon R, Pardo F, Martinez-Monge R, Martin-Algarra S, Manuel Ordonez J, Villafranca E, Moreno M, Cambeiro M, Azinovic I (2003) Surgical resection after preoperative chemoradiotherapy benefits selected patients with unresectable pancreatic cancer. Am J Clin Oncol 26:30–36

Ashamalla H, Zaki B, Mokhtar B, et al. (2003) Hyperfractionated radiotherapy and paclitaxel for locally advanced/unresectable pancreatic cancer. Int J Radiat Oncol Biol Phys 55:679–687

Azria D, Ychou M, Jacot W, Thezenas S, Lemanski C, Senesse P, Prost P, Delard R, Masson B, Dubois JB (2002) Treatment of unresectable, locally advanced pancreatic adenocarcinoma with combined radiochemotherapy with 5-fluorouracil and cisplatin. Pancreas 25:360–365

Ben-Josef E, Shields AF, Vaishampayan U, Vaitkevicius V, El-Rayes BF, McDermott P, Burmeister J, Bossenberger T, Philip PA (2004) Intensity-modulated radiotherapy (IMRT) and concurrent capecitabine for pancreatic cancer. Int J Radiat Oncol Biol Phys 159:454–459

Berlin JD, Catalano P, Thomas JP, Kugler JW, Haller DG, Benson AB 3rd (2002) Phase III study of gemcitabine in combination with fluorouracil versus gemcitabine alone in patients with advanced pancreatic carcinoma: Eastern Cooperative Oncology Group Trial E2297. J Clin Oncol 120:3270–3275

Birkmeyer JD, Siewers AE, Finlayson EV, Stukel TA, Lucas FL, Batista I, Welch HG, Wennberg DE (2002) Hospital volume and surgical mortality in the United States. N Engl J Med 11346:1128–1137

Blackstock AW, Bernard SA, Richards F, Eagle KS, Case LD, Poole ME, Savage PD, Tepper JE (1999) Phase I trial of twice-weekly gemcitabine and concurrent radiation in patients with advanced pancreatic cancer. J Clin Oncol 17:2208–2212

Blackstock AW, Tepper JE, Niedwiecki D, Hollis DR, Mayer RJ, Tempero MA (2003) Cancer and Leukemia Group B (CALGB) 89805: phase II chemoradiation trial using gemcitabine in patients with locoregional adenocarcinoma of the pancreas. Int J Gastrointest Cancer 34:107–116

Bramhall S, Dunn J, Neoptolemos JP (1998) Epidemiology of pancreatic cancer. In:Berger HG, Warshaw A, Carr-Locke DL (eds) The pancreas (two volumes). Blackwell Scientific, Boston, pp 889–906

Bramhall SR, Allum WH, Jones AG, Allwood A, Cummins C, Neoptolemos JP (1995) Treatment and survival in 13,560 patients with pancreatic cancer, and incidence of the disease, in the West Midlands: an epidemiological study. Br J Surg 82:111–115

Bruckner HW, Kalnicki S, Dalton J, et al. (1993) Survival after combined modality therapy for pancreatic cancer. J Clin Gastroenterol 16:199–203

Bruckner HW, Snady HW, Dalton H (1998) Split course radiotherapy and simultaneous chemotherapy effectively downstage and facilitate resection of unresectable pancreatic cancer. Eigth International Congress on Anti-Cancer Treatment SOMPS-O 97

Brunner TB, Grabenbauer GG, Klein P, Baum U, Papadopoulos T, Bautz W, Hohenberger W, Sauer R (2003) Phase I trial of strictly time-scheduled gemcitabine and cisplatin with concurrent radiotherapy in patients with locally advanced pancreatic cancer. Int J Radiat Oncol Biol Phys 155:144–153

Burris HA 3rd, Moore MJ, Andersen J, Green MR, Rothenberg ML, Modiano MR, Cripps MC, Portenoy RK, Storniolo AM, Tarassoff P, Nelson R, Dorr FA, Stephens CD, Von Hoff DD (1997) Improvements in survival and clinical benefit with gemcitabine as first-line therapy for patients with advanced pancreas cancer: a randomized trial. J Clin Oncol 15:2403–2413

Calvo FA, Santos M, Abuchaibe O, Azinovic I, Ortiz de Urbina D, Pardo F, Hernandez JL, Voltas J, Cienfuegos JA (1991) Intraoperative radiotherapy in gastric and pancreatic carcinoma: a European experience. Front Radiat Ther Oncol 25:270–283

Carmichael J, Fink U, Russell RC, et al. (1996) Phase II study of gemcitabine in patients with advanced pancreatic cancer. Br J Cancer 73:101–105

Casper ES, Green MR, Kelsen DP, et al. (1994) Phase II trial of gemcitabine (2,2'-difluorodeoxycytidine) in patients with adenocarcinoma of the pancreas. Invest New Drugs 12:29–34

Chauffert B, Morneux F, Bonnetain F, et al. (2006) Phase III trial comparing initial chemoradiotherapy (intermittent cisplatin and infusional 5-FU) followed by gemcitabine vs gemcitabine alone in patients with locally advanced non metastatic pancreatic cancer: a FFCD-SFRO study. J Clin Oncol 24:4008

Cohen SJ, Dobelbower R, Lipsitz S, et al. (2005) A randomized phase III study of radiotherapy alone or with 5-fluorouracil and mitomycin-C in patients with locally advanced adenocarcinoma of the pancreas: Eastern Cooperative Oncology Group study E8282. Int J Radiat Oncol Biol Phys 62:1345–1350

Crane CH, Janjan NA, Evans DB, Wolff RA, Ballo MT, Milas L, Mason K, Charnsangavej C, Pisters PW, Lee JE, Lenzi R, Vauthey JN, Wong A, Phan T, Nguyen Q, Abbruzzese JL (2001) Toxicity and efficacy of concurrent gemcitabine and radiotherapy for locally advanced pancreatic cancer. Int J Pancreatol 29:9–18

Crane CH, Wolff RA, Abbruzzese JL, Evans DB, Milas L, Mason K, Charnsangavej C, Pisters PW, Lee JE, Lenzi R, Lahoti S, Vauthey JN, Janjan NA (2001) Combining gemcitabine with radiation in pancreatic cancer: understanding important variables influencing the therapeutic index. Semin Oncol 28:25–33

Crane CH, Abbruzzese JL, Evans DB, Wolff RA, Ballo MT, Delclos M, Milas L, Mason K, Charnsangavej C, Pisters PW, Lee JE, Lenzi R, Vauthey JN, Wong AB, Phan T, Nguyen Q, Janjan NA (2002) Is the therapeutic index better with gemcitabine-based chemoradiation than with 5-fluorouracil-based chemoradiation in locally advanced pancreatic cancer? Int J Radiat Oncol Biol Phys 152:1293–1302

Cullinan S, Moertel CG, Wieand HS, Schutt AJ, Krook JE, Foley JF, Norris BD, Kardinal CG, Tschetter LK, Barlow JF (1990) A phase III trial on the therapy of advanced pancreatic carcinoma. Evaluations of the Mallinson regimen and combined 5-fluorouracil, doxorubicin, and cisplatin. Cancer 1565:2207–2212

de Lange SM, van Groeningen CJ, Meijer OW, Cuesta MA, Langendijk JA, van Riel JM, Pinedo HM, Peters GJ, Meijer S, Slotman BJ, Giaccone G (2002) Gemcitabine-radiotherapy in patients with locally advanced pancreatic cancer. Eur J Cancer 38:1212–1217

Epelbaum R, Rosenblatt E, Nasrallah S, Faraggi D, Gaitini D, Mizrahi S, Kuten A (2002) Phase II study of gemcitabine combined with radiation therapy in patients with localized, unresectable pancreatic cancer. J Surg Oncol 81:138–143

Evans DB, Rich TA, Byrd DR, Cleary KR, Connelly JH, Levin B, Charnsangavej C, Fenoglio CJ, Ames FC (1992) Preoperative chemoradiation and pancreaticoduodenectomy for adenocarcinoma of the pancreas. Arch Surg 127:1335–1339

Fisher BJ, Perera FE, Kocha W, Tomiak A, Taylor M, Vincent M, Bauman GS (1999) Analysis of the clinical benefit of 5-fluorouracil and radiation treatment in locally advanced pancreatic cancer. Int J Radiat Oncol Biol Phys 145:291–295

Fossati V, Cattaneo GM, Zerbi A, Galli L, Bordogna G, Reni M, Parolini D, Carlucci M, Bissi A, Staudacher C, et al. (1995) The role of intraoperative therapy by electron beam and combination of adjuvant chemotherapy and external radiotherapy in carcinoma of the pancreas. Tumori 81:23–31

German Cancer Association (2002) Guidelines of the German Cancer Association

Gilly FN, Romestaing PJ, Gerard JP, Braillon GG, Sayag AC, Sentenac IJ, Roche MM, Carry PY (1990) Experience of three years with intra-operative radiation therapy using the Lyon intra-operative device. Int Surg 75:84–88

Glimelius B, Hoffman K, Sjoden PO, Jacobsson G, Sellstrom H, Enander LK, Linne T, Svensson C (1996) Chemotherapy improves survival and quality of life in advanced pancreatic and biliary cancer. Ann Oncol 7:593–600

GITSG (1985) Gastrointestinal Tumor Study Group. Radiation therapy combined with adriamycin or 5-fluorouracil for the treatment of locally unresectable pancreatic carcinoma. Cancer 56:2563–2568

GITSG (1988) Gastrointestinal Tumor Study Group. Treatment of locally unresectable carcinoma of the pancreas: comparison of combined-modality therapy (chemotherapy plus radiotherapy) to chemotherapy alone. J Natl Cancer Inst 80:751–755

Goldson AL (1991) Intraoperative radiotherapy for pancreatic cancer—requiem or revival? Int J Radiat Oncol Biol Phys 21:1389

Haycox A, Lombard M, Neoptolemos J, Walley T (1998) Review article: current treatment and optimal patient management in pancreatic cancer. Aliment Pharmacol Ther 12:949–964

Heinemann V, Schermuly MM, Stieber P, Schulz L, Jungst D, Wilkowski R, Schalhorn A (1999a) CA19-9: a predictor of response in pancreatic cancer treated with gemcitabine and cisplatin. Anticancer Res 19:2433–2435

Heinemann V, Wilke H, Possinger K (1999b) Gemcitabine and cisplatin in the treatment of advanced and metastatic pancreatic cancer. Final results of a phase II study. Proc Am Soc Clin Oncol 18:1052

Heinemann V, Wilke H, Mergenthaler HG, Clemens M, Konig H, Illiger HJ, Arning M, Schalhorn A, Possinger K, Fink U (2000) Gemcitabine and cisplatin in the treatment of advanced or metastatic pancreatic cancer. Ann Oncol 11:1399–1403

Hoffman JP, Lipsitz S, Pisansky T, Weese JL, Solin L, Benson AB 3rd (1998) Phase II trial of preoperative radiation therapy and chemotherapy for patients with localized, resectable adenocarcinoma of the pancreas: an Eastern Cooperative Oncology Group Study. J Clin Oncol 16:317–323

Ikeda M, Okada S, Tokuuye K, Ueno H, Okusaka T (2002) A phase I trial of weekly gemcitabine and concurrent radiotherapy in patients with locally advanced pancreatic cancer. Br J Cancer 2086:1551–1554

Ishikawa O (1996) Surgical technique, curability and postoperative quality of life in an extended pancreatectomy for adenocarcinoma of the pancreas. Hepatogastroenterology 43:320–325

Ishikawa O, Ohigashi H, Sasaki Y, Furukawa H, Kabuto T, Kameyama M, Nakamori S, Hiratsuka M, Imaoka S (1994) Liver perfusion chemotherapy via both the hepatic artery and portal vein to prevent hepatic metastasis after extended pancreatectomy for adenocarcinoma of the pancreas. Am J Surg 168:361–364

Ishikawa O, Ohigashi H, Sasaki Y, Masao K, Kabuto T, Furukawa H, Imaoka S (1998) Adjuvant therapies in extended pancreatectomy for ductal adenocarcinoma of the pancreas. Hepatogastroenterology 45:644–650

Jeekel J, Treurniet-Donker AD (1991) Treatment perspectives in locally advanced unresectable pancreatic cancer. Br J Surg 78:1332–1334

Jessup JM, Steele G Jr, Mayer RJ, Posner M, Busse P, Cady B, Stone M, Jenkins R, Osteen R (1993) Neoadjuvant therapy for unresectable pancreatic adenocarcinoma. Arch Surg 128:559–564

Joensuu TK, Kiviluoto T, Karkkainen P, Vento P, Kivisaari L, Tenhunen M, Westberg R, Elomaa I (2004) Phase I-II trial of twice-weekly gemcitabine and concomitant irradiation in patients undergoing pancreaticoduodenectomy with extended lymphadenectomy for locally advanced pancreatic cancer. Int J Radiat Oncol Biol Phys 160:444–452

Kachnic LA, Shaw JE, Manning MA, Lauve AD, Neifeld JP (2001) Gemcitabine following radiotherapy with concurrent 5-fluorouracil for nonmetastatic adenocarcinoma of the pancreas. Int J Cancer 2096:132–139

Kamthan AG, Morris JC, Dalton J, et al. (1997) Combined modality therapy for stage II and stage III pancreatic carcinoma. J Clin Oncol 15:2920–2927

Kasperk R, Klever P, Andreopoulos D, Schumpelick V (1995) Intraoperative radiotherapy for pancreatic carcinoma. Br J Surg 82:1259–1261

Kawamura M, Kataoka M, Fujii T, Itoh H, Ishine M, Hamamoto K, Yokoyama S, Takashima S, Satoh M, Inoue K (1992) Electron beam intraoperative radiation therapy (EBIORT) for localized pancreatic carcinoma. Int J Radiat Oncol Biol Phys 23:751–757

Kim HJ, Czischke K, Brennan MF, Conlon KC (2002) Does neoadjuvant chemoradiation downstage locally advanced pancreatic cancer? J Gastrointest Surg 6:763–769

Klaasen DJ, MacIntyre JM, Catton GE (1985) Treatment of locally unresectable cancer of the stomach and pancreas: a randomized comparison of 5-fluorouracil alone with radiation plus concurrent and maintenance 5-fluorouracil—an Eastern Cooperative Oncology Group study. J Clin Oncol 3:373–378

Kojima Y, Kimura T, Yasukawa H, Katayama K, Note M, Isobe Y, Fujita H, Nakagawara G, Nakatsugawa S, Shiraishi T (1991) Radiotherapy-centered multimodal treatment of unresectable pancreatic carcinoma. Int Surg 76:87–90

Komaki R, Wadler S, Peters T, Byhardt RW, Order S, Gallagher MJ, Herskovic A, Pederson J (1992) High-dose local irradiation plus prophylactic hepatic irradiation and chemotherapy for inoperable adenocarcinoma of the pancreas. A preliminary report of a multi-institutional trial (Radiation Therapy Oncology Group Protocol 8801). Cancer 169:2807–2812

Kornek GV, Schratter-Sehn A, Marczell A, Depisch D, Karner J, Krauss G, Haider K, Kwasny W, Locker G, Scheithauer W (2000) Treatment of unresectable, locally advanced pancreatic adenocarcinoma with combined radiochemotherapy with 5-fluorouracil, leucovorin and cisplatin. Br J Cancer 82:98–103

Kornek GV, Potter R, Selzer E, Schratter A, Ulrich-Pur H, Rogy M, Kraus G, Scheithauer W (2001) Combined radiochemotherapy of locally advanced unresectable pancreatic adenocarcinoma with mitomycin C plus 24-hour continuous infusional gemcitabine. Int J Radiat Oncol Biol Phys 149:665–671

Kudrimoti M, Regine W, John W, Hanna N (1999) Concurrent infusional gemcitabine and radiation in the treatment of advanced unresectable GI malignancy: a phase I/II study. Proc Am Soc Clin Oncol 18:A928

Lawrence TS, Chang EY, Hahn TM, et al. (1996) Radiosensitization of pancreatic cancer cells by 2',2'-difluoro-2'-deoxycytidine. Int J Radiat Oncol Biol Phys 134:867–872

Li CP, Chao Y, Chi KH, Chan WK, Teng HC, Lee RC, Chang FY, Lee SD, Yen SH (2003) Concurrent chemoradiotherapy treatment of locally advanced pancreatic cancer: gemcitabine versus 5-fluorouracil, a randomized controlled study. Int J Radiat Oncol Biol Phys 157:98–104

Luderhoff EC, Gonzalez Gonzalez D, Bakker P (1996) Pilot study in locally advanced unresectable pancreas carcinoma using a combination of accelerated radiotherapy and continuous infusion of 5-fluorouracil. Radiother Oncol 40:241–243

Magee CJ, Greenhalf W, Howes N, Ghaneh P, Neoptolemos JP (2001) Molecular pathogenesis of pancreatic ductal adenocarcinoma and clinical implications. Surg Oncol 10:1–23 Review

Mallinson CN, Rake MO, Cocking JB, Fox CA, Cwynarski MT, Diffey BL, Jackson GA, Hanley J, Wass VJ (1980) Chemotherapy in pancreatic cancer: results of a controlled, prospective, randomised, multicentre trial. Br Med J 13281:1589–1591

Manabe T, Baba N, Nonaka A, Asano N, Yamaki K, Shibamoto Y, Takahashi M, Abe M, Tobe T (1988) Combined treatment using radiotherapy for carcinoma of the pancreas involving the adjacent vessels. Int Surg 73:153–156

Martenson JA, Vigliotti AP, Pitot HC, Geeraerts LH, Sargent DJ, Haddock MG, Ghosh C, Keppen MD, Fitch TR, Goldberg RM (2003) A phase I study of radiation therapy and twice-weekly gemcitabine and cisplatin in patients with locally advanced pancreatic cancer. Int J Radiat Oncol Biol Phys 155:1305–1310

McGinn CJ, Shewach DS, Lawrence TS (1996) Radiosensitizing nucleosides. J Natl Cancer Inst 88:1193–1203

McGinn CJ, Zalupski MM, Shureiqi I, Robertson JM, Eckhauser FE, Smith DC, Brown D, Hejna G, Strawderman M, Normolle D, Lawrence TS (2001) Phase I trial of radiation dose escalation with concurrent weekly full-dose gemcitabine in patients with advanced pancreatic cancer. J Clin Oncol 1519:4202–4208

Mehta VK, Fisher G, Ford JA, Poen JC, Vierra MA, Oberhelman H, Niederhuber J, Bastidas JA (2001) Preoperative chemoradiation for marginally resectable adenocarcinoma of the pancreas. J Gastrointest Surg 5:27–35

Moertel CG, Childs DS Jr, Reitemeier RJ, Colby MY Jr, Holbrook MA (1969) Combined 5-fluorouracil and supervoltage radiation therapy of locally unresectable gastrointestinal cancer. Lancet 252:865–867

Moertel CG, Frytak S, Hahn RG, O'Connell MJ, Reitemeier RJ, Rubin J, Schutt AJ, Weiland LH, Childs DS, Holbrook MA, Lavin PT, Livstone E, Spiro H, Knowlton A, Kalser M, Barkin J, Lessner H, Mann-Kaplan R, Ramming K, Douglas HO Jr, Thomas P, Nave H, Bateman J, Lokich J, Brooks J, Chaffey J, Corson JM, Zamcheck N, Novak JW (1981) Therapy of locally unresectable pancreatic carcinoma: a randomized comparison of high dose (6000 rads) radiation alone, moderate dose radiation (4000 rads + 5-fluorouracil), and high dose radiation + 5-fluorouracil: The Gastrointestinal Tumor Study Group. Cancer 48:1705–1710

Mohiuddin M, Cantor RJ, Biermann W, Weiss SM, Barbot D, Rosato FE (1988) Combined modality treatment of localized unresectable adenocarcinoma of the pancreas. Int J Radiat Oncol Biol Phys 14:79–84

Moore M, Andersen J, Burris H, et al. (1995) A randomized trial of gemcitabine versus 5FU as first-line therapy in advanced pancreatic cancer. Proc Am Soc Oncol 14 [Suppl]:199a

Morganti AG, Trodella L, Valentini V, Macchia G, Alfieri S, Smaniotto D, Luzi S, Costamagna G, Doglietto GB, Cellini N (2003) Concomitant gemcitabine (Gemzar) and extended nodes irradiation in the treatment of pancreatic and biliary carcinoma: a phase I study. Onkologie 26:325–329

Mose S, Karapetian M, Jüling-Pohlit L, et al. (1999) Verstärkung der radiotherapeutischen Wirkung auf HeLa-Zellen durch Gemcitabine. Strahlenther Onkol 175:78–83

Muler JH, McGinn CJ, Normolle D, Lawrence T, Brown D, Hejna G, Zalupski MM (2004) Phase I trial using a time-to-event continual reassessment strategy for dose escalation of cisplatin combined with gemcitabine and radiation therapy in pancreatic cancer. J Clin Oncol 22:238–243

Neoptolemos JP, Russell RC, Bramhall S, Theis B (1997) Low mortality following resection for pancreatic and periampullary tumours in 1026 patients: UK survey of specialist pancreatic units. UK Pancreatic Cancer Group. Br J Surg 84:1370–1376

Neoptolemos JP, Stocken DD, Friess H, Bassi C, Dunn JA, Hickey H, Beger H, Fernandez-Cruz L, Dervenis C, Lacaine F, Falconi M, Pederzoli P, Pap A, Spooner D, Kerr DJ, et al. (2004) A randomized trial of chemoradiotherapy and chemotherapy after resection of pancreatic cancer. N Engl J Med 18350:1200–1210

Niederhuber JE, Brennan MF, Menck HR (1995) The National Cancer Data Base report on pancreatic cancer. Cancer 176:1671–1677

Nishimura A, Sakata S, Iida K, Iwasaki Y, Takeshima T, Todoroki T, Ohara K, Hata K, Miyoshi M, Seo Y, et al. (1988) Evaluation of intraoperative radiotherapy for carcinoma of the pancreas: prognostic factors and survival analyses. Radiat Med 6:85–91

Nishimura Y, Hosotani R, Shibamoto Y, Kokubo M, Kanamori S, Sasai K, Hiraoka M, Ohshio G, Imamura M, Takahashi M, Abe M (1997) External and intraoperative radiotherapy for resectable and unresectable pancreatic cancer: analysis of survival rates and complications. Int J Radiat Oncol Biol Phys 139:39–49

Okamoto A, Tsuruta K, Isawa T, Kamisawa T, Tanaka Y, Onodera T (1994) Intraoperative radiation therapy for pancreatic carcinoma. The choice of treatment modality. Int J Pancreatol 16:157–164

Okamoto A, Tsuruta K, Karasawa K, Miyanari N, Matsumoto G, Kamisawa T, Egawa N (2003) Resection versus palliation: treatment of stage III and IVA carcinomas of the pancreas employing intraoperative radiation. World J Surg 27:599–605

Okamoto A, Matsumoto G, Tsuruta K, Baba H, Karasawa K, Kamisawa T, Egawa N (2004) Intraoperative radiation therapy for pancreatic adenocarcinoma: the Komagome hospital experience. Pancreas 28:296–300

Okusaka T, Okada S, Tokuuye K, Wakasugi H, Saisho H, Ishikawa O, Matsuno S, Sato T, et al. (2001) Lack of effectiveness of radiotherapy combined with cisplatin in patients with locally advanced pancreatic carcinoma. Cancer 191:1384–1389

Okusaka T, Ito Y, Ueno H, Ikeda M, Takezako Y, Morizane C, Kagami Y, Ikeda H (2004) Phase II study of radiotherapy combined with gemcitabine for locally advanced pancreatic cancer. Br J Cancer 1691:673–677

Palmer KR, Kerr M, Knowles G, Cull A, Carter DC, Leonard RC (1994) Chemotherapy prolongs survival in inoperable pancreatic carcinoma. Br J Surg 81:882–885

Pedrazzoli S, DiCarlo V, Dionigi R, Mosca F, Pederzoli P, Pasquali C, Kloppel G, Dhaene K, Michelassi F (1998) Standard versus extended lymphadenectomy associated with pancreatoduodenectomy in the surgical treatment of adenocarcinoma of the head of the pancreas: a multicenter, prospective, randomized study. Lymphadenectomy Study Group. Ann Surg 228:508–517

Pipas JM, Mitchell SE, Barth RJ Jr, Vera-Gimon R, Rathmann J, Meyer LP, Wagman RS, Lewis LD, McDonnell C, Colacchio TA, Perez RP (2001) Phase I study of twice-weekly gemcitabine and concomitant external-beam radiotherapy in patients with adenocarcinoma of the pancreas. Int J Radiat Oncol Biol Phys 150:1317–1322

Poggi MM, Kroog GS, Russo A, Muir C, Cook J, Smith J, Mitchell JB, Herscher LL (2002) Phase I study of weekly gemcitabine as a radiation sensitizer for unresectable pancreatic cancer. Int J Radiat Oncol Biol Phys 154:670–676

Rich TA, Evans DB (1995) Preoperative combined modality therapy for pancreatic cancer. World J Surg 19:264–269

Rich TA, Lokich JJ, Chaffey JT (1985) A pilot study of protracted venous infusion of 5-fluorouracil and concomitant radiation therapy. J Clin Oncol 3:402–406

Rothenberg ML, Moore MJ, Cripps MC, Andersen JS, Portenoy RK, Burris HA 3rd, Green MR, Tarassoff PG, Brown TD, Casper ES, Storniolo AM, Von Hoff DD (1996) A phase II trial of gemcitabine in patients with 5-FU-refractory pancreas cancer. Ann Oncol 7:347–353

Saad ED, Machado MC, Wajsbrot D, Abramoff R, Hoff PM, Tabacof J, Katz A, Simon SD, Gansl RC (2002) Pretreatment CA 19-9 level as a prognostic factor in patients with advanced pancreatic cancer treated with gemcitabine. Int J Gastrointest Cancer 32:35–41

Safran H, Dipetrillo T, Iannitti D, Quirk D, Akerman P, Cruff D, Cioffi W, Shah S, Ramdin N, Rich T (2002) Gemcitabine, paclitaxel, and radiation for locally advanced pancreatic cancer: a Phase I trial. Int J Radiat Oncol Biol Phys 154:137–141

Scherer E (1987) Pankreaskarzinome. In: Scherer E (ed) Strahlentherapie, 3 Aufl. Springer, Berlin Heidelberg New York, pp S657–S663

Shewach DS, Hahn TM, Chang E, et al. (1994) Metabolism of 2',2'-difluoro-2'-deoxycytidine and radiation sensitization of human colon carcinoma cells. Cancer Res 1554:3218–3223

Shinchi H, Takao S, Noma H, Matsuo Y, Mataki Y, Mori S, Aikou T (2002) Length and quality of survival after external-beam radiotherapy with concurrent continuous 5-fluorouracil infusion for locally unresectable pancreatic cancer. Int J Radiat Oncol Biol Phys 153:146–150

Shipley WU, Wood WC, Tepper JE, Warshaw AL, Orlow EL, Kaufman SD, Battit GE, Nardi GL (1984) Intraoperative electron beam irradiation for patients with unresectable pancreatic carcinoma. Semin Thorac Cardiovasc Surg Pediatr Card Surg Annu 200:289–296

Spitz FR, Abbruzzese JL, Lee JE, Pisters PW, Lowy AM, Fenoglio CJ, Cleary KR, Janjan NA, Goswitz MS, Rich TA, Evans DB (1997) Preoperative and postoperative chemoradiation strategies in patients treated with pancreaticoduodenectomy for adenocarcinoma of the pancreas. J Clin Oncol 15:928–937

Staley CA, Lee JE, Cleary KR, Abbruzzese JL, Fenoglio CJ, Rich TA, Evans DB (1996) Preoperative chemoradiation, pancreaticoduodenectomy, and intraoperative radiation therapy for adenocarcinoma of the pancreatic head. Am J Surg 171:118–124

Talamonti MS, Catalano PJ, Vaughn DJ, Whittington R, Beauchamp RD, Berlin J, Benson AB 3rd (2000) Eastern Cooperative Oncology Group phase I trial of protracted venous infusion fluorouracil plus weekly gemcitabine with concurrent radiation therapy in patients with locally advanced pancreas cancer: a regimen with unexpected early toxicity. J Clin Oncol 118:3384–3389

Terk M, Turhal N, Mandeli J (1997) Long term follow-up of combined modality therapy for unresectable pancreatic cancer. Proc Am Soc Clin Oncol 16:307

Todd KE, Gloor B, Lane JS, Isacoff WH, Reber HA (1998) Resection of locally advanced pancreatic cancer after downstaging with continuous-infusion 5-fluorouracil, mitomycin-C, leucovorin, and dipyridamole. J Gastrointest Surg 2:159–166

Tuckson WB, Goldson AL, Ashayeri E, Halyard-Richardson M, DeWitty RL, Leffall LD Jr (1988) Intraoperative radiotherapy for patients with carcinoma of the pancreas. The Howard University Hospital experience, 1978–1986. Ann Surg 207:648–654

Van Laethem JL, Demols A, Gay F, Closon MT, Collette M, Polus M, Houbiers G, Gastelblum P, Gelin M, Houtte PV, Closset J (2003) Postoperative adjuvant gemcitabine and concurrent radiation after curative resection of pancreatic head carcinoma: a phase II study. Int J Radiat Oncol Biol Phys 1556:974–980

Whittington R, Solin L, Mohiuddin M, Cantor RI, Rosato FE, Biermann WA, Weiss SM, Pajak TF (1984) Multimodality therapy of localized unresectable pancreatic adenocarcinoma. Cancer 54:1991–1998

Wiegel T, Runkel N, Frommhold H, Rube C, Hinkelbein W (2000) Radiotherapeutic strategies in the multimodal therapy of resectable and nonresectable pancreatic carcinoma. Strahlenther Onkol 176:299–306

Wilkowski R, Heinemann V, Rau H (2000) Locally advanced pancreatic carcinoma. Radiochemotherapy prolongs survival. MMW Fortschr Med 19142:31–32

Wilkowski R, Heinemann V, Stoffregen C (2002) Gemcitabine (Gemzar) and radiotherapy—is it feasible? Front Radiat Ther Oncol 37:78–83

Wilkowski R, Thoma M, Duhmke E, Rau HG, Heinemann V (2004) Concurrent chemoradiotherapy with gemcitabine and cisplatin after incomplete (R1) resection of locally advanced pancreatic carcinoma. Int J Radiat Oncol Biol Phys 158:768–772

Wilkowski R, Thoma M, Bruns C, Wagner A, Heinemann V (2006) Chemoradiotherapy with gemcitabine and continuous 5-FU in patients with primary inoperable pancreatic cancer. JOP 7:349–360

Wolff RA, Chiao P, Lenzi R, Pisters PW, Lee JE, Janjan NA, Crane CH, Evans DB, Abbruzzese JL (2000) Current approaches and future strategies for pancreatic carcinoma. Invest New Drugs 18:43–56

Wolff RA, Evans DB, Gravel DM, Lenzi R, Pisters PW, Lee JE, Janjan NA, Charnsangavej C, Abbruzzese JL (2001) Phase I trial of gemcitabine combined with radiation for the treatment of locally advanced pancreatic adenocarcinoma. Clin Cancer Res 7:2246–2253

Wood WC, Shipley WU, Gunderson LL, Cohen AM, Nardi GL (1982) Intraoperative irradiation for unresectable pancreatic carcinoma. Cancer 1549:1272–1275

Yavuz AA, Aydin F, Yavuz MN, Ilis E, Ozdemir F (2001) Radiation therapy and concurrent fixed dose amifostine with escalating doses of twice-weekly gemcitabine in advanced pancreatic cancer. Int J Radiat Oncol Biol Phys 1551:974–981

Yeo CJ, Abrams RA, Grochow LB, Sohn TA, Ord SE, Hruban RH, Zahurak ML, Dooley WC, Coleman J, Sauter PK, Pitt HA, Lillemoe KD, Cameron JL (1997) Pancreaticoduodenectomy for pancreatic adenocarcinoma: postoperative adjuvant chemoradiation improves survival. A prospective, single-institution experience. Ann Surg 225:621–633

11

Brachytherapy of Liver Metastases

T. Denecke, E. Lopez Hänninen

Recent Results in Cancer Research, Vol. 177

Abstract

Brachytherapy for the treatment of liver metastases is a novel approach. In this procedure, techniques of locally ablative treatment in interventional radiology and radiation therapy are combined. After computed tomography (CT)-guided percutaneous implantation of catheters into the hepatic tumor, the irradiation is performed in an afterloading technique. This minimally invasive procedure offers circumscriptive high-dose rate irradiation of the lesion to treat in a single session, irrespective of breathing motion or potential cooling effects of neighboring vessels. Good local control rates have been achieved in several tumor entities, including both secondary and primary malignancies of the liver. This article gives an overview of the application technique, possible adverse events, and outcome with special attention to the pancreatic cancer scenario.

11.1 Introduction

Locally ablative therapy is an interesting option for patients with irresectable metastatic disease or primary hepatic malignomas confined to the liver. The aim is the complete ablation of all hepatic lesions or at least the achievement of a local tumor control. Specifically, radio-frequency ablation (RFA) has captured increasing interest, since it is easy to use even as an outpatient procedure in selected patients (Meyers et al. 2003). Laser-induced thermotherapy (LITT) offers the opportunity of real-time therapy monitoring by magnetic-resonance thermometry, which is thought to be advantageous to other locally ablative procedures (e.g., RFA) (Nolsoe et al. 1993; Vogl et al. 1995). However, these procedures have limitations concerning number and localization, as well as size and shape, of tumor lesions.

More recently, there is growing interest in applying radiotherapy to hepatic malignancies. Compared to local thermoablative procedures, radiation efficacy is not affected by cooling effects of neighboring vessels or bile ducts, which are known to be a potential source of local tumor progression after RFA or LITT. Adjacent organs such as the colon or the hilar bile ducts play a minor role for possible complications. The size and shape of the radiation target volume is not restricted to less than 5 cm in diameter and spheroid lesions. However, as the tolerance dose of liver parenchyma is lower than that of most tumor tissues, the therapeutic efficacy of percutaneous irradiation interferes with the mandatory maintenance of a sufficient liver function. The main problems are the breathing excursion of the liver and the flat dose shoulder surrounding the target volume, resulting in a relatively high radiation exposure of the normal hepatic parenchyma. Even though there do exist innovations such as respiratory gated irradiation, stereotactic irradiation, or tomotherapy devices, these problems have not generally been solved to date (Herfarth et al. 2004; Wurm et al. 2006).

The drawbacks of external beam radiotherapy can be overcome when irradiation is brought next to or into the tumor, offering a steep dose decrease to the periphery around the irradiated focus and independency from breathing motion. This approach is referred to as brachytherapy. As a high dose rate, hypofractionated radiation therapy, this technique is used, e.g., for endobronchial or endovaginal irradiation of lung and cervical cancer, or interstitial irradiation of superficial tumors (e.g., breast cancer, head and neck cancer). It is usually realized in an afterloading technique, where a radiation source, e.g., iridium-192, is inserted into prepositioned catheters, a technique that offers the opportunity of high dose rate irradiation (HDR, >12 Gy/h) with minimal exposure of neighboring tissues. The sites accessible for traditional noninvasive brachytherapy are limited, as body cavities such as the trachea or the vagina are needed to insert the afterloading catheter, or invasive implantation of catheters is required.

Concerning brachytherapy of hepatic malignomas, intraoperative radiation therapy has been successfully used in the past. However, as most of the indications are palliative approaches, minimally invasive procedures with a low risk of morbidity and mortality are warranted. This can be achieved by employing radiological interventional procedures, which are mainly based on image guidance. To treat hepatic malignancies, the afterloading technique is combined with the procedure of image-guided interventional, locally ablative treatment. Inserting a radiation source into the tumor in an afterloading technique via transhepatic catheters implanted percutaneously under computed tomography (CT) guidance is largely independent of breathing motion and offers a steep dose reduction toward the periphery around the target volume for optimally focused dosing of the tumor. This technique is invasive and thus requires a short radiation time and is therefore applied as a single session HDR brachytherapy (Ricke et al. 2004a).

In the following sections, aspects of interstitial brachytherapy with CT-guided afterloading will be discussed including patient selection, treatment planning, procedures, technical considerations, adverse effects, and clinical outcome.

11.2 CT-Guided High Dose Rate Brachytherapy via Interstitial Afterloading

11.2.1 Background

High dose rate brachytherapy for the treatment of unresectable liver metastases has been used previously in an intraoperative setting. Efficacy and safety have been proved in several studies. In these trials the minimal target doses covering the entire tumor ranged between 15 and 30 Gy; internal dose inhomogeneities inside the target volume, depending on the radiation technique, were tolerated (Nauta et al. 1987; Dritschilo et al. 1988; Thomas et al. 1993). In a study with 22 patients suffering from irresectable liver metastases, irradiation was realized with laparotomy and interstitial HDR brachytherapy using iridium-192 with doses in the tumor periphery ranging from 20 to 30 Gy (Thomas et al. 1993). There was no acute or chronic radiation toxicity observed at a median follow-up of 11 months. Median actuarial local control at irradiated sites was 8 months, with 26% actuarial local control at 26 months by CT or magnetic resonance imaging (MRI). This phase I/II trial demonstrates the feasibility of single fraction HDR brachytherapy in the treatment of liver metastases.

However, as most of these procedures are palliative, a minimally invasive approach without the risk of laparotomy is favorable. This may be achieved by image-guided procedures, e.g., CT-guided percutaneous puncture of the hepatic tumor and catheter placement for subsequent afterloading as described by Ricke et al. (2004a). This interventional radiological approach has been successfully employed for treatment of several secondary and primary hepatic malignomas, and also in malignomas of the lung and other sites (Ricke et al. 2004a, 2005a).

11.2.2 Patient Selection

In general, locally ablative treatment should be preserved for patients with a limited number of tumor deposits, regionally confined disease, or symptomatic lesions. Local overtreatment as an unnecessary risk should be avoided. Whether a patient might profit from locally ablative treatment depends on the tumor entity, tumor spread, and the overall clinical condition. Fluorodeoxyglucose-positron emission tomography (FDG-PET) has proved to be a valuable adjunctive to the conventional staging modalities in the evaluation of patients prior to locally ablative treatment (Amthauer et al. 2006). The indication has to be made individually after thorough examination and careful assessment of alternative treatment options. Clinical and paraclinical parameters such as comorbidity, liver function, and blood coagulation have to be taken into consideration, as well as the patient's wishes.

Theoretically, minimally invasive interstitial afterloading is applicable to many potential tumor localizations. It has already been successfully applied for treatment of pulmonary and hepatic malignomas, but also in the mediastinum, in the retroperitoneum, and bone. The main limitation is of course the technical feasibility of catheter placement, as a minimal risk of the procedure has to be ensured. Additional limitations are surrounding tissues at risk for adverse effects of irradiation, such as bowel, stomach, spinal canal, skin, neuronal tissue, etc. The number and size of the lesions to treat is also an issue. However, the procedure can be adapted to achieve a sufficient dose coverage in target volumes that are much larger than those suitable for thermal ablation techniques (Ricke et al. 2004b). In large tumor volumes or numerous target lesions, the procedure can be completed with several step-by-step sessions. Additionally, it has been shown that CT-guided interstitial brachytherapy is independent from the cooling effects of large vessels or bile ducts in the ablation zone, which have been identified as potential causes of inadequate heating and local recurrent tumor growth in thermal ablation techniques (Ricke et al. 2004b). Furthermore, as one of the major advantages compared to thermal ablation techniques, the shape of the ablation zone can be adapted to the irregular geometries of target lesions after the catheter implantation by modulating the dwell locations and dwell times of the radiation source inside the afterloading sheaths. Thus, the achievable ablation volume is not only defined by the CT-guided puncture, but also by the planning after a contrast-enhanced CT scan is obtained with optimal demarcation of the tumor lesions and the implanted catheters.

The widest experience has been with hepatic malignomas and the following will mainly focus on interstitial HDR brachytherapy of liver metastases via percutaneous transhepatic afterloading. However, these technical aspects of locally ablative treatment apply not only for hepatic malignomas but also for other organs invaded by tumors, such as the lung, where patients may benefit from interstitial therapy, predominantly in a palliative scenario (Ricke et al. 2005a).

11.2.3 Therapy Procedure

The application of CT-guided interstitial brachytherapy consists of five steps. After appropriate patient selection with staging and assessment of the feasibility based on local findings, the steps are (1) planning the access, (2) CT-guided catheter implantation, (3) radiation planning, (4) actual irradiation via afterloading, and (5) removal of applicators.

For access planning, cross sectional imaging (whether CT or MRI) is needed (Fig. 11.1a). The chosen imaging modality must be capable of outlining the tumor precisely against the surrounding tissue, vessels, and central bile ducts. A gross planning of catheter positions is done using the axial slices, as this is the orientation of the fluoroscopic CT monitoring of the intervention. Besides the puncture direction, dose coverage of the clinical target volume and sparing of surrounding tissues at risk has to be respected during catheter placement. It is recommendable to place the needle that way, that a bridge of liver parenchyma lies between the liver capsule and the tumor border. This buffer provides a hold for the catheter and prevents bleeding of commonly hypervascularized tumors and the potential spilling of tumor cells into the abdominal cavity.

The patient is positioned supine in the CT scanner and monitored for blood oxygenation and heart frequency. The intervention is performed under aseptic conditions and CT guidance after intravenous analgosedation as well as local anesthesia at the cutaneous puncture site. The puncture is monitored by CT fluoroscopy. A guide wire is inserted through the needle, and then a flexible catheter sheath replaces the needle (opaque on X-ray). After removal of the guide wire, an afterloading catheter is placed into the catheter sheath. The system is stitched to the skin for fixation. If more than one afterloading catheter is needed, the procedure is repeated.

Upon completion of catheter placement, a contrast-enhanced scan of the liver is acquired

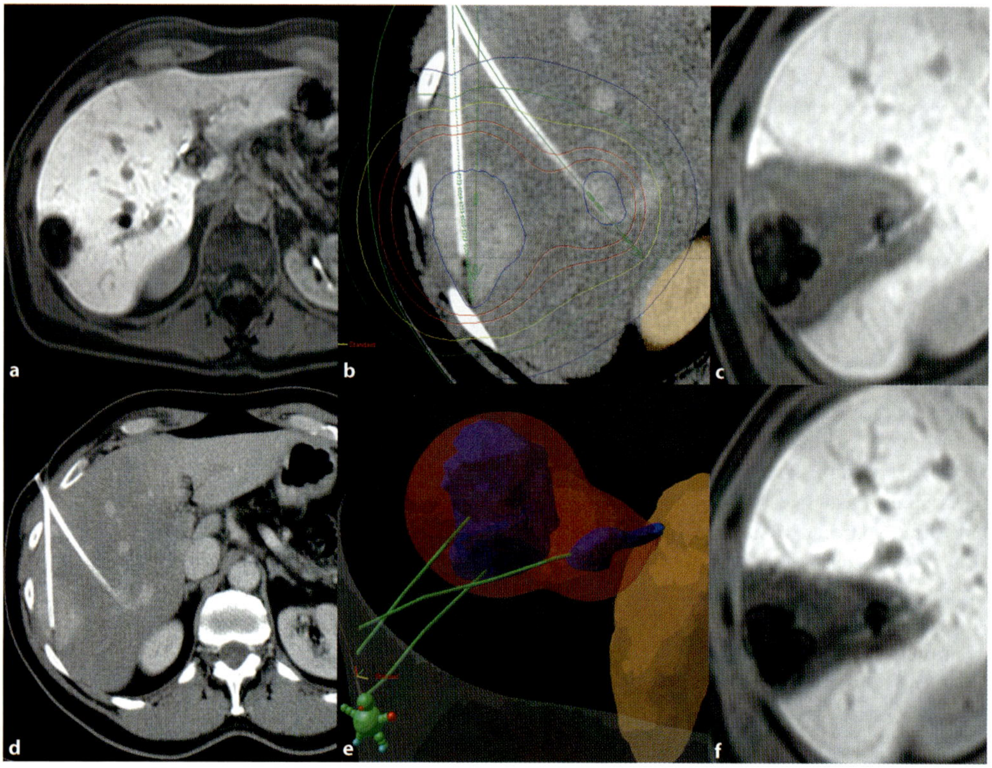

Fig. 11.1a–f A 51-year-old patient with osteoclastic-type giant cell carcinoma of the pancreatic corpus, with portal vein thrombosis to the left liver lobe and two metastases in the right lobe: **a** T1-weighted MRI (hepatocyte specific contrast material) of the liver shows the initial status of the liver lesions and the functional impairment of the left lobe because of the portal vein thrombus in the left main branch. After a chemotherapy course (cisplatin, etoposide, ifosfamide) with stable disease and exclusion of extrahepatic spread, the liver metastases were treated with CT-guided interstitial HDR brachytherapy in a single session. **d** Shows the planning CT scan with the afterloading catheters in place. **b, e** Demonstrates the definition of the gross tumor volume (*blue lines*), the definition of the kidney as a risk organ (*orange area*), and the resulting brachytherapy plan with the minimal dose in the clinical target volume at 20 Gy (*red line*), as well as the steep dose reduction to the periphery (15 Gy isodose, *orange*; 10 Gy isodose, *yellow*; 5 Gy, *green*; 2.5 Gy, *dark blue*). The follow-up MRI scans at 6 weeks (**c**) and 6 months (**f**) after intermittent resection of the primary tumor show the shrinking ablation zone with good local control of the metastases and a spacious safety margin of ablated liver tissue as indicated by the loss of contrast enhancement (hepatocyte-specific contrast material) in the surrounding area

for documentation of the exact catheter location in relation to the tumor (Fig. 11.1d). These data are the basis for 3D reconstructions and radiation therapy planning on a dedicated workstation by outlining the gross tumor volume, the catheters, and the surrounding risk tissues (e.g., bowel, stomach wall, gall bladder, kidney, spinal canal, skin) (Fig. 11.1b, e). This technique with retrospective registration of the catheter positions is highly accurate and less complex as compared to prospectively arranged catheter positions with templates or intraoperative raster placement (Tonus et al. 2001; Kolotas et al. 2003). With a selected minimal target dose, usually 15–25 Gy, an afterloading plan is generated giving dwell locations and dwell times for the iridium-192 source [half-life, 78.8 days; decay, beta (672 keV) and gamma (<469 keV)] inside the afterloading catheters. This plan needs control and can be adjusted manually if necessary. The goal is to modulate a planned target volume covering the entire gross tumor volume and a safety margin while sparing healthy surrounding tissue, especially risk organs, as much as possible. An optimization of target volume definition and consecutively the dose coverage of the tumor can be achieved by registration of the previously acquired FDG-PET images with the CT data (Denecke et al. 2006). Although the number of catheters is theoretically unlimited, it is recommendable not to exceed 6–8 catheters, depending on the tumor size and shape. Because of the stress situation, the radiation time should be limited to a maximum of 1 h, depending on the patient's condition.

Using this plan, the afterloading procedure is performed and subsequently the catheters are slowly removed, sealing the puncture channels with tissue glue or other thrombogenic material to prevent bleeding.

11.2.3 Undesired Side Effects

Complications can be subdivided into acute complications, occurring during or immediately after treatment, and late complications. The inadvertent acute events are mainly due to mechanical alterations caused by the puncture and catheter placement (e.g., bleeding, perforation of bowel, stomach, or gall bladder). These inadvertent events, however, occur very rarely, as CT-guided puncture of the liver is a safe way to avoid severe injuries of nontarget tissues. Major bleeding from the liver is an extremely rare complication and can be prevented by sufficient sealing of the puncture channel during retraction of the catheter sheaths. Other acute side effects are emesis, pain, and shivers, which are to be treated medically.

Delayed side effects besides infectious complications are mainly related to radiation exposure of nontarget tissues. Treating hepatic malignomas, exposure of surrounding healthy liver tissue to a relevant radiation doses is desired as a safety margin. However, a sufficient hepatic reserve has to be ensured before treating hepatic malignomas, particularly in patients with large and/or multiple lesions, preexisting liver disease (e.g., hepatocellular carcinoma in cirrhosis, portal vein thrombosis), previously irradiated liver (dose accumulation), or otherwise impaired liver function reserve due to prior chemotherapy. The tolerance dose of a healthy liver is approximately 30 Gy to the whole organ or 50 Gy to one-third of the liver volume. For external radiotherapy, the clinical endpoints are liver failure and severe hepatitis. If the irradiated volume of normal liver tissue is reduced to approximately 100 ml or less, the tolerated doses are much higher—in principle, without any upper limit with respect to the clinical endpoints mentioned. Additionally, the different radiobiological effects of a single high dose fraction to the tissue compared to fractionated strategies has to be considered. It is well known that healthy tissue tolerates larger doses applied in multiple fractions. The options for the irradiated liver tissue are either destruction or recovery to normal liver function. Additionally, compensative mechanisms of the remaining non-irradiated liver parenchyma has to be taken into account. A recent study showed that for interstitial brachytherapy in an afterloading technique with an iridium-192 source, the tolerance dose causing an early function loss of hepatocytes as determined in MRI with hepatocyte specific contrast material 6 week after irradiation was 9.9 Gy (±2.3 standard deviation) (Ricke et al. 2004b). This and the careful assessment of the hepatic reserve have to be taken into consideration when planning the treatment to avoid posttherapeutic hepatic failure.

Other tissues at risk are, e.g., bile ducts, gall bladder, gastrointestinal tract, skin, kidney, and spinal cord. Previously described complications have included rare events such as strictures of the common bile duct or gastric ulcers (Ricke et al. 2004a; Streitparth et al. 2006). Concerning gastric complications, a threshold dose of 15.5 Gy/ml tissue for the clinical endpoint ulceration of gastric mucosa has been estimated (Streitparth et al. 2006). This in vivo assessment is in accordance with tolerance data by Emami et al. (1991). Regarding the small and large bowel, dose thresholds have not been estimated yet, but it has been hypothesized that they are similar to those described for the gastric wall; overall, however, these complications and late effects are rare, to which patients with repeated irradiation close to the risk tissues are more prone (Ricke et al. 2004a, 2005b). Concerning gastric exposure, a proton pump inhibitor therapy is being recommended as ulcer prophylaxis. Potential risk and benefit have to be thoroughly evaluated before treatment initiation and during radiation planning.

11.2.4 Efficacy

Local tumor ablation has become a valuable tool in oncological treatment concepts. The majority of locally ablative procedures are performed by applying thermal ablation, such as RFA or LITT. However, with respect to the limitations of thermal ablation modalities (i.e., tumor size, tumor shape, tumor location, adjacent risk structures), novel techniques combining brachytherapy with interventional techniques have demonstrated favorable outcomes. In contrast to thermal ablation, CT-guided brachytherapy is independent of complex geometric configurations of the lesions, as dwell times and dwell locations of the source within the applicators can be adjusted to fit the outlines of the tumor (Rühl and Ricke 2006). Furthermore, adjacent ducts and vessels do not influence the ablation zone as brachytherapy is not prone to disturbing cooling effects. In contrast to external beam radiation, breathing motions are not an issue, because the afterloading catheters move with the tumor (Ricke et al. 2004b).

Early studies on CT-guided brachytherapy showed local tumor control rates of 87% after 6 months at minimal dose levels of 12–20 Gy (Ricke et al. 2004a). An analysis of the treatment of 200 colorectal liver metastases between 1 and 11 cm (median 4 cm) recruited for a phase III study revealed a local tumor control rate of 96% after 12 months when applying 25 Gy, and 67% when applying 20 Gy as the minimal tumor dose. Major adverse events were hemorrhage in 3 patients (2%), which ceased after blood transfusion (Ricke et al. 2005c).

The use of interstitial brachytherapy is not limited to its application inside the liver, as treatment of lung malignancies has also demonstrated promising results with respect to local tumor control and side effects. In a phase I trial, 15 patients with 28 lung metastases and nonsmall cell lung cancer in 2 cases were treated with a single fraction of at least 20 Gy inside the entire clinical target volume. No major adverse events were reported. Minor events included radiographically visible local hemorrhage in 2 patients (Ricke et al. 2005a). In contrast to thermal ablation techniques, air cavities in the lung were not seen. Radiobiologically, the cytotoxic effect after single-fraction, high-dose rate irradiation shows within weeks to months, with only moderate acute injury (Manning et al. 2001).

11.3 The Role of CT-Guided Interstitial Brachytherapy in Pancreatic Cancer

The widest experience with CT-guided brachytherapy has been with colorectal cancer, breast cancer, and hepatocellular carcinoma. In contrast, pancreatic neoplasias are less favorable for locally ablative treatment, depending on the histological subtype.

Regarding liver metastases from neuroendocrine gastroenteropancreatic tumors, locally ablative treatment has been used successfully for cell reduction, tumor eradication, and symptom relief in functionally active tumors (Elvin et al. 2005; O'Toole and Ruszniewski 2005). In this context, a special focus of CT-guided brachytherapy is the treatment of lesions unfavorable for LITT or RFA because of size, shape, and location. Even though some of these tumors are known to be less sensitive to radiation therapy, it has to be emphasized that in the setting of single session HDR brachytherapy with doses above 20 Gy and core doses above 50–100 Gy, the criterion radiosensitivity of tumor tissues plays a minor role. Therefore, CT-guided brachytherapy for locally ablative treatment of liver metastases appears to be a promising tool in this subset of pancreatic neoplasias.

Concerning the treatment of pancreatic ductal adenocarcinoma, there are no data available yet assessing the use of this novel technique. Ductal adenocarcinoma represents the majority (90%–95%) of pancreatic malignancies and is known to have a poor prognosis (5-year overall survival, 1%–2%) (Wagner et al. 1999; Tsiotos et al. 1999; Brand and Tempero 1998; Rosewicz and Wiedenmann 1997). The resection of the primary tumor currently being the only potentially curative treatment (5-year overall survival after R0 resection, approximately 20%), most of the affected patients (approximately 80%) are irresectable at the time of first diagnosis, owing to distant metastases or local tumor extent (Lopez-Hänninen et al. 2002; Wagner et al. 1999; Tsiotos et al. 1999; Brand and Tempero 1998; Rosewicz and Wiedenmann 1997). Even though there are promising developments in both surgical technique and chemotherapeutic agents, the outcome remains rather poor. This emphasizes the need for innovative treatment strategies as adjuncts to the traditional therapeutic approach.

The efforts being made toward treating the primary pancreatic ductal adenocarcinoma by locally ablative procedures such as RFA and LITT, as well as external beam irradiation for neoadjuvant or palliative therapy, have met with varying success (Stroszczynski et al. 2001; Varshney et al. 2006). As most adenocarcinomas are located in the pancreatic head (approximately 75%) the lesions are difficult to reach by CT-guided local ablation. Surrounding vessels and risk structures, such as the bile ducts, the duodenum, and the stomach, as well as the pancreatic parenchyma itself, limit the ablation volume for either modality. Even in intraoperative RFA of pancreatic malignancies, there have been severe complications observed, such as necrotizing pancreatitis (Elias et al. 2004). The primary tumor, especially when judged as irresectable, is a diffuse mass with an irregular growth pattern. Therefore, the inclusion of the entire tumor is often impossible and it can be questioned whether local tumor destruction exposes the patient unnecessarily to risks that outweigh the potential benefit. Even though CT-guided brachytherapy is more flexible regarding the configuration of the target volume, these limitations apply here as well. On the other hand, retarding the local tumor progression only by a few months has to be considered a success, as alternative treatment options are rare and offer only moderate response rates and rather poor outcomes.

Referring to hematogenous distant metastases, these are most commonly located in the liver. Even though the progression of the disease is rapid and, in most cases of metachronous liver metastases, further micrometastases are present that are invisible to diagnostic imaging, hepatic metastases in theory can be considered as a limited disease. Thus, it can be considered whether a patient might profit from removal of the metastases if the primary tumor has been resected. There are currently no data showing an advantage of hepatic surgery in such a scenario, and any unnecessary risk has to be kept as low as possible in the palliative setting. Therefore, the use of minimally invasive ablation of liver metastases is a promising alternative to surgery, not only in irresectable patients. Treating hepatic metastases by thermal ablation in pancreatic cancer patients implies an additional issue. As most adenocarcinomas are seated in the pancreatic head, the resection includes a biliodigestive anastomosis. This condition allows ascending bacterial colonization of the biliary tree, which supports the development of abscesses in the necrotic ablation zones after thermal tumor coagulation (Thomas et al. 2004). A similar condition is present in palliative treatment of irresectable patients with stents in the common bile duct. In contrast to thermal ablation, brachytherapy induces a prolonged tumor inactivation along with ongoing organization of the developing necrosis, which is accessible to the immune system, and therefore the rate of abscesses is extremely low compared to thermal tumor destruction. Infection of the ablation zone therefore appears to be a minor problem for interstitial afterloading in this specific patient group.

To create reasonable indications for the use of locally ablative treatment in pancreatic cancer patients, it has to be implemented into a multidisciplinary approach including surgery and chemotherapy in an individualized therapeutic strategy. A possible indication for locally ablative treatment would be the eradication of liver metastases to facilitate resection of the primary tumor. For illustration of this multidisciplinary individualized approach, we present a case with an undifferentiated osteoclastic-type giant cell tumor of the pancreatic corpus (Fig. 11.1).

The patient presented with two liver metastases in the right lobe and a portal vein thrombosis of the left branch at initial diagnosis. Chemotherapy maintained stable disease, but caused intolerable sensory irritation in the hands and the feet. The patient was referred to our department for CT-guided interstitial HDR brachytherapy of the liver metastases in order to retard local tumor progression. Because of inaccessibility and the previously mentioned risks of locally ablative therapy inside the pancreas, the primary tumor was not treated. After ensuring a good local control of the liver metastases by MRI 3 months after brachytherapy of the two liver lesions and exclusion of new intra- and extrahepatic metastases by CT, a R0 resection of the pancreatic tail and corpus with the primary was performed. Eighteen months after brachytherapy the patient is still free of tumor with a good quality of life.

To summarize, CT-guided brachytherapy of liver metastases may be reasonable in patients with local resectability and a limited number of liver metastases, when stable disease is ensured by a sufficient surveillance interval. Here and in previously resected patients with metachronous liver metastases, the palliative use of CT-guided brachytherapy might prove beneficial in the future and appears to be advantageous compared to thermal ablation because of the reduced rate of abscesses in the ablation zone.

11.5 Conclusion

Combining the features of substantially different therapies, such as the safety of CT-guided organ puncture, efficacy of brachytherapy, and the principles of the afterloading technique, a novel therapeutic approach in radiation oncology has been developed. Percutaneous afterloading of hepatic malignomas enables effective treatment, even in those patients who are not suitable to undergo surgical or thermal ablations because of tumor size or location. There are promising data for the treatment of hepatocellular carcinoma and colorectal liver metastases, and further studies are pending. For pancreatic cancer, the potential indications for CT-guided brachytherapy are currently limited to the treatment of liver metastases. Despite the lack of controlled trials, there is probably a role for this therapeutic approach in an individualized multidisciplinary therapeutic approach in a carefully selected patient group.

References

Amthauer H, Denecke T, Hildebrandt B, Rühl R, Miersch A, Nicolaou A, Ruf J, Plotkin M, Lopez Hänninen E, Stroszczynski C, Gutberlet M, Langrehr J, Riess H, Ricke J (2006) Evaluation of patients with liver metastases from colorectal cancer for locally ablative treatment with laser induced thermotherapy: impact of positron emission tomography with fluor-18-fluorodeoxyglucose on therapeutic decision making. Nuklearmedizin 45:177–184

Brand RE, Tempero MA (1998) Pancreatic cancer. Curr Opin Oncol 10:362–366

Denecke T, Grabik W, Steffen I, Amthauer H, Wust P, Rühl R, Rosner C, Ricke J, Felix R, Lopez Hänninen E (2006) Value of FDG-PET and image fusion for optimization of target volume definition in CT guided interstitial high dose rate single fraction brachytherapy of colorectal liver metastases (abstr). Radiology 28:501–512

Dritschilo A, Harter KW, Thomas D, Nauta R, Holt R, Lee TC, Rustgi S, Rodgers J (1988) Intraoperative radiation therapy of hepatic metastases: technical aspects and report of a pilot study. Int J Radiat Oncol Biol Phys 14:1007–1011

Elias D, Baton O, Sideris L, Lasser P, Pocard M (2004) Necrotizing pancreatitis after radiofrequency destruction of pancreatic tumours. Eur J Surg Oncol 30:85–87

Elvin A, Skogseid B, Hellman P (2005) Radiofrequency ablation of neuroendocrine liver metastases. Abdom Imaging 30:427–434

Emami B, Lyman J, Brown A, Coia L, Goitein M, Munzenrider JE, Shank B, Solin LJ, Wesson M (1991) Tolerance of normal tissue to therapeutic irradiation. Int J Radiat Oncol Biol Phys 21:109–122

Herfarth KK, Debus J, Wannenmacher M (2004) Stereotactic radiation therapy of liver metastases: update of the initial phase-I/II trial. Front Radiat Ther Oncol 38:100–105

Kolotas C, Roddiger S, Strassmann G, Martin T, Tselis N, Aebersold DM, Baltas D, Zamboglou N (2003) Palliative interstitial HDR brachytherapy for recurrent rectal cancer. Implantation techniques and results. Strahlenther Onkol 179:458–463

Lopez Hänninen E, Amthauer H, Hosten N, Ricke J, Bohmig M, Langrehr J, Hintze R, Neuhaus P, Wiedenmann B, Rosewicz S, Felix R (2002) Prospective evaluation of pancreatic tumors: accuracy of MR imaging with MR cholangiopancreatography and MR angiography. Radiology 224:34–41

Manning MA, Zwicker RD, Arthur DW, Arnfield M (2001) Biologic treatment planning for high-dose-rate brachytherapy. Int J Radiat Oncol Biol Phys 49:839–845

Meyers MO, Sasson AR, Sigurdson ER (2003) Locoregional strategies for colorectal hepatic metastases. Clin Colorectal Cancer 3:34–44

Nauta RJ, Heres EK, Thomas DS, Harter KW, Rodgers JE, Holt RW, Lee TC, Walsh DB, Dritschilo A (1987) Intraoperative single-dose radiotherapy. Observations on staging and interstitial treatment of unresectable liver metastases. Arch Surg 122:1392–1395

Nolsoe CP, Torp-Pedersen S, Burcharth F, Horn T, Pedersen S, Christensen NE, Olldag ES, Andersen PH, Karstrup S, Lorentzen T, et al. (1993) Interstitial hyperthermia of colorectal liver metastases with a US-guided Nd-YAG laser with a diffuser tip: a pilot clinical study. Radiology 187:333–337

O'Toole D, Ruszniewski P (2005) Chemoembolization and other ablative therapies for liver metastases of gastrointestinal endocrine tumours. Best Pract Res Clin Gastroenterol 19:585–594

Ricke J, Wust P, Stohlmann A, Beck A, Cho CH, Pech M, Wieners G, Spors B, Werk M, Rosner C, Lopez Hänninen E, Felix R (2004a) CT-guided interstitial brachytherapy of liver malignancies alone or in combination with thermal ablation: phase I-II results of a novel technique. Int J Radiat Oncol Biol Phys 58:1496–1505

Ricke J, Wust P, Wieners G, Beck A, Cho CH, Seidensticker M, Pech M, Werk M, Rosner C, Lopez Hänninen E, Freund T, Felix R (2004b) Liver malignancies: CT-guided interstitial brachytherapy in patients with unfavorable lesions for thermal ablation. J Vasc Interv Radiol 15:1279–86

Ricke J, Wust P, Wieners G, Hengst S, Pech M, Lopez Hänninen E, Felix R (2005a) CT-guided interstitial single-fraction brachytherapy of lung tumors: phase I results of a novel technique. Chest 127:2237–2242

Ricke J, Seidensticker M, Ludemann L, Pech M, Wieners G, Hengst S, Mohnike K, Cho CH, Lopez Hänninen E, Al-Abadi H, Felix R, Wust P (2005b) In vivo assessment of the tolerance dose of small liver volumes after single-fraction HDR irradiation. Int J Radiat Oncol Biol Phys 62:776–784

Ricke J, Mohnike K, Pech M, Wieners G, Wust P, Felix R (2005c) CT-guided interstitial HDR-brachytherapy of liver malignancies: results of a prospective phase III trial in colorectal liver metastasis. Radiology 230:164

Rosewicz S, Wiedenmann B (1997) Pancreatic carcinoma. Lancet 349:485–489

Rühl R, Ricke J (2006) Image-guided microtherapy for tumor ablation: from thermal coagulation to advanced irradiation techniques. Onkologie 29:219–224

Streitparth F, Pech M, Bohmig M, Ruehl R, Peters N, Wieners G, Lopez Hänninen E, Felix R, Wust P, Ricke J (2006) In-vivo assessment of the gastric mucosal tolerance dose after single fraction, small volume irradiation of liver malignancies by CT-guided HDR-brachytherapy. Int J Radiat Oncol Biol Phys 65:1479–1486

Stroszczynski C, Hosten N, Puls R, Nagel S, Scholman HJ, Wlodarczyk W, Oettle H, Moesta KT, Schlag PM, Felix R (2001) Histopathological correlation to MRI findings during and after laser-induced thermotherapy in a pig pancreas model. Invest Radiol 36:413–421

Thomas DS, Nauta RJ, Rodgers JE, Popescu GF, Nguyen H, Lee TC, Petrucci PE, Harter KW, Holt RW, Dritschilo A (1993) Intraoperative high-dose rate interstitial irradiation of hepatic metastases from colorectal carcinoma. Results of a phase I-II trial. Cancer 71:1977–1981

Thomas KT, Bream PR Jr, Berlin J, Meranze SG, Wright JK, Chari RS (2004) Use of percutaneous drainage to treat hepatic abscess after radiofrequency ablation of metastatic pancreatic adenocarcinoma. Am Surg 70:496–499

Tonus C, Debertshauser D, Strassmann G, Kolotas C, Walter S, Zamboglou N, Nier H (2001) CT-based navigation systems for intraoperative radiotherapy using the afterloading-flab technique. Dig Surg 18:470–474

Tsiotos GG, Farnell MB, Sarr MG (1999) Are the results of pancreatectomy for pancreatic cancer improving? World J Surg 23:913–919

Varshney S, Sewkani A, Sharma S, Kapoor S, Naik S, Sharma A, Patel K (2006) Radiofrequency ablation of unresectable pancreatic carcinoma: feasibility, efficacy and safety. JOP 7:74–78

Vogl TJ, Müller PK, Hammerstingl R, Wienhold N, Mack MG, Philipp C, Deimling M, Beuthan J, Pegios W, Riess H, et al. (1995) Malignant liver tumors treated with MR imaging-guided laserinduced thermotherapy: technique and prospective results. Radiology 196:257–265

Wagner M, Dikopoulos N, Kulli C, Friess H, Buchler MW (1999) Standard surgical treatment in pancreatic cancer. Ann Oncol 4:247–251

Wurm RE, Gum F, Erbel S, Schlenger L, Scheffler D, Agaoglu D, Schild R, Gebauer B, Rogalla P, Plotkin M, Ocran K, Budach V (2006) Image guided respiratory gated hypofractionated stereotactic body radiation therapy (H-SBRT) for liver and lung tumors: initial experience. Acta Oncol 45:881–889

12 Detection of Disease Recurrence and Monitoring of Therapy

J. Ruf, H. Amthauer

Recent Results in Cancer Research, Vol. 177

Abstract

The detection of disease recurrence and treatment monitoring pose high demands on diagnostic modalities. Whereas serum marker levels in most cases allow an assessment of tumor load and a respective response to therapy, they do not confer information on the localization of disease. Although this diagnostic gap is filled by imaging modalities, most techniques based on morphology will come to a limit when fibrotic tissue alterations have to be differentiated from viable tumor tissue in case of suspected recurrence or when residual masses after chemotherapy have to be assessed. The metabolic information on tumor cells gained by fluorodeoxyglucose-positron emission tomography (FDG-PET) imaging appears not only to be more sensitive and reliable in this respect, but also appears to allow assumptions on response to therapy, and ultimately on patient prognosis.

12.1 Definition of Tumor Recurrence and Epidemiological Aspects

Pancreatic carcinoma is characterized by its poor prognosis. Only a minority of patients are eligible for curative surgery upon tumor detection (Birk et al. 1998).

Even in those patients operated with curative intent, 5-year survival is only 31%–51% (Pantalone et al. 2001). This observation can partly be explained by the fact that even in patients with small tumors (<2 cm), lymph-node metastases are present in about 50% of all cases (Cleary et al. 2004; Meyer et al. 2003). Similarly, in a recent analysis of the Japanese National Pancreas Cancer Registry, only 16.5% of all patients with tumors smaller than 2 cm did not have an infiltration of adjacent tissue or vessels, lymph node, or distant metastases (Egawa et al. 2004). As a consequence, a small size of the primary tumor does not necessarily signify an early stage of disease. Unfortunately, even a more radical surgical approach often fails to lead to an improvement of survival rate, and at the cost of a reduced quality of life (Riall et al. 2005). Therefore, disease recurrence has to be expected even in the small subgroup of patients operated with curative intent.

12.2 Disease Recurrence

Apart from clinical symptoms such as pain, weight loss, or jaundice, the increase in serum tumor markers is usually a sensitive indicator for disease recurrence. Probably the most important of these markers is the carbohydrate antigen CA 19-9. Although it is not specific for pancreatic cancer and may also be elevated in other cancers of the gastrointestinal tract, serial assessments have shown its usefulness as a parameter for the monitoring of therapy and the assessment of prognosis (Micke et al. 2003). Whereas factors such as bile retention have to be taken into consideration when assessing high tumor marker levels, a greater problem is probably caused by the fact that CA 19-9 is not expressed in all patients with pancreatic cancer. It has been shown that individuals who are negative for the expression of the Lewis (Lea and Leb) blood antigen (accounting for approx. 10% of the general population) also do not synthesize CA 19-9. Thus, they cannot not be monitored by its serum determination (Goggins 2005).

Moreover, a drawback of serological tumor markers is the lack of information they provide on the localization of disease recurrence. Locally confined recurrence might be treatable by surgery or interventional procedures in conjunction with systemic chemotherapy. Moreover, even in case of disseminated disease an assessment of tumor response to therapy is desirable. Thus, imaging modalities do play a crucial role in recurrence detection.

Most recurrences occur locally due to lymphatic spread or microscopic perineural invasion (Griffin et al. 1990). In contrast to the good results achieved with endoscopic/endoluminal procedures in the assessment of suspicious pancreatic masses prior to surgery (Harewood and Wiersema 2002), changes in intestinal continuity and the respective anastomoses may limit their use for recurrence detection in patients after Whipple's operation or pylorus preserving pancreatoduodenectomy (PPPD).

Although cross-sectional morphologic imaging by computed tomography (CT) or magnetic resonance imaging (MRI) is of great value for the assessment of postoperative complications and immediate follow-up (Scialpi et al. 2005), there are problems in the interpretation of findings in the former pancreas bed, where the differentiation of fibrotic scar tissue from tumor recurrence is often difficult (Mortele et al. 2000). Functional imaging by positron emission tomography (PET) offers a solution to these negative or indeterminate findings in morphological imaging (Fig. 12.1). Unfortunately, the general scarcity of studies on recurrence detection is also true for PET studies, as only a few preliminary studies have addressed this issue (Franke et al. 1999; Jadvar and Fischman 2001; Rose et al. 1999; Higashi et al. 2003).

In a recent study, our group demonstrated the value of fluorodeoxyglucose-positron emission tomography (FDG-PET) for the assessment of suspected pancreas cancer recurrence (Ruf et al. 2005). Included were 31 patients with suspected recurrence after surgery who either showed weight-loss, pain, increased CA 19-9 levels, or a combination of these symptoms. All patients were examined by whole-body FDG-PET and contrast-enhanced multidetector CT ($n = 14$) or MR ($n = 17$) imaging. In accordance with the literature, 25/31 patients had local recurrences upon follow-up, which had been diagnosed by imaging modalities in 23/25 patients. FDG-PET detected 96% (22/23) of these cases, whereas morphological imaging by CT or MRI was positive in only 39% (9/23). Liver metastases were, in contrast, better depicted by MRI and CT imaging, with a detection rate of 92% (11/12) vs 42% (5/12) for FDG-PET. The possible explanation for this observation is the improved detection of small hepatic lesions made possible by dynamic multiphase MRI/CT examinations in contrast to PET, which in the case of small lesions suffers from partial volume effects that make tumor-specific FDG uptake indiscernible from physiologic hepatic activity. Despite the drawback of

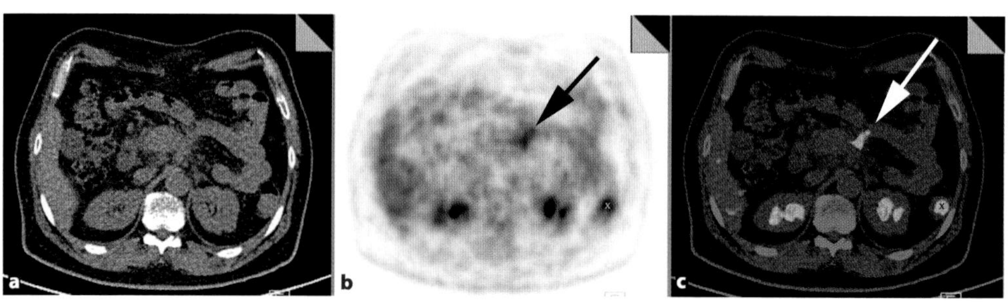

Fig. 12.1a–c A 58-year-old man presenting with newly diagnosed diabetes and unspecific abdominal pain 8 years after left-sided pancreas resection (pT1a pN0 G2 R0). Whereas the contrast-enhanced CT scan showed no suspicious mass, fluorodeoxyglucose-positron emission tomography (FDG-PET) (a low-dose PET-CT scan) showed focal tracer uptake at the resection margin of the pancreatic corpus (*arrow*), indicating local recurrence. Also note the physiologic gut activity in the descending colon (*x*)

limited anatomical orientation, FDG-PET was again superior to MRI/CT with regards to abdominal lymph-node involvement, as focal uptake was more indicative of tumor recurrence than the mere size assessment of lymph nodes by morphologic imaging. Moreover, as FDG-PET is routinely performed in a whole-body technique, unknown extra-abdominal metastases were detected in 2 patients.

Since FDG-PET was superior to morphological imaging, it is imaginable that it allows for an earlier detection of recurrence and therefore an earlier initiation of therapy. However, other potential influential factors on FDG uptake have to be addressed (please also refer to Chap. 3). As pancreatic surgery may lead to a diabetic metabolic state (if not already present prior to surgery), a potential decrease in FDG sensitivity has to be considered especially in those patients with a low compliance with regards to antidiabetic medication or in which euglycemia is difficult to achieve (Diederichs et al. 1998). Moreover, as in the initial assessment of pancreatic masses, cellularity, the expression of glucose transporters and enzymatic activity of glycolytic enzymes, has to be heeded (Higashi et al. 2002).

12.3 Response to Therapy and Prognosis

Apart from the clinical patient reexamination, the response to radiation treatment or chemotherapy is usually assessed by morphological imaging modalities such as ultrasound, CT or MRI, using both the number of lesions and their respective size as parameters. However, whereas an increase or decrease of the number lesions is relatively easy to discern, changes in lesion size as assessed either by WHO (perpendicular diameter) or the EORTC's area measurement approach (response evaluation criteria in solid tumors, RECIST) may be rendered more difficult by necrotic, fibrotic, and/or cystic transformation of metastases under therapy (Miller et al. 1981; Therasse et al. 2000). The value of metabolic imaging for the differentiation of residual vital tumor tissue vs necrotic or fibrotic residue has been demonstrated, e.g., in the neoadjuvant treatment of colorectal cancer, where FDG-PET correlated far better than morphological imaging to the histopathology of the resected tumor (Amthauer et al. 2004). In concordance with morphological imaging, attempts have also been made to standardize the response to therapy by the use of quantification measurements (Young et al. 1999).

Interestingly, apart from the determination of the primary diagnosis, prognosis rather than response to therapy has been assessed by the majority of FDG-PET studies (Table 12.1). A possible reason for this is the simple fact that response to therapy requires at least two studies of the at the time of the rather costly PET examination. In 1997, Nakata and coworkers pioneered with a study on 14 patients suffering from pancreatic cancer that received conventional imaging as well as FDG-PET prior to treatment. FDG uptake was semiquantified by the determination of the standardized uptake value (SUV) of the primary tumor, which was correlated to patient survival. Using a cut-off SUV of 3.0 for high and low glucose uptake respectively, they observed a significant difference in the patient group with low uptake (14 months) and high uptake (5 months). Using a SUV of 6.1, Zimny and coworkers (2000) were able to reproduce these results in 52 patients with 5 months survival in case of an SUV exceeding 6.1 vs 9 months survival in the case of an SUV below 6.1 ($p=0.0321$), with multivariate analysis revealing the SUV as an independent prognostic factor. These results were strengthened by an Italian study on 60 patients, which came to a similar conclusion using a cut-off for SUV of 4 (Sperti et al. 2003).

Although the wide range of cut-offs for SUV in these studies can be explained by differing examination protocols utilized at the respective institutions, it is doubtful that there actually is an "ideal" SUV threshold (please also refer to Chap. 3). Moreover, only the glucose avidity of the primary tumor has been primarily assessed, whereas the correlation of SUV to tumor stage or the SUV of metastases has only been poorly investigated (Higashi et al. 2003).

Nevertheless, these studies indicate the potential of metabolic imaging by FDG-PET in patients diagnosed with pancreatic cancer, leaving aside the pitfalls associated with the primary diagnosis of pancreatic cancer, i.e., the differentiation of glucose-avid inflammation from glucose-avid cancer (please refer to Chap. 3). With regards to one-time examinations, dual-phase imaging, i.e., the measurement of glucose uptake at two time-points during one imaging session, not only appears to improve the differentiation of benign from malignant disease, but potentially allows for a more precise assessment of prognosis, more appropriately reflecting the kinetics of glucose metabolism. Using a dual-phase approach, Lyshchik and coworkers (2005) determined an intraindividual retention index (RI) based on the respective SUVs measured 1 h (1) and 2 h (2) after tracer injection ($RI = SUV2 - SUV1 / SUV1 \times 100\%$) for each of their 65 patients. RI was an independent marker for survival in the multivariate analysis, and showed the strongest prognostic difference for an RI cut-off of 10% (UICC stage I–III: 15.3 months vs 11.5 months; stage IV: 9.5 months vs 4.9 months).

Moreover, it is imaginable that a more appropriate estimation of prognosis can be derived not from a single examination upon tumor detection but rather when the response to therapy is assessed (Table 12.1). In one study, nine patients underwent FDG imaging both before and 4 weeks after chemoradiation therapy. Instead of the determination of a cut-off for SUV, the change in SUV was assessed. The group observed that a decrease in SUV larger than 50% was present in all patients that showed good histological response to therapy (Rose et al. 1999). Another study examined 11 patients both before and 1 month after chemotherapy (Maisey et al. 2000). Although their evaluation of PET data was rather simple, as only visual analysis was performed, they saw a significantly extended survival in those patients that showed no FDG uptake in the control scan as opposed to the group in which tumor activity was still visible (mean survival: 318 vs 139 days).

Both studies draw their conclusions from serial PET examinations that, just as with dual-phase imaging, might deliver more robust results, since they are based on intraindividual comparisons in which the biological factor, the patient, remains a constant.

Furthermore, as metabolic changes usually occur earlier than morphological changes, it might be possible to estimate the response of a patient undergoing (rather than after) therapy and to switch to a another therapeutic regimen in case of nonresponse. The potential of FDG-PET in this setting has been demonstrated e.g., in esophageal cancer. In one study on patients with carcinoma of the gastroesophageal junction, the change in FDG uptake between baseline

Table 12.1 Summary of FDG-PET studies according to FDG uptake/SUV and survival

Author	Year	Journal	Pt.	FDG-PET	PET-parameters	Survival
Nakata et al.	1997	*Cancer*	14	Pretreatment scan	SUV < 3	14 (months)
					SUV ≥ 3	5 (months)
Zimny et al.	2000	*Scand J Gastroenterol*	52	Pretreatment scan	SUV < 6.1	9 (months)
					SUV ≥ 6.1	6 (months)
Maisey et al.	2000	*Br J Cancer*	11	Pre- and post-treatment scan	FDG uptake pos.	139 (days)
					FDG uptake neg.	318.5 (days)
Sperti et al.	2003	*J Gastrointest Surg*	60	Pretreatment scan	SUV ≤ 4	265 (days)
					SUV > 4	178 (days)
Lyshchik et al.	2005	*Eur J Nucl Med Mol Imaging*	65	Dual-phase scan 1 and 2 h p.i.	RI > 10%	Stage I–III: 15.3 months
						Stage IV: 11.5 months
					RI > 10%	Stage I–III: 9.5 months
						Stage IV: 4.9 months

RI, retention index; SUV, standard uptake value, Pt., patients examination and a control examination as early as 14 days after initiation of neoadjuvant chemotherapy was indicative for the differentiation of patients who profited from therapy vs those who did not according to conventional follow-up and postoperative histology (Weber et al. 2001). With regards to pancreatic cancer, however, further studies are required.

12.4 Summary

Due to the high percentage of patients with pancreatic carcinoma that can only be palliatively treated and the high rate of recurrence in patients operated with curative intent, reliable imaging modalities for therapy control, the assessment of prognosis, and recurrence detection are desirable.

Whereas MRI and CT will remain the basic imaging modalities for therapy control and patient follow-up due to their availability, metabolic imaging by FDG-PET has the potential to improve both the monitoring of therapy and the assessment of prognosis.

References

Amthauer H, Denecke T, Rau B, Hildebrandt B, Hunerbein M, Ruf J, Schneider U, Gutberlet M, Schlag PM, Felix R, Wust P (2004) Response prediction by FDG-PET after neoadjuvant radiochemotherapy and regional hyperthermia of rectal cancer: correlation with endorectal ultrasound and histopathology. Eur J Nucl Med Mol Imaging 31:811–819

Birk D, Fortnagel G, Formentini A, Beger HG (1998) Small carcinoma of the pancreas. Factors of prognostic relevance. J Hepatobiliary Pancreat Surg 5:450–454

Cleary SP, Gryfe R, Guindi M, Greig P, Smith L, Mackenzie R, Strasberg S, Hanna S, Taylor B, Langer B, Gallinger S (2004) Prognostic factors in resected pancreatic adenocarcinoma: analysis of actual 5-year survivors. J Am Coll Surg 198:722–731

Diederichs CG, Staib L, Glatting G, Beger HG, Reske SN (1998) FDG PET: elevated plasma glucose reduces both uptake and detection rate of pancreatic malignancies. J Nucl Med 39:1030–1033

Egawa S, Takeda K, Fukuyama S, Motoi F, Sunamura M, Matsuno S (2004) Clinicopathological aspects of small pancreatic cancer. Pancreas 28:235–240

Franke C, Klapdor R, Meyerhoff K, Schauman M (1999) 18-FDG positron emission tomography of the pancreas: diagnostic benefit in the follow-up of pancreatic carcinoma. Anticancer Res 19:2437–2442

Goggins MG (2005) The molecular diagnosis of pancreatic cancer. In: Von Hoff DD, Evans DB, Hruban RH (eds) Pancreatic cancer. Jones and Bartiett Publishers, Toronto, pp 251–264

Griffin JF, Smalley SR, Jewell W, Paradelo JC, Reymond RD, Hassanein RE, Evans RG (1990) Patterns of failure after curative resection of pancreatic carcinoma. Cancer 66:56–61

Harewood GC, Wiersema MJ (2002) Endosonography-guided fine needle aspiration biopsy in the evaluation of pancreatic masses. Am J Gastroenterol 97:1386–1391

Higashi T, Saga T, Nakamoto Y, Ishimori T, Mamede MH, Wada M, Doi R, Hosotani R, Imamura M, Konishi J (2002) Relationship between retention index in dual-phase (18)F-FDG PET, and hexokinase-II and glucose transporter-1 expression in pancreatic cancer. J Nucl Med 43:173–180

Higashi T, Saga T, Nakamoto Y, Ishimori T, Fujimoto K, Doi R, Imamura M, Konishi J (2003) Diagnosis of pancreatic cancer using fluorine-18 fluorodeoxyglucose positron emission tomography (FDG PET)—usefulness and limitations in "clinical reality". Ann Nucl Med 17:261–279

Jadvar H, Fischman AJ (2001) Evaluation of pancreatic carcinoma with FDG PET. Abdom Imaging 26:254–259

Lyshchik A, Higashi T, Nakamoto Y, Fujimoto K, Doi R, Imamura M, Saga T (2005) Dual-phase 18F-fluoro-2-deoxy-D-glucose positron emission tomography as a prognostic parameter in patients with pancreatic cancer. Eur J Nucl Med Mol Imaging 32:389–397

Maisey NR, Webb A, Flux GD, Padhani A, Cunningham DC, Ott RJ, Norman A (2000) FDG-PET in the prediction of survival of patients with cancer of the pancreas: a pilot study. Br J Cancer 83:287–293

Meyer W, Jurowich C, Reichel M, Steinhauser B, Wunsch PH, Gebhardt C (2003) Pathomorphological and histological prognostic factors in curatively resected ductal adenocarcinoma of the pancreas. Surg Today 30:582–587

Micke O, Bruns F, Kurowski R, Horst E, deVries AF, Hausler JW, Willich N, Schafer U (2003) Predictive value of carbohydrate antigen 19-9 in pancreatic cancer treated with radiochemotherapy. Int J Radiat Oncol Biol Phys 57:90–97

Miller AB, Hoogstraten B, Staquet M, Winkler A (1981) Reporting results of cancer treatment. Cancer 47:207–214

Mortele KJ, Lemmerling M, de Hemptinne B, De Vos M, De Bock G, Kunnen M (2000) Postoperative findings following the Whipple procedure: determination of prevalence and morphologic abdominal CT features. Eur Radiol 10:123–128

Nakata B, Chung YS, Nishimura S, Nishihara T, Sakurai Y, Sawada T, Okamura T, Kawabe J, Ochi H, Sowa M (1997) 18F-fluorodeoxyglucose positron emission tomography and the prognosis of patients with pancreatic adenocarcinoma. Cancer 79:695–699

Pantalone D, Ragionieri I, Nesi G (2001) Improved survival in small pancreatic cancer. Dig Surg 18:41–46

Riall TS, Cameron JL, Lillemoe KD, Campbell KA, Sauter PK, Coleman J, Abrams RA, Laheru D, Hruban RH, Yeo CJ (2005) Pancreaticoduodenectomy with or without distal gastrectomy and extended retroperitoneal lymphadenectomy for periampullary adenocarcinoma—part 3: update on 5-year survival. J Gastrointest Surg 9:1191–1204

Rose DM, Delbeke D, Beauchamp RD, Chapman WC, Sandler MP, Sharp KW, Richards WO, Wright JK, Frexes ME, Pinson CW, Leach SD (1999) 18Fluorodeoxyglucose-positron emission tomography in the management of patients with suspected pancreatic cancer. Ann Surg 229:729–737

Ruf J, Lopez Hanninen E, Oettle H, Plotkin M, Pelzer U, Stroszczynski C, Felix R, Amthauer H (2005) Detection of recurrent pancreatic cancer: comparison of FDG-PET with CT/MRI. Pancreatology 5:266–272

Scialpi M, Scaglione M, Volterrani L, Lupattelli L, Ragozzino A, Romano S, Rotondo A (2005) Imaging evaluation of post pancreatic surgery. Eur J Radiol 53:417–424

Sperti C, Pasquali C, Chierichetti F, Ferronato A, Decet G, Pedrazzoli S (2003) 8-Fluorodeoxyglucose positron emission tomography in predicting survival of patients with pancreatic carcinoma. J Gastrointest Surg 7:953–959

Therasse P, Arbuck SG, Eisenhauer EA, Wanders J, Kaplan RS, Rubinstein L, Verweij J, Van Glabbeke M, van Oosterom AT, Christian MC, Gwyther SG (2000) New guidelines to evaluate the response to treatment in solid tumors. European Organization for Research and Treatment of Cancer, National Cancer Institute of the United States, National Cancer Institute of Canada. J Natl Cancer Inst 92:205–216

Weber WA, Ott K, Becker K, Dittler HJ, Helmberger H, Avril NE, Meisetschlager G, Busch R, Siewert JR, Schwaiger M, Fink U (2001) Prediction of response to preoperative chemotherapy in adenocarcinomas of the esophagogastric junction by metabolic imaging. J Clin Oncol 19:3058–3065

Young H, Baum R, Cremerius U, Herholz K, Hoekstra O, Lammertsma AA, Pruim J, Price P (1999) Measurement of clinical and subclinical tumor response using [18F]-fluorodeoxyglucose and positron emission tomography: review and 1999 EORTC recommendations. European Organization for Research and Treatment of Cancer PET Study Group. Eur J Cancer 35:1773–1778

Zimny M, Fass J, Bares R, Cremerius U, Sabri O, Buechin P, Schumpelick V, Buell U (2000) Fluorodeoxyglucose positron emission tomography and the prognosis of pancreatic carcinoma. Scand J Gastroenterol 35:883–888

13 Surgical Palliation of Advanced Pancreatic Cancer

M. Bahra, D. Jacob

Recent Results in Cancer Research, Vol. 177

Abstract

In about 80% of patients with pancreatic cancer surgical resection is not feasible at the time of diagnosis. Therefore, palliative treatment plays a key role in the treatment of pancreatic cancer. The defined goals of palliative treatment are: reduction of symptoms, reduction of in-hospital stays, and an adequate control of pain. In patients with nonresectable pancreatic carcinoma the leading goal of palliative strategies should be the control of biliary and duodenal obstructions such as jaundice-associated pruritus or sustained nausea and vomiting due to gastric outlet obstruction. Although the role of endoscopy for palliation has been increasing, operative palliation is still indicated in selected cases. Obstructive jaundice is found in approximately 70% of patients suffering from carcinoma of the pancreatic head at diagnosis and has to be eliminated to avoid progressive liver dysfunction and liver failure. In up to 50% of patients with pancreatic cancer, clinical symptoms such as nausea and vomiting occur. For the treatment of malignant biliary obstructions in patients with pancreatic carcinoma, endoscopic biliary drainage is the option of first choice. In case of persistent stent-problems such as occlusion or recurrent cholangitis, a hepaticojejunostomy should be considered. The role of a prophylactic gastroenterostomy is still under discussion. In patients with combined biliary and gastric obstruction a combined bypass should be performed to avoid a second operation. The significance of laparoscopic biliary bypass is not yet clear. A surgical, minimally invasive approach for treating bile duct obstruction is not the standard nowadays. The role of surgical pain relief is mostly negligible today. Computed tomography (CT)- or EUS-guided celiac plexus neurolysis has replaced surgical intervention today. The significance of palliative resections is currently a controversial topic. However, beyond controlled randomized studies, a palliative pancreaticoduodenectomy in patients with advanced pancreatic carcinoma cannot be recommended at this time.

13.1 Introduction

Considerable advances in the treatment of patients with pancreatic cancer have been reached during recent decades and surgical results after pancreatic head resection have clearly improved in the majority of patients, yet the disease is diagnosed too late for a curative surgical approach [1]. This fact and the aggressiveness of the pancreatic adenocarcinoma are the reasons for the poor overall 5-year survival rate, which has only moderately increased from less than 5% to approx. 7% nowadays. In about 80% of the patients coming to diagnosis with pancreatic carcinoma, palliative therapy is the only treatment option.

Palliative strategies in patients with pancreatic carcinoma focus on three symptoms: pain, duodenal obstruction, and obstructive jaundice, whereby the palliative treatment of these symptoms is primarily directed at reducing the clinical symptoms, reducing the hospital stay, and last but not least ensuring as much overall quality of life as possible. Currently both nonoperative endoscopic procedures and surgical techniques are available to provide palliation of the leading symptoms, and the principal goal of a palliative treatment plan should be tailored to most effectively suit the patients' clinical presentation and their overall physical and mental condition; it should also incorporate the estimated prognosis.

In the past, surgery has been the only treatment option for effective palliation in patients with pancreatic carcinoma. But with the rapid advances in the development of endoscopic techniques, the significance of surgical palliation has declined. The main consideration for avoiding surgical palliation is the morbidity and mortality associated with surgical procedures such as gastroenterostomy, hepaticojejunostomy, and even laparotomy, although the latter occurs only in advanced cancer patients. It remains, however, unclear as to how the value of surgical palliation vs endoscopic palliation may be appropriately judged, and neither life quality investigations nor purely outcome-centered evaluations have so far succeeded in establishing a useful therapeutic algorithm for this severely ill patient population. Hence, decision-making on a palliative strategy for an individual patient remains difficult and may have to be based on an interdisciplinary discussion between the patient, oncologist, therapeutic radiologist, and surgeon.

13.2 Palliative Therapy of Biliary Obstruction: Stent or Surgery?

The surgical options for palliative therapy in biliary obstruction include operative placement of biliary drains such as a T-drainage, choledochoduodenostomy, hepaticojejunostomy, or, in rare cases, a peripheral or distal hepaticojejunostomy (Fig. 13.1). It is important to note that the

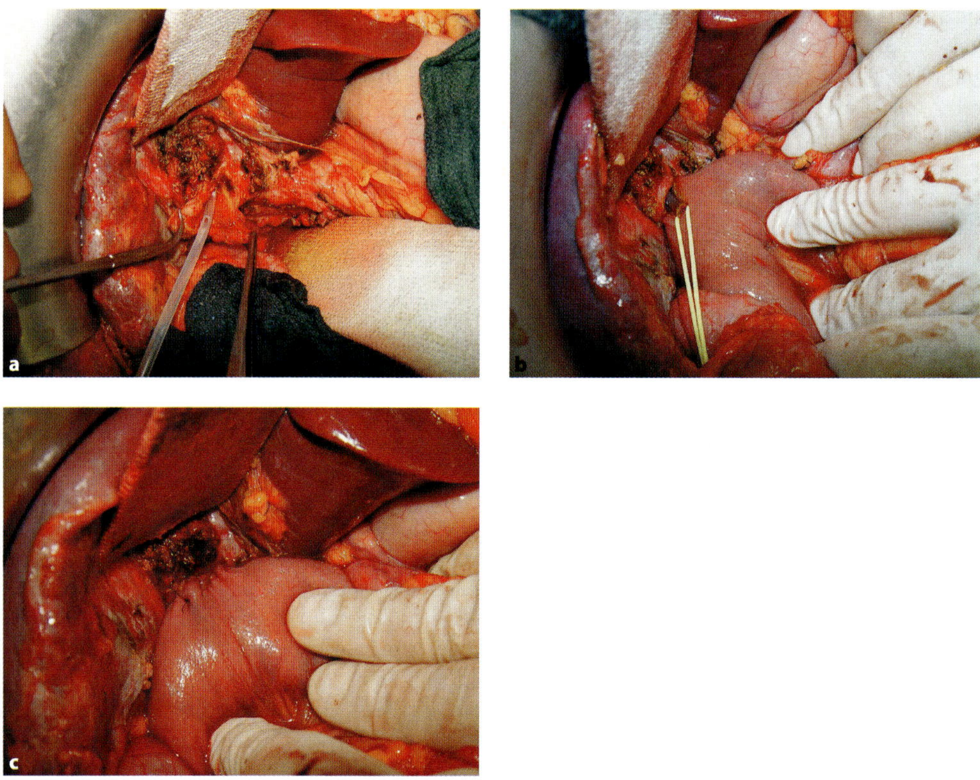

Fig. 13.1a–c In the case of a malignant biliary obstruction associated with persistent stent-problems such as occlusions or recurrent cholangitis, a hepatico-jejunostomy should be considered. The common bile duct has to be anastomosed end-to-side into a jejunal loop. After that, the gastrointestinal continuity has to be restored by standard Roux-Y-reconstruction

often-discussed argument that the placement of a T-drainage is a very small surgical procedure with a low complication rate is, on one hand, correct; however, it has to be considered that this procedure creates an external biliary fistula with all its possible complications and implications for life quality. It should therefore be considered only when other measures of palliative treatment of obstructive jaundice have failed or cannot be undertaken for technical reasons. In addition, the amount of bile loss through such an external biliary fistula may lead to a profound electrolyte and fluid imbalance; hence, in such cases we advocate a simple anastomosis between jejunum and the gallbladder to provide relief of biliary obstruction. The cholecystogastrostomy described in earlier reports may lead to bile gastritis, increased gastrin release, and secondary acid hypersecretion, as well as food entry into the biliary system and subsequent recurrent obstruction or cholangitis (or both) [2]. We therefore have abandoned this procedure along with most other centers experienced in pancreatic surgery.

Hence, the cholecystojejunostomy remains the standard surgical procedure for palliation when the surgical dissection of the hepatoduodenal ligament has to be avoided. If cholecystojejunostomy is chosen, the cystic duct ought to attach a common bile duct and the distance to the tumor mass needs to be at least 2–3 cm to prevent early reobstruction by continuing tumor growth. Several trials have compared cholecystojejunostomy and hepatic enterostomy to evaluate whether the risk of bile duct injuries due to resection of the hepatoduodenal ligament may be avoided. Watanapa et al. [36] found that cholecystoenterostomy yielded a success rate of 89%, which was not significantly different from a success rate of 97% in patients receiving a hepaticoenterostomy. In addition, the authors found that cholangitis and recurrent jaundice were observed in 20% of the cholecystojejunostomy cases, whereas the complication rate in the group with hepaticoenterostomy was higher. The authors concluded that there may be a slightly increased risk of surgical complications when dissecting the hepatoduodenal ligament for hepaticojejunostomy. Furthermore, other authors have indicated that the possible troublesome dissection of the hepatoduodenal ligament may often be avoided when the common bile duct is transected in the middle or lower section and a side-to-side choledochoenterostomy is performed rather than the standard end-to-side hepaticojejunostomy.

Some authors have evaluated the choledochoduodenostomy, which has been proved to be an effective surgical method for treating obstructive jaundice in benign conditions and also has been used in selected cases for biliary reconstruction after orthotopic liver transplantation [3]. However, in the case of pancreatic carcinoma, which has led to jaundice, many surgeons today feel that, in the advanced stages of pancreatic carcinoma (when patients are receiving palliative surgical treatment), an anastomosis in close proximity to the tumor may lead to early restenosis and occurrence of jaundice. Additionally, the peritumoral inflammation usually leads to stiff duodenum, which will not allow attention-free anastomosis, thereby increasing the risk for anastomotic leakage. However, other authors have utilized the choledochoduodenostomy routinely and have shown that the procedure is associated with a lower complication rate, a short length of postoperative hospital stay, and a very low recurrence rate of obstructive jaundice (below 2%). Therefore, since the overall complications rate for the other methods of biliary bypass were higher, they advocate the choledochojejunostomy as the standard method for surgical palliation in obstructive jaundice caused by advanced pancreatic carcinoma [4].

The introduction and development of endoscopic methods of biliary reconstruction reaching from papillotomy to placements of intraductal stents in patients has revolutionized the palliative treatment of patients with obstructive jaundice due to pancreatic cancer. Today endoscopic placement of biliary stents is accepted as a standard treatment in patients with unresectable pancreatic carcinoma. However, the controversy regarding the abdominal palliative treatment—stent or surgery—is still ongoing and undecided. Several prospective randomized trials have compared nonoperative biliary stenting with operative procedures such as hepaticojejunostomy or others. The study by Shepherd et al. did not show a significant difference in complication rate, 30-day mortality rate, incidence of postoperative gastric outlet obstruction, or median survival [5]. However, the rate of recurrent jaundice was significantly higher after biliary stenting compared to the surgical bypass procedure (43% vs. 0%). Furthermore, in a randomized trial Smith et al. demonstrated that recurrent jaundice occurred more often in patients after stent placement than in patients after surgical biliary bypass [6] (Table 13.1).

The main argument for surgical bypass is that the surgical procedure is thought to be a definitive treatment avoiding the regular endoscopic procedures for changing of stents or treating stent complications, which are frequent in this patient population. In addition, many surgeons feel that the definitive palliative surgical procedure is more cost-effective for the same reason. However, a recent study by Artifon and coworkers shows that endoscopic biliary drainage carries lower costs and provides better quality of life when compared to palliative surgical procedures [7]. Again, as in most other studies comparing surgical endoscopic bypass, no difference in the median survival of the investigated groups was found.

Taken together it is still unclear whether there is a standard treatment algorithm to be advocated, since all studies carry the problem of bias in patient selection and the lack of acceptable and validated quality-of-life data. Nevertheless, endoscopic biliary drainage has become the gold standard for palliation of malignant bile duct obstructions in patients with pancreatic carcinoma, and the numbers of surgical palliative procedures have clearly declined. However, surgical options still carry significance. For example, in the case of refractory stent problems such as stent occlusion or recurrent cholangitis, operative stent withdraw and hepaticojejunostomy may be indicated. Furthermore, primary hepaticojejunostomy should be performed in cases of endoscopically impassable tumor masses; finally, if an advanced pancreatic tumor is judged to be nonresectable at laparotomy, a prophylactic hepaticojejunostomy should be considered in patients with obstructive jaundice or in the case of threatening obstructive jaundice. To decide on the optimal treatment strategy for a patient with biliary obstruction due to pancreatic carcinoma, a close collaboration between the surgeon, the endoscopist, and the oncologic specialist is necessary; complicated cases should be managed based on interdisciplinary approaches.

13.3 Palliative Surgery for Gastric Outlet Obstruction Alone or in Combination with Biliary Bypass?

The standard palliative surgical procedure for gastric outlet obstruction due to upper abdominal malignancies is a retro- or antecolic end-to-side or side-to-side gastrojejunostomy. While

Table 13.1 Comparison of nonsurgical and surgical palliative treatment in patients with advanced pancreatic head carcinoma and malignant biliary obstruction. Prospective randomized trials

	Bornman et al. [34]		Shepherd et al. [5]		Andersen et al. [35]		Smith et al. [6]	
	Stent	Surgical bypass	Stent	Surgical bypass	Stent	Surgical bypass	Stent	Surgical bypass
	($n=25$)	($n=25$)	($n=23$)	($n=25$)	($n=25$)	($n=25$)	($n=101$)	($n=100$)
Complications (%)	28	32	24	40	36	20	11	29
30-day mortality	8	20	9	20	20	24	8	15
Median hospital stay (days)	18	14	5	13	26	27	19	26
Recurrent jaundice/ cholangitis (%)	38	16	30	0	28	16	36	2
Median survival (weeks)	19	14	22	18	12	14	21	26

this is normally a simple surgical procedure due to the often marginal clinical condition of the patients in advanced tumor stages, the gastrojejunostomy shows high morbidity and mortality rates [8]. The question of whether a prophylactic gastroenterostomy is rational and should be performed when a normal resectable situation in patients with pancreatic head carcinoma is found at laparotomy is undecided as of yet and under discussion. A recent study by Egrari et al. shows that the mean time to obstruction was 15.7 months compared to a mean overall survival of approx. 13 months in patients with advanced pancreatic carcinoma. The authors demonstrated that due to the rapid natural progression of pancreatic adenocarcinoma, most patients do not survive long enough to obstruct and therefore do not need a prophylactic gastroenterostomy [9].

Today many investigators feel that, due to possible morbidity and mortality, prophylactic gastroenterostomy is unnecessary, and only a selective use of gastroenterostomy should be exercised in the case of present or impending duodenal obstruction that has already led to clinical symptoms. A second area of discussion is the question whether a combination of biliary and gastric bypass is reasonable and profitable for the patient with pancreatic carcinoma in the palliative situation. A French study analyzing 2,493 patients with unresected cancer of the pancreas demonstrated that the mortality in patients with a combination of biliary and gastric bypass was similar [10]. However, they also observed that 16% of the patients undergoing biliary bypass alone developed a gastric obstruction. This finding was confirmed by other groups [11, 12]. Therefore, a number of authors concluded that a combination of biliary and gastric bypass as the initial procedure should be performed, since it minimizes the risk of reoperation and provides definitive palliation [10, 13]. To create a gastrojejunostomy in addition to a surgical bypass of biliary obstruction is not a technical challenge for experienced general surgeons and today is associated with low morbidity and mortality rates. However, the decision for an initial combination of biliary and gastric bypass depends on several factors such as preexisting gastric outlet obstruction at the time of operation, imminent gastric obstruction, the overall condition of the patient, tumor stage, and tumor biology (Fig. 13.2).

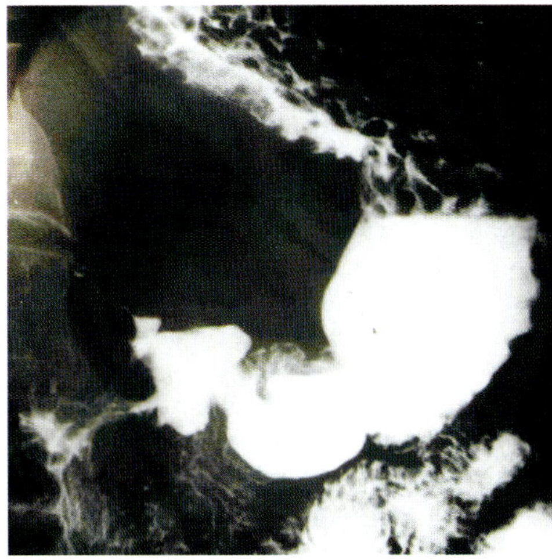

Fig. 13.2 Gastric outlet obstruction due to duodenal stenosis in a patient with advanced nonresectable pancreatic carcinoma. This patient will benefit from a gastroenteric bypass. If the obstruction is diagnosed prior to an intended hepaticojejunostomy, an initial combined biliary and gastric bypass should be considered

As stated above, the best therapeutic strategy and the surgical method chosen for an individual patient should be discussed with consideration for all clinical factors defining the individual patient; when surgical options are considered, it seems important to underline that for patients with unresectable pancreatic cancer who present clinically manifest gastric obstruction at admission, the median survival often may be as little as 4 weeks, even when newer oncologic treatment concepts are initiated [14]. This may be an important argument for an initial combined biliary and gastric bypass to ensure that such patients have the chance to leave the hospital with immediately effected palliation.

13.4 Minimally Invasive Procedures for Surgical Palliation

Throughout the last few decades, minimally invasive procedures for palliative surgery have been reported in increasing numbers. This holds true also for palliative biliary and gastric bypass procedures, and today a considerable number laparoscopic gastric and biliary bypasses for periampullary carcinomas have been reported in the literature [15, 16]. In these studies, laparoscopic techniques are either performed as cholecystojejunostomies or hepaticojejunostomies to create a biliary bypass. The possible advantages of minimally invasive surgical approaches seem obvious since especially in those severely ill patients the trauma of the surgical procedure and the time of hospital stay are very important factors. However, some possible disadvantages of the minimally invasive procedures have to be considered. The mean operating time seems to be significantly longer compared to standard open surgical procedures, thereby increasing the surgical trauma. Furthermore, special laparoscopic expertise is required to ensure a low complication rate, since both a hepaticojejunostomy and gastroenterostomy are considered advanced laparoscopic procedures. Today, endoscopic stenting via endoscopic retrograde cholangiography is the gold standard for palliation in patients with malignant bile duct obstruction due to carcinoma of the pancreatic head, and although several authors reported results for laparoscopic biliary bypass in single patients, no prospective randomized study comparing laparoscopic surgery vs stenting has yet been reported. The first choice of treatment in patients with bile duct obstruction due to pancreatic cancer should therefore be the endoscopic stenting. If indicated (based on repeated stent occlusions or recurrent cholangitis), surgical intervention regardless of the surgical technique should be discussed. During this discussion it has to be considered that the laparoscopic biliary bypass is not a standard minimally invasive procedure and only experts in the field of laparoscopy should perform such operations in this very ill patient population.

In a small group of patients, Kazanjian et al. demonstrated that laparoscopic gastrojejunostomy is a safe and effective palliation for patients with gastric outlet obstruction due to pancreatic carcinoma. In their analysis it was especially significant in a group of patients with a very limited survival [17]. In addition, a group from Norway compared open vs laparoscopic gastrojejunostomy for palliation in advanced pancreatic cancer retrospectively and found that laparoscopic gastrojejunostomy in advanced cases offered a reduced estimated blood loss and a shortened hospital stay when compared to open gastrojejunostomy [18]. Hence, at this time minimally invasive procedures using standardized techniques should be considered for relief of gastric outlet obstruction due to pancreatic carcinoma when the laparoscopic expertise is present. In this situation a low complication rate can be ensured and the minimally invasive techniques might be a viable alternative for open surgical procedures, especially in patients with a very limited prognosis [19].

13.5 Role of Surgical Pain Relief

The surgeons treating patients with advanced pancreatic head carcinoma have to keep in mind that quality of life is the most important factor for these patients who have such a dire prognosis. In this context, pain is the most feared symptom for a majority of the patients and for many of them pain constitutes a clinically significant problem until death; pain management is troublesome.

Pain fibers from the pancreatic gland (the celiac ganglion) run within the major and minor splanchnic nerves to the spinal column. An interruption of this pathway can provide pain relief, and such a disruption can be accomplished by either targeting the abdominal or the thoracic cavity. The first intraoperative chemical splanchnicectomy was introduced by Copping and colleagues in 1969 [20]. In their clinical experience reported almost 10 year later, approximately 90% of patients with pain at diagnosis experienced significant relief after intraoperative chemical splanchnicectomy [21]. Since then many investigators have utilized this method, and Lillemoe and coworkers reported in a randomized controlled trial that intraoperative chemical splanchnicectomy with 50% alcohol significantly reduced or prevented pain in patients with unresectable pancreatic cancer [22]. In contrast, van Geenen and coworkers from Amsterdam could not confirm these findings. In their randomized study, patients were divided into three groups: (1) palliative bypass surgery receiving intraoperative celiac plexus blockade, (2) palliative bypass surgery without celiac plexus blockade but followed by high-dose conformal radiotherapy, and (3) palliative bypass surgery with both (celiac plexus blockade, followed by high-dose conformal radiotherapy). They concluded that celiac plexus blockade for pain management did not result in an increase to pain medication-free survival and therefore presumed that celiac plexus blockade could not demonstrate a positive effect on pain management for the patients with advanced pancreatic carcinoma [23]. To disrupt the pain neuropathway, splanchnic nerves within the thorax could also be interrupted. This can be accomplished either via thoracotomy or via video-assisted thoracoscopy (VATS) [24, 25]. In recent times, the plexus blockade has been reached via nonsurgical interventions, namely using endoscopic ultrasound (EUS) or wild-guided techniques. A prospective study of the EUS-guided celiac plexus neurolysis for pain treatment in patients with advanced pancreatic head cancer showed that the technique is safe and yields pain control [26]. In light of such nonsurgical alternatives for celiac plexus blockage, the role of surgical pain relief seems to be marginal nowadays. However, in selected patients, namely who are not responding to noninvasive methods of plexus blockade, a surgical intervention may still be indicated.

13.6 Palliative Resection: Does It Play a Role?

Adenocarcinoma of the pancreatic head is considered one of the gastrointestinal malignancies with the worst prognosis. If no standardized operative procedures have been established (classical Kausch-Whipple resection, pylorus preserving pancreatic head resection) the overall 5-year survival rate of patients with pancreatic head carcinoma today is estimated to be approx. 5%, and the 5-year survival rate after curative resection reaches approx. 20% in specialized centers around the world [27, 28]. However, differing from earlier reports, the perioperative mortality has decreased significantly during the last few decades, and today morbidity rates around 15% and mortality rates below 3% for standardized pancreatic head resection have been reached in high-volume centers. This fact and the consideration that the patient with pancreatic head carcinoma in the majority of cases presents in stage 3, in which advanced disease is present and undetected further tumor spread has to be expected, many investigators today believe that real curative resections are rare events. Further arguments on this line are supported by the results of recent multicenter trials in adjuvant chemotherapy after R0 or R1 resections for pancreatic head carcinoma showing that even the patients with R1 resection profit considerably from postoperative adjuvant therapy [29]. Therefore, oncologists have long proposed that the pancreatic head resection for a defined tumor no longer be termed a curative resection, since in most of the cases advanced stages of the disease are present. Many investigators today believe that all resections for pancreatic head carcinoma are, in principle, palliative. Following this argument, the goal of the resection may change much more toward reaching quality of life for the patients, as with other palliative procedures.

At present no prospective data are available in which a palliative resection was investigated in a randomized fashion. Several authors have reported about retrospective data comparing palliative procedures (biliary and gastric bypasses combined or alone) with pancreatic resections [30]. Lillemoe et al. investigated the role of palliative resection compared to combined biliary and gastric bypass, showing a significant improved overall survival for patients undergoing palliative pancreaticoduodenectomy. All patients were patients in which, after transecting the pancreas (passing the point of no return during pancreatic head surgery), nonresectability was found in the retro-pancreatico-duodenal plane [31]. However, in this study no further subdivisions regarding the R-status was accomplished. In another study, Reinders et al. compared patients after a microscopically nonradical pancreaticoduodenectomy with patients after surgical bypass [32]. Both studies neither evaluated the quality of life nor the long-term follow-up criteria and only showed that the so-called palliative pancreaticoduodenectomy procedures yield significantly better results and longer survival than ones in which patients received surgical bypass, leaving their primary tumor mass in place. In one recent study the investigators compared patients in a palliative situation undergoing double loop bypass surgery with patients undergoing palliative pancreaticoduodenectomy. Special emphasis was laid on the investigation of quality of life in this study. All patients undergoing bypass were subgrouped into those with locally advanced disease and those with metastasized diseased. The 1-year survival was 25% in the palliative resected group vs 20% in the locally advanced and 15% in the metastasized disease group. The quality-of-life data were favorable for the patients after bypass surgery; however, the morbidity and mortality rates in patients after palliative resection were elevated [33].

These results prompted us to propose a study in which the role of the palliative resection itself should be evaluated. Following extensive interdisciplinary discussions with gastroenterologists and oncologists, we derived a protocol in which patients with carcinomas of the pancreatic head that had already metastasized into the liver at diagnosis and revealed a resectable situation were randomized into two groups. One group would receive standard gemcitabine chemotherapy until tumor progression, whereas the other group would receive a pancreatic head resection with or without liver resection and subsequently standard gemcitabine treatment until tumor progression. The liver resection was only to be performed when resections could provide a significant tumor mass reduction because the additional surgical risk to the pancreatic head procedure was to be avoided This study is now underway (and hopefully open for recruitment) and we will be able to analyze the results in the near future.

Palliative pancreatic head resections outside of accepted study protocols should not be performed since the significant additional clinical risk of complications for morbidity and mortality is not acceptable; they must only be performed in the framework of randomized prospective trails.

13.7 Summary

For the treatment of malignant biliary obstructions in patients with pancreatic carcinoma, endoscopic biliary drainage is the option of first choice. In case of persistent stent-problems such as occlusion or recurrent cholangitis, a hepaticojejunostomy should be considered. The role of a prophylactic gastroenterostomy is still under discussion. In selected patients with duodenal stenosis present at the time of operation, or patients with impending duodenal obstruction, a prophylactic gastroenteric bypass may be indicated. The same should be considered for patients showing a duodenal stenosis during an operation for biliary obstruction. In such patients an initial combined biliary and gastric bypass should be performed to avoid a second operation for gastric outlet obstruction. The significance of laparoscopic biliary bypass is not yet clear. A surgical, minimally invasive approach for treating bile duct obstruction is not the standard nowadays, and it should be reserved for experts in the field of laparoscopy. Otherwise, laparoscopic gastrojejunostomy is a standardized surgical procedure that offers significant advantages in regards to morbidity and mortality compared to open surgical techniques. The role of surgical pain relief is mostly negligible today. Computed tomography (CT)- or EUS-guided celiac plexus neurolysis have replaced surgical interventions. The significance of palliative resections is a controversial topic nowadays. However, beyond controlled randomized studies, a palliative pancreaticoduodenectomy in patients with advanced pancreatic carcinoma cannot be recommended at this time.

References

1. Flanders TY, Foulkes WD (1996) Pancreatic adenocarcinoma: epidemiology and genetics. J Med Genet 33:889–898
2. Cagetti M, Nicolosi A, Dazzi C (1984) Cholecystogastrostomy versus choledochoduodenostomy in non-resectable carcinoma of the head of the pancreas [in Italian]. Minerva Chir 39:1069–1072
3. Schmitz V, Neumann UP, Puhl G, et al. (2006) Surgical complications and long-term outcome of different biliary reconstructions in liver transplantation for primary sclerosing cholangitis-choledochoduodenostomy versus choledochojejunostomy. Am J Transplant 6:379–385
4. Potts JR 3rd, Broughan TA, Hermann RE (1990) Palliative operations for pancreatic carcinoma. Am J Surg 159:72–77

5. Shepherd HA, Royle G, Ross AP, et al. (1988) Endoscopic biliary endoprosthesis in the palliation of malignant obstruction of the distal common bile duct: a randomized trial. Br J Surg 75:1166–1168
6. Smith AC, Dowsett JF, Russell RC, et al. (1994) Randomised trial of endoscopic stenting versus surgical bypass in malignant low bileduct obstruction. Lancet 344:1655–1660
7. Artifon EL, Sakai P, Cunha JE, et al. (2006) Surgery or endoscopy for palliation of biliary obstruction due to metastatic pancreatic cancer. Am J Gastroenterol 101:2031–2037
8. Weaver DW WM, Bowmann DL, Walt A (1987) Gastrojejunostomy: is it helpful for patients with pancreatic cancer? Surgery 102:608–613
9. Egrari S, O'Connell TX (1995) Role of prophylactic gastroenterostomy for unresectable pancreatic carcinoma. Am Surg 61:862–864
10. Huguier M, Baumel H, Manderscheid JC, et al. (1993) Surgical palliation for unresected cancer of the exocrine pancreas. Eur J Surg Oncol 19:342–347
11. Nardi GL (1984) Pancreatic cancer and palliative gastroenterostomy. Am J Surg 147:839–840
12. Singh SM, Reber HA (1989) Surgical palliation for pancreatic cancer. Surg Clin North Am 69:599–611
13. Neuberger TJ, Wade TP, Swope TJ, et al. (1993) Palliative operations for pancreatic cancer in the hospitals of the U.S. Department of Veterans Affairs from 1987 to 1991. Am J Surg 166:632–636
14. Thomson BN, Banting SW, Gibbs P (2006) Pancreatic cancer—current management. Aust Fam Physician 35:212–217
15. Kuriansky J, Saenz A, Astudillo E, et al. (2000) Simultaneous laparoscopic biliary and retrocolic gastric bypass in patients with unresectable carcinoma of the pancreas. Surg Endosc 14:179–181
16. Rhodes M, Nathanson L, Fielding G (1995) Laparoscopic biliary and gastric bypass: a useful adjunct in the treatment of carcinoma of the pancreas. Gut 36:778–780
17. Kazanjian KK, Reber HA, Hines OJ (2004) Laparoscopic gastrojejunostomy for gastric outlet obstruction in pancreatic cancer. Am Surg 70:910–913
18. Bergamaschi R, Marvik R, Thoresen JE, et al. (1998) Open versus laparoscopic gastrojejunostomy for palliation in advanced pancreatic cancer. Surg Laparosc Endosc 8:92–96
19. Adler DG, Baron TH (2002) Endoscopic palliation of malignant gastric outlet obstruction using self-expanding metal stents: experience in 36 patients. Am J Gastroenterol 97:72–78
20. Copping J, Willix R, Kraft R (1969) Palliative chemical splanchnicectomy. Arch Surg 98:418–420
21. Flanigan DP, Kraft RO (1978) Continuing experience with palliative chemical splanchnicectomy. Arch Surg 113:509–511
22. Lillemoe KD, Cameron JL, Kaufman HS, et al. (1993) Chemical splanchnicectomy in patients with unresectable pancreatic cancer. A prospective randomized trial. Ann Surg 217:447–455
23. van Geenen RC, Keyzer-Dekker CM, van Tienhoven G, et al. (2002) Pain management of patients with unresectable peripancreatic carcinoma. World J Surg 26:715–720
24. Giraudo G, Kazemier G, Van Eijck CH, Bonjer HJ (1999) Endoscopic palliative treatment of advanced pancreatic cancer: thoracoscopic splanchnicectomy and laparoscopic gastrojejunostomy. Ann Oncol 10 [Suppl 4]:278–280
25. Krishna S, Chang VT, Shoukas JA, Donahoo J (2001) Video-assisted thoracoscopic sympathectomy-splanchnicectomy for pancreatic cancer pain. J Pain Symptom Manage 22:610–616
26. Gunaratnam NT, Sarma AV, Norton ID, Wiersema MJ (2001) A prospective study of EUS-guided celiac plexus neurolysis for pancreatic cancer pain. Gastrointest Endosc 54:316–324
27. Geer RJ, Brennan MF (1993) Prognostic indicators for survival after resection of pancreatic adenocarcinoma. Am J Surg 165:68–72
28. Yeo CJ, Cameron JL, Lillemoe KD, et al. (1995) Pancreaticoduodenectomy for cancer of the head of the pancreas. 201 patients. Ann Surg 221:721–731
29. Neuhaus P, Oettle H, Post S, et al. (2005) A randomised, prospective, multicenter, phase III trial of adjuvant chemotherapy with gemcitabine vs. observation in patients with resected pancreatic cancer. ASCO Abstr LBA4013
30. Sohn TA, Lillemoe KD, Cameron JL, et al. (1999) Surgical palliation of unresectable periampullary adenocarcinoma in the 1990s. J Am Coll Surg 188:658–666
31. Lillemoe KD, Sauter PK, Pitt HA, et al. (1993) Current status of surgical palliation of periampullary carcinoma. Surg Gynecol Obstet 176:1–10

32. Reinders ME, Allema JH, van Gulik TM, et al. (1995) Outcome of microscopically nonradical, subtotal pancreaticoduodenectomy (Whipple‘s resection) for treatment of pancreatic head tumors. World J Surg 19:410–414
33. Schniewind B, Bestmann B, Kurdow R, et al. (2006) Bypass surgery versus palliative pancreaticoduodenectomy in patients with advanced ductal adenocarcinoma of the pancreatic head, with an emphasis on quality of life analyses. Ann Surg Oncol 13:1403–1411
34. Bornman PC, Harries-Jones EP, Tobias R, et al. (1986) Prospective controlled trial of transhepatic biliary endoprosthesis versus bypass surgery for incurable carcinoma of head of pancreas. Lancet 1:69–71
35. Andersen JR, Sorensen SM, Kruse A, et al. (1989) Randomised trial of endoscopic endoprosthesis versus operative bypass in malignant obstructive jaundice. Gut 30:1132–1135
36. Watanapa P, Williamson RC (1992) Surgical palliation for pancreatic cancer: developments during the past two decades. Br J Surg 79:8–20

Part III New Treatment Strategies and Outlook

14 Antiangiogenic Strategies in Pancreatic Cancer

H. Riess

Recent Results in Cancer Research, Vol. 177

Abstract

Since the introduction of gemcitabine in the treatment of pancreatic cancer, progress in the use of combination chemotherapies has been very limited. Of the different novel options, antiangiogenic treatment strategies are among those being intensively studied in preclinical and clinical settings of adenocarcinoma of the pancreas. Phase I and limited-size phase II studies using drugs with antiangiogenic properties have reported encouraging results. Overall, the results of phase III studies with some metalloprotease inhibitors and bevacizumab have so far failed to demonstrate a survival benefit for these drugs. Further investigations that will take into account the heterogeneity of pancreatic cancer are warranted using these or other antiangiogenic active substances.

14.1 Introduction

Targeted therapies inhibiting specific pathways that facilitate the growth and progress of malignant tumors are under intensive investigation in oncology. So far, several agents developed to inhibit tumor angiogenesis have been evaluated in clinical studies [11, 20]. In this context advanced adenocarcinoma of the pancreas represents a malignancy worth studying.

The highly aggressive nature of pancreatic cancer may be due to the expression of growth factors, resulting in high intrinsic tyrosine kinase activities that stimulate cell proliferation, dissemination, and neoangiogenesis. A number of studies have indicated that angiogenesis involves several cytokines such as vascular endothelial growth factor (VEGF), basic fibroblast growth factor (bFGF), and angiopoietin 1 [1, 4, 21, 28]. VEGF and bFGF are clearly overexpressed in pancreatic cancer and result in accelerated tumor growth [29, 46]. The cellular effects of these factors are mediated by specific cell surface receptors with intrinsic tyrosine kinase activities.

The results of qualitative and semiquantitative assessments of VEGF and VEGF receptor expressions in pancreatic cancer have been confirmed by quantitative methods, demonstrating that VEGF and its two principal receptors were expressed in adenocarcinomas of the pancreas [8, 9]. These expressions vary in different individual tumors, but a significant association was found between expression of VEGF-R2 and poor prognosis, suggesting that VEGF-R2 expression is a marker of more aggressive disease [8]. Both VEGF and VEGF-receptors are overexpressed in pancreatic cancer, and the degree of expression correlates with microvessel density and poor prognosis [40]. This is true not only in advanced metastatic pancreatic adenocarcinoma but also for early recurrences after curatively intended resection [37].

In preclinical models, inhibition of VEGF decreased pancreatic cancer growth by inhibition of neovascularization and lymphangiogenesis [4, 9, 31]. In addition, VEGF inhibition decreases interstitial pressure within the tumor and thereby increases the delivery of chemotherapeutic agents, suggesting an additive effect of antiangiogenic and conventional cytotoxic therapies [4, 50].

In addition to synergistic interactions with other treatment modalities, inhibition of tumor angiogenesis theoretically offers several benefits such as a lack of severe toxicities familiar to cytotoxic therapies, a lack of tumor resistance, and thus a potent antitumor effect. It has been demonstrated that a disruption of VEGF signaling, for example by the use of neutralizing antibodies, slows tumor growth in preclinical models. It is important to realize that the antiangiogenetic suppression of VEGF signaling targets the nutritional support of tumor cells by inhibiting blood vessel formation.

Treatment with inhibitors of angiogenesis most likely will prevent tumor progression, facilitate tumor cell killing by cytotoxic agents, radiation, or immunological strategies, and may induce tumor cell senescence and stimulate apoptosis. In addition to the antitumor efficacy of antiangiogenic agents demonstrated in patients with different tumor types and the antitumor effect of cytotoxic drugs, the combination may result in a supra-additive effect.

While an increasing number of new drugs for antiangiogenetic strategies have been developed, it has become clear that the classical cytotoxic drug that is effective in the treatment of patients with pancreatic cancer, gemcitabine, may have antiangiogenetic effects too.

14.2 Results in Preclinical Models or Phase I Studies in Patients

Small molecule tyrosine kinase inhibitors such as PD173074 block VEGF-R2 as well as bFGF-R1 signaling, thus showing antiangiogenetic and antimitogenic activities and abrogating two important pathways in cancer growth and metastasis [9]. In human pancreatic cancer cell lines, PD173074 inhibited cell growth in correlation with the level of bFGF-R1 expression of the tumor cells. This resulted in the inhibition of cell cycle progression at the G0/G1 transmission point with a consecutive increase in apoptosis [9, 11, 20]. In a model of xenografted human pancreatic cancer cells, inhibition of orthotopic tumor growth was achieved most likely by a combination of inhibited mitogenesis, increased apoptosis, and reduced angiogenesis in PD173074-treated animals. This study showed that a high-dose single drug treatment may have clinically relevant therapeutic activity, but data in patients are not yet available.

The concept of creating synergistic antitumor effects by the combined inhibition of several pathways through the use of combination therapies [such as by inhibiting the epidermal growth factor receptor (EGFR) and the VEGF-receptor pathways using different drugs] represents an attractive approach. Indeed, clinical studies in patients with advanced colorectal cancer have shown an additive affect of such a combination with regard to response, progression-free survival, and overall survival using the anti-VEGF bevacizumab and the anti-EGFR cetuximab. This approach has been clinically tested in patients with pancreatic cancer too, but results are not yet available [33].

Using multikinase inhibitors such as sorafenib—thus targeting several pathways, including VEGF signaling, via a single molecule, and thus showing antiangiogenetic properties in preclinical models—is an alternative treatment strategy to the combination of drugs. The treatment option with sorafenib has been demonstrated in preclinical models and in early clinical studies to have activity against several tumor types including adenocarcinoma of the pancreas.

Matrix metalloproteinases (MMP) are different proteolytic enzymes responsible for the breakdown of connective tissue proteins [12]. They play an important role in growth regulation, differentiation, tumor cell spread, and tissue repair. The activity of MMP is highly regulated at different levels. Preclinical and clinical data show that MMP overexpression correlates with increased tumor cell growth and spread in several malignancies [26, 38, 41]. Inhibition of MMP and restoring the normal balance of proteolytic activity may prevent tumor growth and metastasis [13, 18, 49]. A low molecular weight MMPinhibitor, marimastat, has been demonstrated to inhibit tumor growth and spread in preclinical cancer models [48, 49] including human pancreatic cancer.

The mammalian target of rapamycin (mTOR) is a serine-threonine kinase with important effects on the regulation of cell growth and proliferation [17]. In a preclinical model of human pancreatic cancer rapamycin alone and, more actively, its combination with an anti-VEGF antibody strongly inhibited primary and metastatic tumor growth [42]. In this investigation combination therapy improved the effect of single agent treatments. Rapamycin in combination with anti-VEGF antibody inhibited pancreatic tumor cell proliferation, induced apoptosis, and decreased tumor angiogenesis. A clinical trial with rapamycin in pancreatic cancer is ongoing.

14.3 Clinical Studies in Patients with Pancreatic Adenocarcinoma

There are several different antiangiogenic treatment strategies that have been investigated in patients with pancreatic cancer. These include the matrix metalloproteinase inhibitors, agents interfering with the VEGF signaling pathway, and several others such as thalidomide, cyclooxygenase II inhibitors, and EGFR inhibitors.

14.3.1 Matrix Metalloproteinase Inhibitors

A randomized dose-finding study [5] comparing single agent marimastat, a low molecular weight, broad-spectrum MMP inhibitor, with gemcitabine demonstrated a clear dose-response effect for marimastat, with 1-year survival rates of marimastat at a dose of 25 mg b.i.d. similar to that of gemcitabine, whereas the lower doses (5 and 10 mg b.i.d.) were clearly less effective than gemcitabine.

Another prospective randomized study [6] comparing marimastat (10 mg b.i.d.) in combination with gemcitabine to gemcitabine plus placebo in 269 patients with advanced pancreatic cancer failed to demonstrate a significant survival benefit by the addition of marimastat (median survival 165.5 vs 164 days; 1-year survival 18% vs 17%). Grade 3 or 4 musculoskeletal toxicity, a well-known adverse event of marimastat therapy, was reported in less than 5% of the patients.

Due to this study, the further development of marimastat in this indication was stopped.

BAY 12-9566, another MMP inhibitor with antiangiogenetic properties, is well tolerated and showed antitumor activity in a phase I study in pancreatic adenocarcinoma [19, 22, 24, 25]. A phase III study [36] comparing head-to-head BAY 12-9566 (800 mg b.i.d.) with gemcitabine enrolled 277 patients. In this study the median survival of the MMP inhibitor was demonstrated to be significantly inferior to gemcitabine (3.74 vs 6.59 months).

14.3.2 VEGF Pathway Inhibition

Bevacizumab, a recombinant anti-VEGF monoclonal antibody, first demonstrated significant improvement in response, progression-free survival, and overall-survival in a phase III randomized trial in patients with advanced colorectal cancer, when combined with cytotoxic drugs (bevacizumab 5 mg/kg every second week, together with folinic acid, 5-fluorouracil and irinotecan) [27]. Based on these findings and some evidence of clinical efficacy in pancreatic cancer but without a cancer-specific dose-finding investigation, a phase II study [32] in 52 patients with advanced pancreatic adenocarcinoma combining bevacizumab (10 mg/kg every second week) with gemcitabine as the first-line treatment was initiated. Of the patients, 21% achieved a partial response and another 46% of patients had stable disease resulting in a median progression-free survival of 5.4 months and a median overall survival of 8.8 months—results clearly better than those usually reported for single-agent gemcitabine. Grade 3 and 4 toxicities included hypertension and thrombosis in 19% and 13% of the patients, respectively. Intestinal perforations occured in 8% and bleeding in 2%. There was no correlation observed between pretreatment VEGF plamsa levels and response to anti-VEGF therapy.

Due to these results, a phase III trial [34] of gemcitabine plus bevacizumab as compared to gemcitabine plus placebo was initiated by the cancer and leukemia group B (CALGB) but stopped recruitment after an interim analysis showing that there was no chance of reaching the primary study endpoint of a significant prolongation of overall survival due to the addition of bevacizumab. Accordingly, the first study results presented at the American Society of Clinical Oncology (ASCO)-GI 2007 symposium do not support the superiority of bevacizumab plus gemcitabine: median survival of the 302 patients on bevacizumab and gemcitabine was 5.7 months as compared to 6.0 months for the 300 patients on placebo and gemcitabine.

There is some discussion with regard to the 10 mg/kg of bevacizumab given every 2 weeks used in this trial, as studies in colorectal cancer had demonstrated clinical activity with lower doses (5 mg/kg every 2 weeks) of bevacizumab. On the other hand (interestingly too) there was no increase in gastrointestinal perforations (0% vs 0%) or grade 3/4 bleedings (3% vs 2%) reported for the experimental arm.

Despite the fact that single agent gemcitabine is standard therapy for patients with advanced pancreatic cancer [10], there are several hints in favor of combination chemotherapy in this indication too. This is true especially for the combination of gemcitabine with platin or fluoropyrimidine derivates. Premature results of ongoing multicenter phase II studies reported response rates of 11%–22% and median overall survival times of 7.5 to 8.9 months when bevacizumab was added to gemcitabine/oxaliplatin, gemcitabine/cisplatin, or gemcitabine/capecitabine chemotherapy [30, 35, 44]. In these studies severe toxicities with regard to perforations, bleeding, and thromboembolism have been reported. Final study results will be reported soon and may warrant new phase III studies.

Due to the risk of visceral perforation, bleeding, and thrombosis, most likely due to the comedication with bevacizumab, patients with locally advanced pancreatic cancer with duodenal involvement are excluded in most phase II study of bevacizumab plus radiation therapy in locally advanced nonmetastasized pancreatic cancer. A dose-finding study [14] for bevacizumab together with capecitabine (825 mg/m^2 b.i.d. 5 days a week) and concomitant to radiation therapy with 50 Gy was initiated in patients with locally advanced pancreatic adenocarcinoma. The addition of bevacizumab did not increase the acute toxicity of this radiochemotherapy as compared to historical controls. An overall response rate of 19% was obtained with 6 out of 12 patients, demonstrating a partial response at the 5 mg/kg level of bevacizumab.

14.3.3 Other Antiangiogenic Strategies

14.3.3.1 Thalidomide

Thalidomide has shown antitumor activities in several malignancies, especially hematological neoplasms such as multiple myeloma [45]. In addition, in renal cell carcinoma, prostate cancer, and hepatocellular cancer, antitumor effects have been reported [43]. The antitumor effect of thalidomide is not clearly understood [16]. In addition to inhibition of tumor necrosis factor alpha, clinical efficacy may be mediated, at least in part, by anti-VEGF effects. A phase I/II clinical study [15] of combination therapy with gemcitabine, celecoxib (400 mg b.i.d.), and thalidomide (200–300 mg o.d.) resulted in no tumor regression, but a mean overall survival of 10 months was reported. Treatment was clinically tolerable with skin rash in 25% of the patients.

Another 50 patients with advanced pancreatic adenocarcinoma who had a weight loss of at least 10% were randomized to receive thalidomide (200 mg daily) or placebo in a single-center double-blind randomized controlled trial [23]. At 4 weeks, 17 patients on thalidomide gained an average of 0.37 kg compared to a loss of 2.21 kg in 16 controls. At 8 week, 12 patients on thalidomide lost 0.06 kg vs 3.62 kg in 8 controls. In this study, data on tumor response are not available.

14.3.3.2 Inhibition of Epidermal Growth Factor Receptor

EGFR is a well-recognized target of anticancer therapy [2]. Monoclonal antibodies and small molecule tyrosine kinase inhibitors have been shown to be active in different cancers and have obtained approval. Results obtained with this treatment strategy are reported elsewhere in this issue of *Recent Results in Cancer Research.* Furthermore, the first results of a randomized phase II study [33] comparing gemcitabine/bevacizumab together with erlotinib or cetuximab suggest an increase in response rate (ca. 20%) by the use of triple drug therapies.

If this holds true will soon become evident, as the results of a major phase III study, the combination of gemcitabine/erlotinib together with bevacizumab or placebo, will be reported.

14.3.3.3 Cyclooxygenase 2 Inhibition

Cyclooxygenase (Cox 2) stimulates tumor growth by its proangiogenic and apoptosis-inhibiting effects. Celecoxib, a specific Cox 2 inhibitor, has antitumor activity against several human cancers in preclinical models, including pancreatic cancer xenograft [3, 39, 47, 53].

There were 28 patients included in a phase II study [52] evaluating the role of celecoxib in addition to gemcitabine in advanced pancreatic cancer. The results of 20 patients were presented on the annual meeting of the ASCO in 2006 and showed a median overall survival of 6.2 months—not dramatically different from results expected for gemcitabine alone. Grade 3 or 4 nonhematological toxicities included nausea, vomiting, supraventricular arrhythmias, dyspnea, pleural effusions, and hyponatremia, as well as gastrointestinal bleeding in one patient.

Further evaluation of this agent has been stopped due to cardiac toxicity possibly caused by celecoxib [7].

14.4 Conclusions

Adenocarcinoma of the pancreas remains a major cause of cancer morbidity and mortality worldwide. Recent results confirm that the dismal prognosis of patients can be improved by small steps. Still, there is an urgent need for novel treatment strategies. In contrast to anti-EGFR targeted, small-molecule therapy, the first large clinical trials failed to prove the effectivity of other antiangiogenic strategies in combination with gemcitabine in this indication. Nevertheless, stimulated by the results with erlotinib, antiangiogenic treatment options continue to be among those most likely to further improve the prognosis in this tumor entity.

References

1. Bachelder RE, Lipscomb EA, Lin X, Wendt MA, Chadborn NH, Eickholt BJ, Mercurio AM (2003) Competing autocrine pathways involving alternative neuropilin-1 ligands regulate chemotaxis of carcinoma cells. Cancer Res 63:5230–5233
2. Baker CH, Solorzano CC, Fidler IJ (2002) Blockade of vascular endothelial growth factor receptor and epidermal growth factor receptor signaling for therapy of metastatic human pancreatic cancer. Cancer Res 2002 62:1996–2003
3. Blanquicett C, Saif MW, Buchsbaum DJ, Eloubeidi M, Vickers SM, Chhieng DC, et al. (2005) Antitumor efficacy of capecitabine and celecoxib in irradiated and lead-shielded, contralateral human BxPC-3 pancreatic cancer xenografts: clinical implications of abscopal effects. Clin Cancer Res 11:8773–8781
4. Bockhorn M, Tsuzuki Y, Xu L, et al. (2003) Differential vascular and transcriptional responses to anti-vascular endothelial growth factor antibody in orthotopic human pancreatic cancer xenografts. Clin Cancer Res 9:4221–4226
5. Bramhall SR, Rosemurgy A, Brown PD, Bowry C, et al. (2001) Marimastat as first-line therapy for patients with unresectable pancreatic cancer: a randomized trial. J Clin Oncol 19:3447–3455
6. Bramhall SR, Schulz J, Nemunaitis J, Brown PD, Baillet M, Buckels JA (2002) A double-blind placebo-controlled, randomised study comparing gemcitabine and marimastat with gemcitabine and placebo as first line therapy in patients with advanced pancreatic cancer. Br J Cancer 87:161–167
7. Brophy JM (2005) Celecoxib and cardiovascular risks. Expert Opin Drug Saf 4:1005–1015
8. Buchler P, Reber HA, Buchler MW, et al. (2002) VEGF-RII influences the prognosis of pancreatic cancer. Ann Surg 236:738–749
9. Buchler P, Reber HA, Ullrich A, et al. (2003) Pancreatic cancer growth is inhibited by blockade of VEGF-RII. Surgery 134:772–782
10. Burris HA 3rd, Moore MJ, Andersen J, Green MR, Rothenberg ML, Modiano MR, et al. (1997) Improvements in survival and clinical benefit with gemcitabine as first-line therapy for patients with advanced pancreas cancer: a randomized trial. J Clin Oncol 15:2403–2413
11. Carmeliet P (2003) Angiogenesis in health and disease. Nat Med 9:653–669
12. Chambers AF, Matrisian LM (1997) Changing views of the role of matrix metalloproteinases in metastasis. J Natl Cancer Inst 89:1260–1270
13. Chirivi RG, Garofalo A, Crimmin MJ, Bawden LJ, Stoppacciaro A, Brown PD, Giavazzi R (1994) Inhibition of the metastatic spread and growth of B16-BL6 murine melanoma by a synthetic matrix metalloproteinase inhibitor. Int J Cancer 58:460–464
14. Crane CH, Ellis M, Abbruzzese JL, Douglas EB, Henry X, Ho L, et al. (2005) Phase I trial of bevacizumab (BV) with concurrent radiotherapy (RT) and capecitabine (CAP) in locally advanced pancreatic adenocarcinoma (PA). J Clin Oncol 23 [Suppl]:4033

15. Densmore JJ, Fox JR, Kannarkat G, Morgan JK, Petroni G, Blount T, et al. (2005) A Phase I/II trial of weekly gemcitabine with celecoxib and thalidomide for patients with advanced pancreatic cancer. J Clin Oncol 23 [Suppl]:4241
16. Dredge K, Marriott JB, Dalgleish AG (2002) Immunological effects of thalidomide and its chemical and functional analogs. Crit Rev Immunol 22:425–437
17. Dutcher JP (2004) Mammalian target of rapamycin inhibition. Clin Cancer Res 10:6382S–6387S
18. Eccles SA, Box GM, Court WJ, Bone EA, Thomas W, Brown PD (1996) Control of lymphatic and hematogenous metastasis of a rat mammary carcinoma by the matrix metalloproteinase inhibitor batimastat (BB-94). Cancer Res 56:2815–2822
19. Erlichman C, Adjei AA, Alberts SR, Sloan JA, Goldberg RM, Pitot HC, et al. (2001) Phase I study of the matrix metalloproteinase inhibitor, BAY 12-9566. Ann Oncol 12:389–395
20. Folkman J (2003) Fundamental concepts of the angiogenic process. Curr Mol Med 3:643–651
21. Fujimoto K, Hosotani R, Wada M, Lee JU, Koshiba T, Miyamoto Y, et al. (1998) Expression of two angiogenic factors, vascular endothelial growth factor and platelet-derived endothelial cell growth factor in human pancreatic cancer, and its relationship to angiogenesis. Eur J Cancer 34:1439–1447
22. Gatto C, Rieppi M, Borsotti P, Innocenti S, Ceruti R, Drudis T, et al. (1999) BAY 12-9566, a novel inhibitor of matrix metalloproteinases with antiangiogenic activity. Clin Cancer Res 5:3603–3607
23. Gordon JN, Trebble TM, Ellis RD, Duncan HD, Johns T, Goggin PM (2005) Thalidomide in the treatment of cancer cachexia: a randomised placebo controlled trial. Gut 54:540–545
24. Heath EI, O'Reilly S, Humphrey R, Sundaresan P, Donehower RC, Sartorius S, et al. (2001) Phase I trial of the matrix metalloproteinase inhibitor BAY 12-9566 in patients with advanced solid tumours. Cancer Chemother Pharmacol 48:269–274
25. Hirte H, Goel R, Major P, Seymour L, Huan S, Stewart D, et al. (2000) A phase I dose escalation study of the matrix metalloproteinase inhibitor BAY 12-9566 administered orally in patients with advanced solid tumours. Ann Oncol 11:1579–1584
26. Honda M, Mori M, Ueo H, Sugimachi K, Akiyoshi T (1996) Matrix metalloproteinase-7 expression in gastric carcinoma. Gut 39:444–448
27. Hurwitz H, Fehrenbacher L, Novotny W, Cartwright T, Hainsworth J, Heim W, et al. (2004) Bevacizumab plus irinotecan, fluorouracil, and leucovorin for metastatic colorectal cancer. N Engl J Med 350:2335–2342
28. Itakura J, Ishiwata T, Friess H, Fujii H, Matsumoto Y, Buchler MW, Korc M (1997) Enhanced expression of vascular endothelial growth factor in human pancreatic cancer correlates with local disease progression. Clin Cancer Res 3:1309–1316
29. Itakura J, Ishiwata T, Shen B, et al. (2000) Concomitant over-expression of vascular endothelial growth factor and its receptors in pancreatic cancer. Int J Cancer 85:27–34
30. Javle MM, Iyer RV, Yu J, et al. (2006) Phase II study of gemcitabine, capecitabine and bevacizumab for advanced pancreatic cancer (APC) with ECOG PS 0-1 (abstr). Proc Am Soc Clin Oncol 24:4117
31. Kato H, Ishikura H, Kawarada Y, Furuya M, Kondo S, Kato H, Yoshiki T (2001) Anti-angiogenic treatment for peritoneal dissemination of pancreas adenocarcinoma: a study using TNP-470. Jpn J Cancer Res 92:67–73
32. Kindler HL, Friberg G, Singh DA, Locker G, Nattam S, Kozloff M, Taber DA, Karrison T, Dachman A, Stadler WM, Vokes E (2005) Phase II trial of bevacizumab plus gemcitabine in patients with advanced pancreatic cancer. J Clin Oncol 23:8033–8804
33. Kindler HL, Bylow KA, Hochster HS, et al. (2006) A randomized phase II study of bevacizumab (B) and gemcitabine (G) plus cetuximab (C) or erlotinib (E) in patients (pts) with advanced pancreatic cancer (PC): a preliminary analysis (abstr). Proc Am Soc Clin Oncol 24:4040
34. Kindler HL, Niedzwiecki D, Hollis D, et al. (2007) A double-blind, placebo-controlled, randomized phase III trial of gemcitabine (G) plus bevacizumab (B) vs gemcitabine plus placebo (P) in patients (pts) with advanced pancreatic cancer (PC): a preliminary analysis of Cancer and Leukemia Group B (CALGB) 80 303 (abstr). Proc Gastrointest Cancers Symp 139:108
35. Ko AH, Dito E, Schillinger B, et al. (2006) A phase II study of gemcitabine (GEM) given at fixed-dose rate (FDR) infusion, low-dose cisplatin (CDDP), and bevacizumab in metastatic pancreatic cancer (PanCa) (abstr). Proc Am Soc Clin Oncol 24:4041
36. Moore MJ, Hamm J, Dancey J, Eisenberg PD, Dagenais M, Fields A, et al. (2003) Comparison of

gemcitabine versus the matrix metalloproteinase inhibitor BAY 12-9566 in patients with advanced or metastatic adenocarcinoma of the pancreas: a phase III trial of the National Cancer Institute of Canada Clinical Trials Group. J Clin Oncol 21:3296–3302
37. Niedergethmann M, Hildenbrand R, Wostbrock B, Hartel M, Sturm JW, Richter A, Post S (2002) High expression of vascular endothelial growth factor predicts early recurrence and poor prognosis after curative resection for ductal adenocarcinoma of the pancreas. Pancreas 25:122–129
38. Nomura H, Sato H, Seiki M, Mai M, Okada Y (1995) Expression of membrane-type matrix metalloproteinase in human gastric carcinomas. Cancer Res 55:3263–3266
39. Raut CP, Nawrocki S, Lashinger LM, Davis DW, Khanbolooki S, Xiong H, et al. (2004) Celecoxib inhibits angiogenesis by inducing endothelial cell apoptosis in human pancreatic tumor xenografts. Cancer Biol Ther 3:1217–1224
40. Seo Y, Baba H, Fukuda T, Takashima M, Sugimachi K (2000) High expression of vascular endothelial growth factor is associated with liver metastasis and a poor prognosis for patients with ductal pancreatic adenocarcinoma. Cancer 88:2239–2245
41. Sier CF, Kubben FJ, Ganesh S, Heerding MM, Griffioen G, Hanemaaijer R, et al. (1996) Tissue levels of matrix metalloproteinases MMP-2 and MMP-9 are related to the overall survival of patients with gastric carcinoma. Br J Cancer 74:413–417
42. Stephan S, Datta K, Wang E, Li J, Brekken RA, Parangi S, Thorpe PE, Mukhopadhyay D (2004) Effect of rapamycin alone and in combination with antiangiogenesis therapy in an orthotopic model of human pancreatic cancer. Clin Cancer Res 15:6993–7000
43. Teo SK, Stirling DI, Zeldis JB (2005) Thalidomide as a novel therapeutic agent: new uses for an old product. Drug Discov Today 10:107–114
44. Tonra JR, Deevi DS, Corcoran E, Li H, Wang S, Carrick FE, Daniel JH (2006) Synergistic antitumor effects of combined epidermal growth factor receptor and vascular endothelial growth factor receptor-2 targeted therapy. Clin Cancer Res 1:2197–2207
45. Vacca A, Scavelli C, Montefusco V, Di Pietro G, Neri A, Mattioli M, et al. (2005) Thalidomide downregulates angiogenic genes in bone marrow endothelial cells of patients with active multiple myeloma. J Clin Oncol 23:5334–5346
46. Von Marshall Z, Cramer T, Hocker M, et al. (2000) De novo expression of vascular endothelial growth factor in human pancreatic cancer: evidence for an autocrine mitogenic loop. Gastroenterology 119:1358–1372
47. Wang HX, Chen QK (2003) Expression and significance of cyclooxygenase-2 in human pancreatic carcinomas. Ai Zheng 22:649–652
48. Watson SA, Morris TM, Collins HM, Bawden LJ, Hawkins K, Bone EA (1999) Inhibition of tumour growth by marimastat in a human xenograft model of gastric cancer: relationship with levels of circulating CEA. Br J Cancer 81:19–23
49. Whittaker M, Floyd CD, Brown P, Gearing AJ (1999) Design and therapeutic application of matrix metalloproteinase inhibitors. Chem Rev 99:2735–2776
50. Wildiers H, Guetens G, De Boeck G, Verbeken E, Landuyt B, Landuyt W, et al. (2003) Effect of antivascular endothelial growth factor treatment on the intratumoral uptake of CPT-11. Br J Cancer 88:1979–1986
51. Willett CG, Boucher Y, di Tomaso E, Duda DG, Munn LL, Tong RT, et al. (2004) Direct evidence that the VEGF-specific antibody bevacizumab has antivascular effects in human rectal cancer. Nat Med 10:145–147
52. Xiong HQ, Hess KR, Kayaleh OR, Goodwin JW, Banerjee T, Sinclair SS, et al. (2005) A phase II trial of gemcitabine and celecoxib for metastatic pancreatic cancer. J Clin Oncol 23:4174
53. Zhou XC, Tang CW, Liu CL, Wang CH (2004) Effects of rofecoxib on angiogenesis of pancreatic cancer xenograft in nude mice. Ai Zheng 23:376–380

15

Targeted Therapy of the Epidermal Growth Factor Receptor in the Treatment of Pancreatic Cancer

S. Heeger

Recent Results in Cancer Research, Vol. 177

Abstract

The epidermal growth factor receptor (EGFR)-mediated pathway is one of the most promising targets for the development of new strategies in anticancer treatments. The so-called "small molecule" tyrosine kinase inhibitor erlotinib has gained marketing authorization in the United States for advanced adenocarcinoma of the lung and for pancreatic cancer, whereas the antibody cetuximab is registered for metastatic colorectal cancer and cancers of the head and neck. Ongoing studies are evaluating the impact of EGFR-targeting therapy in the treatment of locally advanced and metastatic pancreatic cancer.

15.1 Introduction

Epidermal growth factor receptor (EGFR) is known to be of high importance in the development of tumors and their survival in the organism. It belongs to the family of protein tyrosine kinases that have a big influence on the cellular regulation of growth, differentiation, and apoptosis (Ullrich and Schlessinger 1990). Located on the cellular surface, the molecule mediates signal transduction pathways by responding to extracellular signals. Via signal transduction cascades it interacts with different molecules regulating cell proliferation, survival, differentiation and migration (Prenzel et al. 2001; Sonenshein 1997; Alessi and Cohen 1998). Finally, the signal reaches the nucleus, regulating gene expression and transcription (Bromberg and Darnell 2000). Furthermore, EGFR interacts with other members of its receptor family, such as e.g. HER2neu/ErB2 (Gschwind et al. 2001; Earp et al. 1995).

In normal tissue, EGFR is largely controlled by a diversity of regulating mechanisms. In cancer tissue, however, these control mechanisms fail, resulting in overexpression and activation (Salomon et al. 1995; Xu et al. 1984). As in other epithelial tumor types, in pancreatic cancer overexpression of EGFR is correlated with bad clinical outcomes due to increased tumoral aggressiveness (Yamanaka et al. 1993).

EGFR plays an important role in the development of pancreatic cancer. In over 90% of cases EGFR is overexpressed (Lemoine et al. 1992), stimulating pancreatic tumor cell growth (Funatomi et al. 1997).

Another important EGFR activity concerns angiogenesis. EGF induces vascular endothelial growth factor and so, in addition to its direct tumor growth induction, it enhances tumor growth by supporting vascularization (Goldman et al. 1993).

Taking into account all these activities induced by EGFR—regulation of cell growth, tumorigenesis, and angiogenesis—it is obvious that blocking EGFR activity represents an attractive anticancer treatment approach.

Two ways of EGFR blockade have been developed. One class is represented by small molecule tyrosine kinase (TK) inhibitors, which block adenosine triphosphate binding and so inhibit TK activity. Many of these TK inhibitors have been synthesized, some have been developed clinically, such as gefitinib, lapatinib, and erlotinib. For pancreatic cancer, erlotinib is the most developed compound.

The other strategy is inhibiting ligand binding to EGFR by monoclonal antibodies and thereby blocking the following signal transduction cascade, including, e.g., cetuximab or matuzumab. As for pancreatic cancer, the most important compound is cetuximab.

15.2 Preclinical Studies

The above-mentioned findings were investigated on a cellular level in several preclinical studies to evaluate EGFR-targeted therapy for human pancreatic cancer. Ng et al. (2002) showed a significant increase in apoptosis in SCID (severely combined immunodeficient) mice bearing a pancreatic cancer xenograft. Animals were treated with a combination of gemcitabine, wortmannin (phosphatidylinositol 3′-kinase inhibitor), and erlotinib given intravenously.

In another experiment erlotinib alone showed a significant decrease of proliferation of human pancreatic cancer cells (HPAC) in vitro. Orthotopically human pancreatic cancer (HPAC)-implanted nude mice showed reduced tumor implantation, size, weight, and jaundice when treated with erlotinib (Durkin et al. 2006).

Additional effects could be shown in experiments performed with cetuximab alone or in a combination of cetuximab with gemcitabine. In L3.6pl tumors implanted in the pancreas of nude mice, growth inhibition and tumor regression up to complete tumor disappearance was documented for either cetuximab alone or in combination with gemcitabine. No liver metastases were seen in the combination group whereas 50% of the control group (no therapy) showed hepatic spread of the disease. Interestingly, therapy using cetuximab decreased the production of vascular endothelial growth factor and interleukin-8 significantly. Consequently, cetuximab reduced microvessel density and increased the percentage of apoptotic endothelial cancer cells. These effects were potentiated when combined with gemcitabine.

Preclinical investigations demonstrated a strong rationale for EGFR-targeting strategies against cancer of the pancreas and were therefore translated into a variety of clinical protocols in combination with chemotherapy or radiotherapy (or both).

15.3 Clinical Trials in Pancreatic Cancer

Standard of care in pancreatic cancer is chemotherapeutic treatment with gemcitabine. However, response rates and survival data are poor (Burris et al. 1997) and there is a strong clinical need for improved systemic therapy. Few data are available on compounds interfering with EGFR in pancreatic cancer. These clinical studies will be discussed here.

15.3.1 Clinical Trials with TKIs

15.3.1.1 Erlotinib (Tarceva) in First-Line Treatment of Pancreatic Cancer

Moore et al. (2007) compared gemcitabine plus erlotinib (Tarceva, Roche Pharmaceuticals, Basel) versus gemcitabine plus placebo in a phase III trial. From 176 sites in 17 countries, 569 patients were randomized to receive either gemcitabine 1,000 mg/m^2 weekly on days 1 to 43 (i.e., for 6 weeks), followed by 1 week's rest and then, on days 1, 8, and 15 of a 4-week cycle with erlotinib, given at a dose of 100 or 150 mg/day orally or plus placebo. The primary endpoint of the trial was overall survival; secondary endpoints included progression-free survival (PFS), response rate, response duration, toxicity, and quality of life. Response was evaluated every 8 weeks using Response Evaluation Criteria In Solid Tumors (RECIST) criteria.

An interim safety analysis was performed once 50 patients had shown no major increase in toxicity after receiving gemcitabine plus erlotinib at 100 mg/day. Thus, accrual at 150 mg/day was opened. However, recruitment in the 100-mg/day group was so fast that by the time of the interim analysis for the 150-mg/day group the trial was almost completed with patients on 100 mg/day. It was therefore decided to include the appropriate number of patients for 80% statistical power for the 100-mg/day group.

Survival analysis included 486 and showed a significantly longer overall survival for the gemcitabine plus erlotinib group than for gemcitabine alone with an estimated hazard ratio of 0.82 (95% CI 0.69–0.99, $p=0.038$). Median survival times were 6.24 vs 5.91 months, 1-year survival rates were 23% (95% CI 18%–28%) and 17%

(95% CI 12%–21%), respectively. Progression-free survival was also longer in the gemcitabine-erlotinib arm (median 3.75 vs 3.55 months, HR 0.77, $p = 0.004$). Response rates slightly favored gemcitabine-erlotinib (ORR 8.6% vs 8%) with a duration of response of 163 days in both arms.

The treatment was generally well tolerated and comparable in both treatment arms. Known EGFR-induced side effects (Shepherd et al. 2005) included rash, diarrhea, and ILD-like symptoms were more common in the gemcitabine-erlotinib arm, but usually mild to moderate. Hematotoxicity did not differ between treatment arms (Grade 3/4 neutropenia 24% vs 27%, thrombocytopenia 10% vs 11%). The toxicity profile of both compounds did not differ to that known as single agents.

Quality of life was comparable between both treatment arms.

As seen before with EGFR inhibitors (Xiong and Abbruzzese 2002), the presence of rash in the gemcitabine-erlotinib arm was correlated with a greater likelihood of treatment response.

This significant improvement in overall survival of 22% compared to gemcitabine plus placebo led to marketing authorization in the USA for erlotinib in combination with gemcitabine in 2006.

At the ASCO 2007 Gastrointestinal Cancer Symposium, a phase I of a triple therapy combining erlotinib, the monoclonal VEGF receptor antibody bevacizumab, and gemcitabine was reported. In 12 patients the combination seemed to be well tolerated, and the maximum tolerated dose (MTD) has not yet been reached. Two patients showed partial response, 4 had stable disease (Gomez-Martin et al. 2007).

15.3.1.2 Erlotinib (Tarceva) in the Treatment of Relapsed Pancreatic Cancer

As patients who fail standard first-line treatment with gemcitabine have no standard treatment options, the impact of new compounds is being examined in this population.

At the ASCO 2007 Gastrointestinal Cancer Symposium, a trial of single-agent erlotinib for patients with relapsed pancreatic cancer has been reported. In 13 patients having received two prior lines of chemotherapy (1–5), erlotinib showed clinical activity in 5 patients, resulting in stabilization or improvement for up to 12 months. No grade IV toxicity was described; 4 patients had grade 2 rash, 2 had grade 3 diarrhea (Epelbaum et al. 2007).

Another trial examined the impact of capecitabine plus erlotinib after failure of a gemcitabine-based chemotherapy in pancreatic cancer. Receiving capecitabine, 2,000 mg/m^2, plus erlotinib, 150 mg per day, were 28 patients. The toxicity profile met the expectations with grade 3/4 rash and diarrhea (14% each), hand-foot syndrome (11%), and stomatitis (7%). Partial response was reported in 11% and stable disease in 57% of patients. The median survival was 6.7 months (Blaszkowsky et al. 2005).

15.3.1.3 TK-Inhibitors in Combination with Radiation Therapy in Pancreatic Cancer

The combination of the TK inhibitor gefitinib, capecitabine, and radiotherapy led to an increased toxicity in 10 patients with pancreatic cancer without responses in a phase I dose-finding study (Czito et al. 2006). When given simultaneously to radiation therapy, 825 mg/m^2 capecitabine plus 250 mg/day gefitinib induced dose-limiting toxicity in all 3 patients on this dose level (grade 3 nausea, diarrhea), resulting finally in patient withdrawal. On dose level 1 (capecitabine 650 mg/m^2 + gefitinib 250 mg/day) DLTs appeared in 3/7 patients. As for efficacy, no responses have been reported; stable disease was reported for 6 out of 7 patients on dose level 1, and 1 out of 3 patients on dose level 2. No patient was converted to resectable status.

15.3.2 Clinical Trials with Anti-EGFR Antibodies

15.3.2.1 Cetuximab (Erbitux) in the First-Line Treatment of Pancreatic Cancer

Cetuximab (Erbitux, Merck, Darmstadt, Germany) has also been combined with standard gemcitabine chemotherapy as a first-line treatment of pancreatic cancer. A phase II trial has been performed in 41 patients, receiving cetuximab (initial dose 400 mg/m^2, then 250 mg/m^2 weekly) followed by gemcitabine 1,000 mg/m^2 weekly for 7 weeks plus 1 week's rest. Subsequent cycles were 4 weeks long with gemcitabine given on days 1, 8 and 15 and a rest on day 22. Patients were treated until progression or intolerable toxicity.

Patients had a median Karnofski score of 80%; 85.4% had metastatic disease.

Out of 41 patients, 5 (12.2%) showed partial response, and a further 26 (63.4%) had stable disease, resulting in a disease control rate of 75.6%.

As discussed above, the effect of EGFR blockade combines the reduction of tumor growth with antiangiogenesis, both of which in the short run do not result in tumor shrinkage but appear clinically as disease stabilization. Furthermore, the accurate assessment of pancreatic tumor imaging is difficult due to its anatomic location. Therefore, time to progression, which includes objective response plus stable disease, and overall survival may be more appropriate parameters for tumor response assessment in pancreatic cancer.

Median time to best response was 1.7 months, median duration of response was 3.8 months, duration of disease control was 5.4 months, and median time to progression 3.8 months. Median survival duration was 7.1 months; the 1-year overall survival rate was 31.7% and the 1-year PFS rate 12% (Xiong et al. 2004).

These data clearly exceed the results of gemcitabine monotherapy, which showed a 1-year survival rate of 18% and a 1-year PFS of 9%. Also, median TTP and overall survival (3.8 and 7.1 months, respectively) favor the combination of cetuximab and gemcitabine (Burris et al. 1997).

Response data, PFS, and overall survival of the combination cetuximab plus gemcitabine are also comparable to those of other EGF-targeted therapies combined with gemcitabine, as mentioned above.

Acne-like rash (85.4%), asthenia (85.4%), nausea (61%), weight loss (58.5%), diarrhea (53.7%), abdominal pain (53.7%), and vomiting (51.2%) were the most common adverse events. As for grades 3 and 4, neutropenia (39%), asthenia (22%), abdominal pain (22%), and thrombocytopenia (17.1%) were the most commonly reported severe toxicities.

One trial explored the efficacy and safety of cetuximab (250 mg/m^2 per week) combined with gemcitabine (1,000 mg/m^2 q2w) and oxaliplatin (100 mg/m^2 q2w) in 43 patients as first-line treatment of metastatic pancreatic cancer (GEMOXCET). Toxicity was mainly hematological with grades 3/4 of leucopenia 10%, anemia 15%, and thrombocytopenia 12%. Nonhematological toxicity involved nausea 17%, infection 16%, diarrhea 7%, and allergy 6%. Of the patients, 71% had skin rash, 5% grade 3. The overall response rate (34 evaluable patients) was 38% with 1 complete and 12 partial responses. In all, 9 patients (26%) had stable disease. GEMOXCET has been shown to be a feasible regimen with moderate toxicity and promising efficacy data (Kullmann et al. 2007).

15.3.2.2 Cetuximab (Erbitux) in Combination with Radiation Therapy in Pancreatic Cancer

For locally advanced pancreatic cancer, chemoradiation using gemcitabine or 5-fluouracil plus radiotherapy, is standard care, but results are poor with overall survival of between 7 and 12 months and 1-year survival rates of 30%–45% (Tsai et al. 2003). Given the promising results of EGFR targeting therapy in pancreatic cancer, the introduction of cetuximab in this setting as a novel treatment strategy was a stringent therapeutic demand.

Two phase II trials examined the combination of gemcitabine, cetuximab, and radiotherapy as a preoperative induction treatment (Pipas et al. 2006; Krempien et al. 2006) (PARC trial ISRCTN56652283). Though still small in number and preliminary (10 and 20 patients, respectively), the first data report shows promising results, with tumor control rates of 80% and 85%, rendering 60% of patients operable by tumor downstaging. The toxicity profile did not differ from that known for gemcitabine and cetuximab, with rash, diarrhea, and hematotoxicity as the main adverse events. Therefore, even as a neoadjuvant approach, the combination of gemcitabine plus cetuximab is feasible and warrants efficacy. The PARC trial will include 66 patients with locally advanced nonresectable pancreatic cancer, evaluating feasibility via the toxicity profile as its primary study aim, and response rates, time to progression, downstaging of tumor size, post-therapy resectability, and quality of life will be its secondary study aims.

15.4 Conclusion

EGFR-targeting therapies with TK inhibitors and monoclonal antibodies such as cetuximab represent a substantial improvement in the treatment options for patients with pancreatic cancer and probably will enhance the chances and the prognosis of those patients.

References

Alessi DR, Cohen P (1998) Mechanism of activation and function of protein kinase B. Curr Opin Genet Dev 8:55–62

Blaszkowsky LS, Kulke KH, Ryan DP, Clark JW, Meyerhardt J, Zhu AX, Lawrence C, Fuchs CS (2005) A phase II study of erlotinib in combination with capecitabine in previously treated patients with metastatic pancreatic cancer. Proc ASCO 2005. J Clin Oncol 23:4099

Bromberg J, Darnell JE Jr (2000) The role of STATs in transcriptional control and their impact on cellular function. Oncogene 1519:2468–2473

Burris HA 3rd, Moore MJ, Andersen J, Green MR, Rothenberg ML, Modiano MR, Cripps MC, Portenoy RK, Storniolo AM, Tarassoff P, Nelson R, Dorr FA, Stephens CD, Von Hoff DD (1997) Improvements in survival and clinical benefit with gemcitabine as first-line therapy for patients with advanced pancreas cancer: a randomized trial. J Clin Oncol 15:2403–2413

Czito BG, Willett CG, Bendell JC, Morse MA, Tyler DS, Fernando NH, Mantyh CR, Blobe GC, Honeycutt W, Yu D, Clary BM, Pappas TN, Ludwig KA, Hurwitz HI (2006) Increased toxicity with gefitinib, capecitabine, and radiation therapy in pancreatic and rectal cancer: phase I trial results. J Clin Oncol 124:656–662

Durkin AJ, Osborne DA, Yeatman TJ, Rosemurgy AS, Armstrong C, Zervos EE (2006) EGF receptor antagonism improves survival in a murine model of pancreatic adenocarcinoma. J Surg Res 135:195–201

Earp HS, Dawson TL, Li X, Yu H (1995) Heterodimerization and functional interaction between EGF receptor family members: a new signaling paradigm with implications for breast cancer research. Breast Cancer Res Treat 35:115–132

Epelbaum R, Schnaider J, Gluzman A, Figer A (2007) Erlotinib as a single-agent therapy in patients with advanced pancreatic cancer. ASCO Gastrointest Cancers Symp, abstr 202

Funatomi H, Itakura J, Ishiwata T, Pastan I, Thompson SA, Johnson GR, Korc M (1997) Amphiregulin antisense oligonucleotide inhibits the growth of T3M4 human pancreatic cancer cells and sensitizes the cells to EGF receptor-targeted therapy. Int J Cancer 2972:512–517

Goldman CK, Kim J, Wong WL, King V, Brock T, Gillespie GY (1993) Epidermal growth factor stimulates vascular endothelial growth factor production by human malignant glioma cells: a model of glioblastoma multiforme pathophysiology. Mol Biol Cell 4:121–133

Gomez-Martin C, Camara ,J, Rubio B, Amador H, Cortes Funes H, Gravalos C, Hidalgo M (2007) A phase I study of erlotinib, bevacizumab, and gemcitabine in patients with advanced pancreatic cancer. ASCO Gastrointest Cancers Symp, abstr 199

Gschwind A, Zwick E, Prenzel N, Leserer M, Ullrich A (2001) Cell communication networks: epidermal growth factor receptor transactivation as the paradigm for interreceptor signal transmission. Oncogene 20:1594–1600

Krempien RC, Münter MW, Timke C, Huber PE, Friess H, Heeger S, Herfarth KK, Abdollahi A, Hartung G, Buchler MW, Debus J (2006) Phase II study evaluating trimodal therapy with cetuximab intensity modulated radiotherapy (IMRT) and gemcitabine for patients with locally advanced pancreatic cancer (ISRCTN56652283). Proc ASCO Annual Meeting 2006. J Clin Oncol 24:4100

Kullmann F, Hollerbach S, Dollinger MM, Harder J, Fuchs M, Messmann H, Trojan J, Gäbele E, Hinke A, Endlicher E (2007) Cetuximab plus gemcitabine/oxaliplatin (GEMOXCET) in 1st line metastatic pancreatic cancer. First results from a multicenter phase II study. ASCO Gastrointest Cancers Symp, abstr 128

Lemoine NR, Hughes CM, Barton CM, Poulsom R, Jeffery RE, Kloppel G, Hall PA, Gullick WJ (1992) The epidermal growth factor receptor in human pancreatic cancer. J Pathol 166:7–12

Moore MJ, Goldstein D, Hamm J, Figer A, Hecht JR, Gallinger S, Au HJ, Murawa P, Walde D, Wolff RA, Campos D, Lim R, Ding K, Clark G, Voskoglou-Nomikos T, Ptasynski M, Parulekar W (2006) Erlotinib plus gemcitabine compared with gemcitabine alone in patients with advanced pancreatic cancer: a phase III trial of the National Cancer Institute of Canada Clinical Trials Group. JCO early release, published online ahead of print, 23 April 2007. J Clin Oncol 10.1200/JCO 07.9525

Ng SS, Tsao MS, Nicklee T, Hedley DW (2002) Effects of the epidermal growth factor receptor inhibitor OSI–774, Tarceva, on downstream signaling pathways and apoptosis in human pancreatic adenocarcinoma. Mol Cancer Ther 1:777–783

Pipas JM, Zaki B, Suriwinata AA, Tsapakos MJ, Ripple GH, Colacchio TA, Sutton JE, Gordon SR, Kasibhatla MS, Barth RJ (2006) Cetuximab, intensity-modulated radiotherapy (IMRT), and twice-weekly gemcitabine for pancreatic adenocarcinoma. Proc ASCO Annual Meeting. J Clin Oncol 24:14056

Prenzel N, Fischer OM, Streit S, Hart S, Ullrich A (2001) The epidermal growth factor receptor family as a central element for cellular signal transduction and diversification. Endocr Relat Cancer 8:11–31

Salomon DS, Brandt R, Ciardiello F, Normanno N (1995) Epidermal growth factor-related peptides and their receptors in human malignancies. Crit Rev Oncol Hematol 19:183–232

Shepherd FA, Rodrigues Pereira J, Ciuleanu T, Tan EH, Hirsh V, Thongprasert S, Campos D, Maoleekoonpiroj S, Smylie M, Martins R, van Kooten M, Dediu M, Findlay B, Tu D, Johnston D, Bezjak A, Clark G, Santabarbara P, et al. (2005) Erlotinib in previously treated non-small cell lung cancer. N Engl J Med 14353:123–132

Sonenshein GE (1997) Rel/NF-kappaB transcription factors and the control of apoptosis. Semin Cancer Biol 8:113–119

Tsai JY, Iannitti DA, Safran H (2003) Combined modality therapy for pancreatic cancer. Semin Oncol 30:71–79

Ullrich A, Schlessinger J (1990) Signal transduction by receptors with tyrosine kinase activity. Cell 61:203–212

Xiong HQ, Abbruzzese JL (2002) Epidermal growth factor receptor-targeted therapy for pancreatic cancer. Semin Oncol 29:31–37

Xiong HQ, Rosenberg A, LoBuglio A, Schmidt W, Wolff RA, Deutsch J, Needle M, Abbruzzese JL (2004) Cetuximab, a monoclonal antibody targeting the epidermal growth factor receptor, in combination with gemcitabine for advanced pancreatic cancer: a multicenter phase II Trial. J Clin Oncol 122:2610–2616

Xu YH, Richert N, Ito S, Merlino GT, Pastan I (1984) Characterization of epidermal growth factor receptor gene expression in malignant and normal human cell lines. Proc Natl Acad Sci USA 81:7308–7312

Yamanaka Y, Friess H, Kobrin MS, Buchler M, Beger HG, Korc M (1993) Coexpression of epidermal growth factor receptor and ligands in human pancreatic cancer is associated with enhanced tumor aggressiveness. Anticancer Res 13:565–569

16 Antisense Therapeutics for Tumor Treatment: The TGF-beta2 Inhibitor AP 12009 in Clinical Development Against Malignant Tumors

K.-H. Schlingensiepen, B. Fischer-Blass, S. Schmaus, S. Ludwig

Recent Results in Cancer Research, Vol. 177

Abstract

Overexpression of the cytokine transforming growth factor-beta 2 (TGF-beta2) is a hallmark of various malignant tumors including pancreatic carcinoma, malignant glioma, metastasizing melanoma, and metastatic colorectal carcinoma. This is due to the pivotal role of TGF-beta2 as it regulates key mechanisms of tumor development, namely immunosuppression, metastasis, angiogenesis, and proliferation. The antisense technology is an innovative technique offering a targeted approach for the treatment of different highly aggressive tumors and other diseases. Antisense oligonucleotides are being developed to inhibit the production of disease-causing proteins at the molecular level. The immunotherapeutic approach with the phosphorothioate oligodeoxynucleotide AP 12009 for the treatment of malignant tumors is based on the specific inhibition of TGF-beta2. After providing preclinical proof of concept, the safety and efficacy of AP 12009 were assessed in clinical phase I/II open-label dose-escalation studies in recurrent or refractory high-grade glioma patients. Median survival time after recurrence exceeded the current literature data for chemotherapy. Currently, phase I/II study in advanced pancreatic carcinoma, metastatic melanoma, and metastatic colorectal carcinoma and a phase IIb study in recurrent or refractory high-grade glioma are ongoing. The preclinical as well as the clinical results implicate targeted TGF-beta2 suppression as a promising therapeutic approach for malignant tumor therapy.

16.1 Introduction

Pancreatic cancer is the fourth leading cause of cancer-related deaths in men and women in virtually all industrialized countries (Jemal et al. 2005, 2006). Its incidence cuts across all racial and socio-economic barriers. Outcome is nearly always fatal with a 1-year survival rate of about 20% and a 5-year survival rate of less than 5% (Cardenes et al. 2006; Jemal et al. 2005, 2006). The majority of patients exhibit a very aggressive adenocarcinoma (85%). These tumor types are less aggressive and are often curable. Pancreatic tumors are difficult to detect at early stages and, due to their nonspecific symptoms, extremely hard to diagnose. Therefore, most patients present with locally advanced or metastatic disease resulting in high mortality and very short life expectancy. This is at least partially due to the observed resistance of pancreatic cancer to chemotherapy and radiation therapy. Currently, complete surgical resection remains the only therapeutic option with a potential for cure. However, only a low proportion of patients (only 15%–20%) are suitable candidates for surgical resection (Cardenes et al. 2006; Siech et al. 2001). The median survival of these patients who undergo successful resection is approximately 12–19 months with a 5-year survival rate of 15%–20%. Risk factors for pancreatic cancer include advanced age, obesity, diabetes, and chronic pancreatitis (Li et al. 2004; Lowenfels and Maisonneuve 2006). However, cigarette smoking is considered the most significant and avoidable risk factor, causing more than 25% of the pancreatic cancer cases (Li et al. 2004;

Lowenfels and Maisonneuve 2006). Because of the lethality of this disease and the failure of standard treatment to date, future efforts will be focused on the advances that are being made in the understanding and delineation of the genetic and molecular cell biology of cancer cells.

During the last three decades, the interest in new therapeutics such as those based on antisense technology has strongly increased. Today, the improved technology and ability of chemical synthesis of antisense oligodeoxynucleotides (ODNs) has become a routine process and offers researchers the possibility to target almost any single gene (Schlingensiepen et al. 1993). This technology has become a powerful research tool in molecular biology, biochemistry, and microbiology, and has tremendous potential in the fields of functional genomics, drug discovery, and clinical therapy, especially oncology. A major cause of cancer lies in defective gene regulation. Such mutations can result either in an overproduction or in abnormal production of proteins promoting dysfunctional growth and tumor development. Antisense drugs are able to block the blueprint (messenger ribonucleic acid, mRNA) of a cancer gene and specifically inhibit its conversion into the pathogenic cancer protein. Preventing the formation of such pathogenic factors means combating cancer disease directly at its roots.

Transforming growth factor beta (TGF-beta) is a multifunctional cytokine that has been identified as a key factor in tumor development. TGF-beta is a vital factor controlling several signaling cascades with oncogenic potential, including immunosuppression, epithelial to mesenchymal transition (EMT), metastasis and invasion, angiogenesis, and proliferation. Overexpression of the TGF-beta isoform TGF-beta2 is a hallmark of various malignant tumors, e.g., pancreatic carcinoma, malignant brain tumors, malignant melanoma, and metastatic colorectal carcinoma. Thus, targeting this key factor to suppress several cancer mechanisms simultaneously right at their origin offers a very promising therapeutic approach.

The phosphorothioate oligodeoxynucleotide (S-ODN) AP 12009 is used for the treatment of malignant tumors based on the specific inhibition of TGF-beta2. This chapter describes this antisense technology in general and gives an overview of oligodeoxynucleotide modifications and their delivery to cells. Furthermore, the status of preclinical and clinical trials with AP 12009 for the treatment of pancreatic carcinoma, malignant glioma, malignant melanoma, and metastatic colorectal carcinoma is presented.

16.2 Targeted Therapies

Until recently the traditional therapy for patients with advanced pancreatic cancer was palliative 5-fluorouracil (5-FU)-based chemotherapy (Auerbach et al. 1997; Cardenes et al. 2006). Novel approved chemotherapeutic agents such as gemcitabine (Gemzar, Eli Lilly, Indianapolis) and oxaliplatin (Eloxatin, Sanofi-Aventis, Paris), as well as new therapeutic approaches including tyrosine kinase inhibitors, e.g., erlotinib (Tarceva, Genentech, South San Francisco; Osi Pharmaceuticals, Melville, NY) plus chemotherapy, have demonstrated a survival benefit and improved quality of life in patients with advanced disease (Moore et al. 2005). However, the best combinational therapy still results in median survival of less than 1 year. Furthermore, the high risk of severe side effects and possible resistance to chemotherapeutic agents has evoked considerable interest in molecular pathways of tumors and new treatment strategies such as targeted therapies.

Conventional chemotherapeutic treatments aim at rapidly dividing cells. However, even highly proliferative healthy cells such as blood cells, cells in the hair follicles, and cells lining the gastrointestinal tract are attacked. Similarly, conventional radiation therapy affects some healthy cells surrounding the radiated tumor during treatment. Newer radiation therapy techniques can reduce but not fully eliminate this damage. This treatment-related damage of healthy tissue induces chemotherapy's and radiotherapy's well-known side effects. Targeted therapy acts by interfering with specific molecules needed for carcinogenesis and tumor growth. Monoclonal antibodies are one example for targeted therapy. Targeted cancer therapies can be more effective and may offer the advantage of reduced treatment-related side effects and improved outcomes due to their action restricted only to the target. Recent phase II and III trials with molecular targeted therapies in advanced pancreatic cancer include approaches using monoclonal antibodies [e.g., cetuximab, Erbitux (ImClone Systems, New York; an anti-EGFR), trastuzumab, Herceptin (Genentech, South San Francisco; anti-HER-2), bevacizumab, Avastin (F. Hoffmann-La Roche, Basel; anti-VEGF)], small molecules [e.g., gefitinib, Iressa (Astra Zeneca, London; EGFR inhibitor), erlotinib, Tarceva (EGFR inhibitor)], protein inhibitors (e.g., marimastat or BAY 12–9566, both matrix metalloproteinase inhibitors), and antisense therapeutics (e.g., GTI-2501, complementary to the subunit R1 of ribonucleotide reductase) (Cardenes et al. 2006; Lee et al. 2006).

Herein we report on the antisense therapy using the S-ODN AP 12009 for the treatment of pancreatic carcinoma and other solid tumors overexpressing TGF-beta2.

16.2.1 The Antisense Mechanism

In 1978 Zamecnik and Stephenson published their exciting results on the successful blockade of the replication of the Rous sarcoma virus by adding a synthetic oligodeoxynucleotide directed against a specific sequence of the viral genome (Zamecnik and Stephenson 1978). Only two decades later, in 1998, the first antisense compound named Vitravene (Novartis Ophthalmics Europe, Basel; fomivirsen sodium), an S-ODN, was approved by the Food and Drug Administration (FDA) for the treatment of cytomegalovirus-induced retinitis in patients with acquired immunodeficiency syndrome (AIDS) (Roehr 1998). Especially in the field of oncology, a number of antisense compounds have been developed that are currently in clinical trials for the treatment of different types of tumors (Coppelli and Grandis 2005; Dean and Bennett 2003; Lahn et al. 2005; Schlingensiepen et al. 2006).

In contrast to gene therapy, which aims at replacing, removing, or introducing genes to correct a genetic defect or a mutation, antisense drugs neither alter human genes nor have any effect on genetic information. Antisense molecules are a mirror image of the genetic blueprint or sequence that contains the necessary information for the production of the targeted protein. By binding to the blueprint (mRNA), antisense-molecules render the contained information illegible, thereby inhibiting the protein production (Fig. 16.1).

Different antisense mechanisms are under discussion concerning how the translation of the targeted protein is inhibited; these are (1) sterical blockade of the ribosome (Schlingensiepen et al. 1997), which physically prevents the progression of splicing or translation, and (2) RNase H-induced mRNA cleavage (Akhtar and Agrawal 1997). RNase H is an endoribonuclease that specifically hydrolyzes the phosphodiester bonds of the target RNA.

16.2.1.1 Chemical Modifications of Antisense Oligodeoxynucleotides

Native ODNs contain phosphodiester linkages in their nucleotide backbone making them highly soluble in aqueous solutions but also very susceptible to degradation by exo- and endonucleases within minutes (Shaw et al. 1991; Wickstrom 1986). Established modifications of the ODN chemistry aim at an optimal combination of long half-life due to nuclease resistance, sufficient cellular uptake, good hybridization characteristics, specific binding affinity, and reduction of nonspecific interactions, which could cause toxicities (for review see Mahato 2005). The first chemically synthesized modified ODNs were methylphosphonates (Me-ODNs) with a neutral methyl group replacing the negative charge-bearing oxygen of the phosphodiester bond (Miller et al. 1981). Although Me-ODNs demonstrate an excellent nuclease resistance in biological systems (Tidd and Warenius 1989), their lipophilic nature leads to solubility problems in comparison with other analogs (Brysch and Schlingensiepen 1994; Mahato 2005). Furthermore, this type of oligonucleotides exhibits insufficient duplex formation presumably caused by steric hindrance by the methyl group, resulting in poor antisense activity that cannot activate RNase H activity (Crooke 1999; Miller et al. 1981).

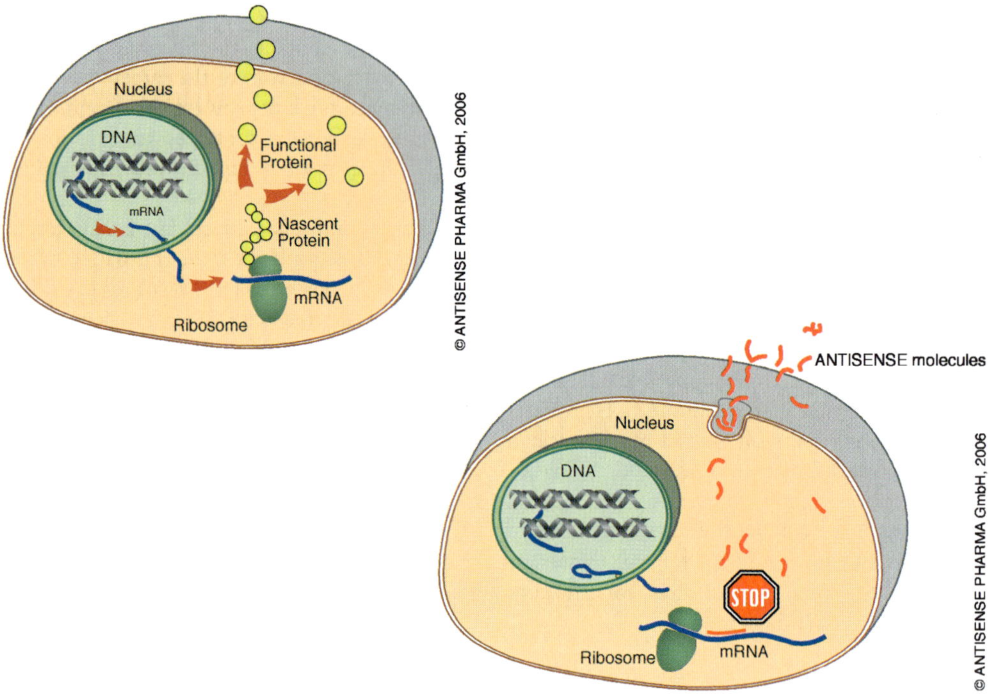

Fig. 16.1 Antisense molecules specifically bind to the mRNA and in consequence block the process of translating the blueprint into a certain pathogenic factor

In S-ODNs, one of the nonbridging oxygens of the phosphate backbone is substituted by a sulfur atom (Eckstein 1983). S-ODNs show analogous characteristics to unmodified ODNs such as their net charge and aqueous solubility, but exhibit a significantly higher stability in vitro and in vivo (Shaw et al. 1991). Furthermore, S-ODNs show excellent antisense activity. Pharmacokinetic experiments in rats, mice, and monkeys have shown that S-ODNs are cleared from plasma biphasically (Agrawal et al. 1995). As observed in preclinical models as well as in humans, the pharmacokinetics of S-ODNs are largely independent of the sequence; thus, different S-ODNs have shown a similar pharmacokinetic profile (Geary et al. 2001). Immediately after administration, they are rapidly distributed into different tissues and organs. Major sites of accumulation are liver and kidney followed by spleen, bone marrow, and lymph nodes (Agrawal et al. 1995, 1991; Mahato 2005). Excretion from the human body occurs primarily via the urine, with up to 30% being excreted within 24 h and 70% within 10 days after a single intravenous administration (Agrawal et al. 1991, 1995). After intravenous administration, S-ODNs are not detectable in the brain since they are not able to pass the blood-brain barrier (BBB) (Agrawal et al. 1991).

Further chemical modifications in ODNs include 2´-*O*-methyl and 2´-*O*-methoxy-ethyl oligonucleotides showing increased nuclease resistance and oligonucleotide:RNA binding affinities (Agrawal et al. 1997). Other chemical modifications of ODNs such as N3´-P5´ phosphoroamidates and morpholino oligonucleotides enhance stability, target affinity, and bioavailability (Kurreck 2003). Another class of oligonucleotide-based compounds consisting of small interfering RNAs has recently become widely used for gene knockdown in vitro and in vivo (Coppelli and Grandis 2005). So far, none of these compounds is in advanced clinical trials. The key factors are cellular uptake, the therapeutic activity of the individual antisense compounds, and the sequences themselves, rather than the chemical modifications alone.

Apart from selecting the optimal gene area, it is crucial to avoid interaction with proteins via certain base sequences, which may result in nonspecific effects. Antisense compounds may contain special motifs such as G-quartets or CG-rich sequences (CpG motif). Four consecutive guanosines exhibit a nonspecific antiproliferative action and inhibit enzymatic activities in several cell types (Burgess et al. 1995; Yaswen et al. 1993). CpG motifs may activate defense mechanisms in humans, leading to a natural and acquired immune response (Krieg 2002).

The future therapeutic success of antisense compounds will depend, as is the case with any targeted therapy, on the careful selection of optimal targets, dosing, schedules, and clinical trial design. The ideal drug candidate should drive tumor progression and should not have redundant pathways, as is case with PKC, for example.

16.2.2 Delivery of Oligodeoxynucleotides into Cells

Antisense ODNs must be internalized into target cells in sufficient amounts to exert their inhibiting effects by targeted downregulation of RNA encoding disease-inducing genes. Owing to their anionic nature and their size, phosphodiester and phosphorothioate ODNs (S-ODNs) are unable to cross the lipophilic cell membrane by passive diffusion. It is well accepted that cellular uptake of S-ODNs is energy-, temperature-, and time-dependent (Levin 1999). The mechanism of cellular uptake can vary depending on the chemical structure and the concentration of the oligonucleotide. Whereas at low concentrations S-ODN uptake is predominantly achieved via a receptor-like mechanism, at higher concentrations adsorptive endocytosis, pinocytosis and caveolar potocytosis are described (Lysik and Wu-Pong 2003; Mahato et al. 2005; Stein et al. 1993; Zamecnik et al. 1994).

In vitro uptake of free antisense ODNs into cultured cell lines is in some cases inefficient. Depending on the cell type, in vitro uptake of ODNs is generally enhanced using different vectors. A variety of viral and nonviral possibilities of oligonucleotide delivery has been developed for basic and clinical research. Viral vectors include retroviral, adenoviral, and adeno-associated viral vectors, which introduce their DNA into the cells with high efficiency. A major obstacle of viral vectors in vivo but not in vitro is the host‘s immune response including both the adaptive response (Yang and Wilson 1995) and the innate immune system (Plank et al. 1996; Sung et al. 2001). Despite the observed limitations on the usage of viral vectors, especially regarding safety, they are still the most used gene transfer vehicles (Gardlik et al. 2005).

Nonviral methods make use of cationic lipid complexes, liposomes (see below), polymers, and other reagents. Furthermore, ODNs may be internalized mechanically, i.e., by generating transient permeabilization of the plasma membrane to allow penetration of naked ODNs into cells by diffusion. However, these methods are not useful in vivo and their relevance for gene function analysis remains questionable. Therefore, plasmid or liposomal complexes are the most commonly used nonviral vectors and represent attractive tools in gene therapy due to their relatively simple production, low toxicity, and low host immunogenicity (Gardlik et al. 2005). Shen and colleagues demonstrated that the use of a cationic liposome elicits enhanced efficacy of ODNs for the inhibition of TGF-beta2 expression in the human promonocytic leukemia cell line U937 (Shen et al. 1999). All of these cationic delivery systems internalize ODNs via an endocytotic mechanism. In contrast to the in vitro situation, many reports have shown that in vivo uptake of S-ODNs does not depend on cationic carrier liposomes (Braasch and Corey 2002; Tari and Lopez-Berestein 2001).

In vitro, most of the ODNs designated for clinical studies were delivered in the presence of carrier liposomes in order to facilitate the ODN uptake. In contrast, during the selection process toward the development of the herein described antisense S-ODN AP 12009, inhibition of TGF-beta2 expression without carriers was crucial. Importantly, in preclinical experiments performed with and without the carrier protein Lipofectin

(Invitrogen, Carlsbad, CA; a transfection reagent) AP 12009 showed similar effects (see below).

16.3 The Target: Transforming Growth Factor-Beta 2

TGF-beta is a multifunctional cytokine playing various roles in cell functions, including morphogenesis, cell proliferation, and migration, and is a key regulator of the immune system. Three isoforms of TGF-beta are described in mammals: TGF-beta1, TGF-beta2, and TGF–beta3. A unique gene on different chromosomes encodes each isoform. All three human isoforms show a different temporal and spatial expression. Major activities of TGF-betas include inhibition of cell proliferation by blocking the cell cycle in late G1 phase, immunosuppressive effects, and enhancing the formation of extracellular matrix. The transcriptional regulation of TGF-beta1 is different from that of TGF-beta2 and TGF-beta3 as the latter are mostly under hormonal and developmental control (Roberts 1998).

TGF-beta is synthesized as homomeric proproteins in vivo, which need to be activated to bind to the signaling receptors (Murphy-Ullrich and Poczatek 2000; Wakefield and Roberts 2002). The so-called latency-associated protein (LAP) is generated by removal of the N-terminus of the mature TGF-beta by a furin-like peptidase. The LAP is noncovalently associated with a homodimer of mature TGF-beta (Li et al. 2006). TGF-beta is secreted as a complex, which consists of the inactive, mature TGF-beta, the LAP, and the latent TGF-beta binding protein (LTBP) (Annes et al. 2003; Oeklue and Hesketh 2000). Extracellular activation of this complex is a critical step in the regulation of TGF-beta function, including plasmin-dependent and plasmin-independent pathways (Derynck and Zhang 2003; Piek et al. 1999; Wakefield and Roberts 2002; Yingling et al. 2004).

Although TGF-beta1 and TGF-beta2 share various similar receptor binding and signaling properties, some crucial differences have been described. In general, the TGF-beta ligand binds to receptors on the cell surface forming a bi-dimeric receptor complex consisting of two pairs of subunits known as receptor type I (TBR-I, usually ALK5) and type II (TBR-II). A membrane-anchored proteoglycan, known as type III receptor (TBR-III or betaglycan), aids this process by capturing TGF-beta for presentation to the signaling receptors I and II. Importantly, the type III receptor is particularly important for TGF-beta2, which cannot bind TBR-II independently and thus depends on the presence of TBR-III to signal—a unique feature that distinguishes TGF-beta2 from TGF-beta1 and TGF-beta3 (Blobe et al. 2001).

The biological activities of TGF-betas are modulated by binding proteins with alpha-2-macroglobulin (A_2M) as the major binding protein for TGF-beta1 and TGF-beta2 in plasma (Danielpour and Sporn 1990; O'Connor-McCourt and Wakefield 1987). A_2M is a homotetrameric glycoprotein that inhibits various proteinases and serves as a regulator and major carrier of various cytokines (Crookston et al. 1994). It is one of the most abundant proteins in human plasma with a concentration of 2–4 mg/ml. Both isoforms, TGF-beta1 and TGF-beta2, bind reversibly and covalently to native A_2M and A_2M-methylamine. It has been shown that A_2M significantly inhibits the receptor binding and biological activity of TGF-betas (O'Connor-McCourt and Wakefield 1987). However, TGF-beta2 is more affected due to a distinctive interaction pattern with A_2M compared to TGF-beta1 and other cytokines (Crookston et al. 1994). First, TGF-beta2 reveals substantially higher affinity to A_2M and therefore an increased complex formation (Danielpour and Sporn 1990; Liu et al. 2001). Second, it is the only growth factor that binds with equivalent affinity to both A_2M and A_2M-methylamine (Crookston et al. 1994). In experiments using native A_2M as well as the activated form A_2M-methylamine, TGF-beta2 shows the highest affinity to both proteins compared to other cytokines including TGF-beta1, nerve growth factor-beta (NGF-beta), platelet-derived growth factor-BB (PDGF-BB), tumor necrosis factor (TNF-alpha), and basic fibroblast growth factor (Crookston et al. 1994).

The significance of TGF-beta has become increasingly evident since it obviously elicits two opposed mechanisms depending on the respective environment (Akhurst and Derynck 2001; Wakefield and Roberts 2002). In normal cells of epithelial origin as well as in early well-differentiated tumor cells of epithelial origin, the TGF-beta pathway restricts cell growth, differentiation, and cell death. However, during progression of cells toward fully malignant tumor cells, these cells undergo changes resulting in reduced expression of TGF-beta receptors, increased expression of TGF-beta ligands, and resistance to growth inhibition by TGF-beta (Moustakas et al. 2002; Wakefield and Roberts 2002).

The crucial role of TGF-beta2 in pancreatic cancer progression and aggressiveness was demonstrated in an animal model consisting of human pancreatic cancer cells grown either ectopically in subcutaneous tissue or orthotopically in the pancreas (Choudhury et al. 2004). In this model, TGF-beta2 expression clearly correlated with tumor aggressiveness and metastatic behavior. The far more aggressive orthotopic tumors not only demonstrated a larger size, shorter latent period, higher metastasis, and more extensive invasion of the stomach, but also a higher expression of TGF-beta2 compared to the less aggressive subcutaneous tumors. In another study on human pancreatic tissue samples, immunohistochemical analysis has shown that all three mammalian isoforms of TGF-beta (TGF-beta1, -beta2, and -beta3) were overexpressed (Friess et al. 1993). However, only the TGF-beta2 isoform was significantly correlated with advanced tumor stage and a more aggressive phenotype. Pancreatic cancer patients bearing TGF-beta2 producing tumors showed the shortest postoperative survival period in contrast to patients with tumors producing TGF-beta1, TGF-beta3, or none of the TGF-beta isoforms (Friess et al. 1993).

16.3.1 Targeted Therapy with the TGF-Beta2 Inhibitor AP 12009

16.3.1.1 Preclinical Experiments

In vitro experiments were performed to evaluate the specificity and efficacy of the TGF-beta2 specific phosphorothioate ODN AP 12009 by employing human tumor cell cultures as well as peripheral blood mononuclear cells (PBMC) from healthy donors and from patients (Schlingensiepen et al. 2006).

The efficacy of AP 12009 in reducing TGF-beta2 secretion of human pancreatic carcinoma cells was determined by measuring the TGF-beta2 concentration in culture supernatants using an enzyme-linked immunosorbent assay (ELISA). Treatment with AP 12009 complexed with the liposomal carrier Lipofectin significantly inhibited TGF-beta2 production compared to Lipofectin alone in all human pancreatic cancer cell lines tested. Importantly, comparable data were obtained in experiments without Lipofectin indicating that AP 12009 alone is able to inhibit TGF-beta induced tumor-promoting effects.

Furthermore, AP 12009 was shown to revert the strong immunosuppressive effects exerted by TGF-beta2. TGF-beta has multiple immunosuppressive properties including inhibition of T cell proliferation and inhibition of T cell differentiation into cytotoxic T lymphocytes (CTLs) and helper T cells (Gorelik and Flavell 2001). TGF-beta inhibits these immune cell functions including cell-dependent cytotoxicity (Weller and Fontana 1995). Treatment with AP 12009 enhances the cytotoxic antitumor response of human lymphokine activated killer (LAK) cells directed against pancreatic carcinoma cells.

The invasion of neoplastic cells into healthy tissue is a pathologic hallmark of highly aggressive tumors such as pancreatic carcinoma, malignant melanoma, or malignant glioma.

The key mechanism for infiltration of tumor cells into healthy tissue leading to metastasis is tumor cell motility. TGF-beta, produced by tumor cells, acts directly on the tumor cells by inducing EMT (Janji et al. 1999), and by increasing motility, invasiveness, and metastasis (Dumont and Arteaga 2000; Oft et al. 1998). AP 12009 inhibits the migration of cancer cells in vitro. The motility of pancreatic cancer cells was measured employing an in vitro spheroid migration model (Nygaard et al. 1998). Tumor cells spontaneously form round shaped clusters (spheroids) when cultured in medium on agar-coated plates, which prevents their adherence to the plastic surface. The spheroids can be transferred into culture medium without agar where the tumor cells start migrating off the spheroids. AP 12009 inhibits migration of the pancreatic tumor cells with the spheroids remaining compact after 24 h. In contrast, untreated and recombinant human (rh-) TGF-beta2 treated cells migrate and, as a consequence, the spheroids dissolve.

Similar results as described for pancreatic cancer cells were obtained for other cancer cells including human malignant glioma and malignant melanoma cell cultures (Jachimczak et al. 1993, 1996; Schlingensiepen et al. 2006). Importantly, all experiments were performed in the presence as well as in the absence of a liposome carrier and showed comparable efficiency to naked and Lipofectin-complexed AP 12009 in various cell lines test.

16.3.1.2 Toxicological Studies

In the current clinical trials of AP 12009 are being developed for the treatment of TGF-beta2-overproducing tumors such as malignant glioma, pancreatic carcinoma, metastatic colorectal carcinoma, and metastatic melanoma. Whereas AP 12009 is administered systemically by intravenous infusion in the indications for pancreatic carcinoma, metastatic colorectal carcinoma, and melanoma, in the case of high-grade glioma the same substance is applied locally by convection-enhanced delivery (CED) directly into the brain tumor tissue.

Local toxicity studies applying AP 12009 by the intrathecal and intracerebral routes were performed in rabbits and monkeys in order to match the intended human mode of application in malignant glioma as close as possible. AP 12009 showed excellent local tolerability in rabbits and monkeys when administered by intrathecal bolus injection. Neither clinical signs of toxicity nor substance-related histomorphological changes were observed. The application of AP 12009 via continuous intracerebral infusion focally resulted in a mild to moderate lymphocytic leptomeningo-encephalitis. Changes are considered a reversible immunological reaction to AP 12009. Local tolerance tests of AP 12009 in rabbits after intravenous, intraarterial, intramuscular, paravenous, and subcutaneous application led neither to macroscopic nor to microscopic changes.

Acute toxicology studies in mice and rats as well as subchronic toxicity studies in rats and in cynomolgus monkeys were performed employing intravenous infusion. Liver and kidney were identified as target organs. The observed changes match the common toxic effects reported for S-ODNs (Henry et al. 1997; Levin et al. 1998). Detailed methods and results were reported by Schlingensiepen et al. (2005).

The pharmacological effects of AP 12009 on the cardiovascular system, complement activation, and hematological parameters corresponded well to the effects reported for other phosphorothioate ODNs as a class of compounds (Mahato 2005).

AP 12009 showed neither mutagenic effect in the *Salmonella typhimurium* strains nor indications of mutagenic properties in cultured human peripheral lymphocytes with respect to chromosomal or chromatid damage. Furthermore, AP 12009 showed no mutagenic properties in the mouse bone marrow micronucleus study using intravenous administration.

16.3.1.3 Clinical Studies: Systemic Application

In pancreatic carcinoma cells, all three mammalian isoforms of TGF-beta (TGF-beta1, TGF-beta2, and TGF-beta3) are expressed. However, only excessive expression of TGF-beta2 is significantly associated with pancreatic cancer progression (Friess et al. 1993).

Spurred by the clinical data in recurrent or refractory high-grade glioma patients (see Sect. 3.1.4) and the impressive antitumor activity in a wide variety of preclinical assays (Schlingensiepen et al. 2006), the clinical studies for other solid tumors were initiated. A multicenter dose-escalation phase I/II trial with AP 12009 in adult patients suffering from advanced pancreatic carcinoma (AJCC stage IVA or IVB) as well as metastatic melanoma (AJCC/UICC stage III or IV) and advanced metastatic colorectal carcinoma (AJCC/UICC stage III or IV), is currently ongoing. The primary endpoint is the assessment of the maximum tolerated dose (MTD) as well as the dose-limiting toxicities. Secondary objectives include safety and tolerability of AP 12009 and its potential antitumor activity. Adult patients (18–75 years) with advanced tumors who are not or no longer amenable to established therapies are eligible for this dose-escalation study. Karnofsky performance status (KPS) should be at least 80%. Patients receive the study drug intravenously via an implanted port system at weekly intervals. Up to ten treatment cycles are to be applied per patient.

The majority of patients already treated received more than the minimum number of two cycles. One of them received ten full cycles. So far, AP 12009 revealed a good safety profile. The MTD has not yet been reached. Further dose escalations are ongoing.

16.3.1.4 Clinical Studies: Local Application in High-Grade Glioma Patients

The TGF-beta2 isoform is specifically overexpressed in malignant gliomas (Frankel et al. 1999; Maxwell et al. 1992). The increased levels of TGF-beta2 are associated with disease stage and causative for the immunodeficient state of patients (Bodmer et al. 1989; Kjellman et al. 2000; Maxwell et al. 1992).

In three phase I/II dose-escalation studies (G001, G002, and G003) a total of 24 adult patients with recurrent or refractory malignant glioma, i.e., anaplastic astrocytoma (AA, WHO grade III) or glioblastoma (GBM, WHO grade IV), and evidence of tumor progression were treated with AP 12009 (Schlingensiepen et al. 2006). In these studies, the drug was administered intratumorally using CED over a 4- or 7-day period. The CED application allows AP 12009 to bypass the BBB. The BBB serves as a natural defense system by blocking the entry of foreign substances, including bacteria and toxins but also many therapeutic agents (Bobo et al. 1994). While conventional diffusion is characterized by a steep drop in drug concentration close to the catheter tip, CED creates a homogeneous drug concentration extending over several centimeters in diameter (Lieberman et al. 1995). To facilitate multiple cycles of AP 12009, the investigational drug was infused through an implanted port system connected to the intratumoral catheter. AP 12009 proved to be well tolerated and revealed a good safety profile. Since two complete remissions in two different dose groups were observed (see below), further dose escalation was not necessary. MTD was not reached. Although the clinical phase I/II trials were primarily designed to assess safety, survival times as well as tumor response data were obtained. Data on antitumor activity from 24 patients included several patients with stabilization of disease and two patients with complete tumor remission, both of them long-lasting without recurrence. One of these two patients, diagnosed with AA, was treated with only one course of AP 12009. At baseline four tumor lesions had been detected, which were spread over both hemispheres. Only one lesion had been infused with one cycle of AP 12009, but all lesions had disappeared several months after start of treatment despite an initial and temporary increase in tumor volume at the beginning of the treatment. The patient died from a myocardial infarction without any signs of tumor, 25 months after start of AP 12009 treatment. The second patient, also diagnosed with AA, received a total of 12 cycles of AP 12009 over the course of the three phase I/II studies (G001, G002, and G003; Fig. 16.2).

Prior to AP 12009 treatment, he had been treated with surgery, radiation, and chemotherapy [temozolomide (TMZ) after the first relapse], followed by a second incomplete surgery. After an initial stabilization following the second cycle, the enhancing lesion continued to increase until 10 months after baseline G001 (Fig. 16.2b), inducing a significant edema. The central reading of the magnetic resonance image (MRI) 20 months after the start of AP 12009 treatment (in G001) was evaluated as partial response (PR, 83% tumor reduction, Fig. 16.2c); there was complete response after 22 months. The patient is known to still be alive today; the MRI in August 2006 (Fig. 16.2d) showed no recurrence. Survival of this patient after the first recurrence is now 307 weeks (71 months); it has been 286 weeks (66 months) since treatment with AP 12009 began (status 01 August 2007).

As of 01 August 2007 the median overall survival after recurrence for AA patients treated with AP 12009 was 146.6 weeks (range 32.0–306.6 weeks), and for GBM patients treated with AP 12009 44.0 weeks (range 18.9–87.9 weeks). The most recent and accurate survival data after start of therapy that clearly distinguish between recurrent AA and GBM are available for the current gold standard treatment TMZ. The re-

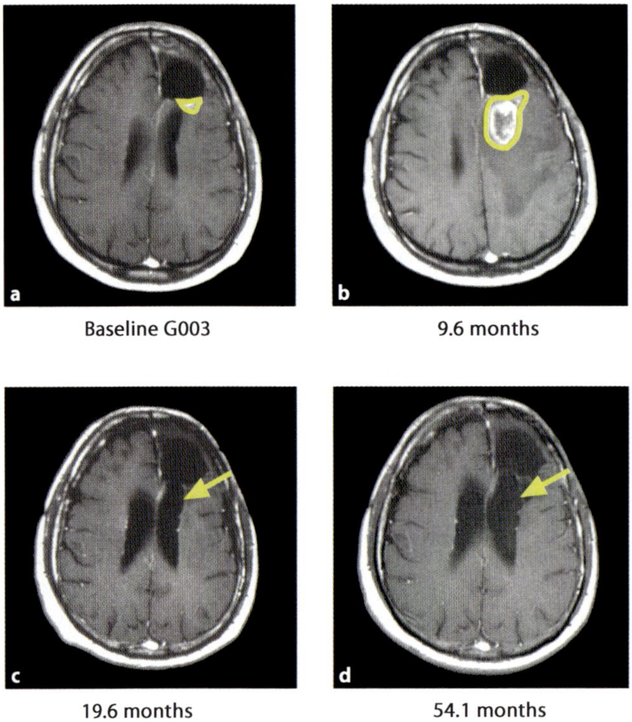

Fig. 16.2a–d MRI scans of a 49-year-old male patient (patient no. 17) diagnosed with anaplastic astrocytoma (AA, WHO grade 3) in 2001 (for details see text)

ported median overall survival for TMZ alone is 42.0 weeks (9.7 months) for recurrent AA (Theodosopoulos et al. 2001), and 31.8 (7.3 months) (Yung 2000; Yung et al. 2000) or 32.0 weeks (7.4 months) (Theodosopoulos et al. 2001) for recurrent GBM. These results were reported for patients with high-grade glioma who received TMZ as first treatment after recurrence. In the adjuvant treatment of newly diagnosed glioma, the combination of TMZ with radiotherapy has improved median overall survival from 12.1 to 14.6 months (Stupp et al. 2005).

The phase IIb clinical trial of AP 12009-G004 is an international, open-label, active-controlled dose-finding study in high-grade glioma patients. The main trial objective is the comparison of two different doses of AP 12009 (10 μM or 80 μM) against standard chemotherapy. In all, 145 patients with either recurrent or refractory AA (WHO grade III) or GBM (WHO grade IV) are receiving either one of the two doses of AP 12009 or standard chemotherapy [TMZ or procarbazine/CCNU (lomustine)/vincristine = PCV, if TMZ was already given]. AP 12009 is applied intratumorally by CED during a 6-month active treatment period at weekly intervals. The primary efficacy endpoint is tumor response after radiological evaluation. The main secondary efficacy endpoints are overall survival and 12-month survival. As in the previous studies, preliminary data show long-lasting responses both in recurrent or refractory AA and GBM patients (Bogdahn et al. 2006; Hau et al. 2006). Especially in recurrent or refractory AA patients, very promising efficacy data have been documented compared to current standard treatment with TMZ or PCV.

16.4 Summary

Despite tremendous advances in cancer research and the development of new therapies, patients with malignant tumors such as advanced pancreatic carcinoma, metastatic melanoma, metastatic colorectal carcinoma, and malignant glioma still face a poor prognosis. The severe morbidity and mortality of these malignant tumor types makes the identification of factors associated with their incidence an important area of both preclinical and clinical research. Antisense technology is a new and innovative method offering a causal approach for the treatment of various highly aggressive diseases. Antisense compounds inhibit the production of disease-causing proteins at the molecular level and combat tumor development directly at its roots. Preclinical experiments using the TGF-beta2 specific phosphorothioate ODN AP 12009 revealed the potential of this compound to reverse TGF-beta2 induced immunosuppression as well as inhibition of tumor cell proliferation and tumor cell migration. Initial clinical studies have demonstrated AP 12009 to be well tolerated and safe. Furthermore, the first evidence of efficacy of AP 12009 antisense therapy in recurrent or refractory high-grade glioma has been provided.

These data confirm that the blockade of TGF-beta2, a key factor in tumorigenesis, in tumor tissue by AP 12009 represents a novel and promising therapeutic approach for malignant tumors such as advanced pancreatic carcinoma and malignant glioma. This approach aims at a reduction of tumor-promoting effects and, most importantly, an enhancement of the antitumor immune response.

Acknowledgements

We thank Drs. D. Fischer and H. Specht for critical reading of the manuscript as well as helpful discussions and suggestions.

References

Agrawal S, Temsamani J, Tang JY (1991) Pharmacokinetics, biodistribution, and stability of oligodeoxynucleotide phosphorothioates in mice. Proc Natl Acad Sci U S A 88:7595–7599

Agrawal S, Temsamani J, Galbraith W, Tang J (1995) Pharmacokinetics of antisense oligonucleotides. Clin Pharmacokinet 28:7–16

Agrawal S, Jiang Z, Zhao Q, Shaw D, Cai Q, Roskey A, Channavajjala L, Saxinger C, Zhang R (1997) Mixed-backbone oligonucleotides as second generation antisense oligonucleotides: in vitro and in vivo studies. Proc Natl Acad Sci U S A 94:2620–2625

Akhtar S, Agrawal S (1997) In vivo studies with antisense oligonucleotides. Trends Pharmacol Sci 18:12–18

Akhurst RJ, Derynck R (2001) TGF-beta signaling in cancer—a double-edged sword. Trends Cell Biol 11:S44–51

Annes JP, Munger JS, Rifkin DB (2003) Making sense of latent TGFbeta activation. J Cell Sci 116:217–224

Auerbach M, Wampler GL, Lokich JJ, Fryer D, Fryer JG, Ahlgren JD (1997) Treatment of advanced pancreatic carcinoma with a combination of protracted infusional 5-fluorouracil and weekly carboplatin: a Mid-Atlantic Oncology Program Study. Ann Oncol 8:439–444

Blobe GC, Schiemann WP, Pepin MC, Beauchemin M, Moustakas A, Lodish HF, O'Connor-McCourt MD (2001) Functional roles for the cytoplasmic domain of the type III transforming growth factor beta receptor in regulating transforming growth factor beta signaling. J Biol Chem 276:24627–24637

Bobo RH, Laske DW, Akbasak A, Morrison PF, Dedrick RL, Oldfield EH (1994) Convection-enhanced delivery of macromolecules in the brain. Proc Natl Acad Sci U S A 91:2076–2080

Bodmer S, Strommer K, Frei K, Siepl C, de Tribolet N, Heid I, Fontana A (1989) Immunosuppression and transforming growth factor-beta in glioblastoma. Preferential production of transforming growth factor-beta 2. J Immunol 143:3222–3229

Bogdahn U, Oliushine VE, Parfenov VE, Kunst M, Mahapatra AK, Sastry KVR, Venkataramana KN, Jachimczak P, Hau P, Schlingensiepen KH (2006) Results of G004, a phase IIb study in recurrent glioblastoma patients with the TGF-b2 targeted compound AP 12009. J Clin Oncol, ASCO Annual Meeting Proceedings 24:1553

Braasch DA, Corey DR (2002) Novel antisense and peptide nucleic acid strategies for controlling gene expression. Biochemistry 41:4503–4510

Brysch W, Schlingensiepen KH (1994) Design and application of antisense oligonucleotides in cell culture, in vivo, and as therapeutic agents. Cell Mol Neurobiol 14:557–568

Burgess TL, Fisher EF, Ross SL, Bready JV, Qian YX, Bayewitch LA, Cohen AM, Herrera CJ, Hu SS, Kramer TB, et al. (1995) The antiproliferative activity of c-myb and c-myc antisense oligonucleotides in smooth muscle cells is caused by a nonantisense mechanism. Proc Natl Acad Sci U S A 92:4051–4055

Cardenes HR, Chiorean EG, Dewitt J, Schmidt M, Loehrer P (2006) Locally advanced pancreatic cancer: current therapeutic approach. Oncologist 11:612–623

Choudhury A, Moniaux N, Ulrich AB, Schmied BM, Standop J, Pour PM, Gendler SJ, Hollingsworth MA, Aubert JP, Batra SK (2004) MUC4 mucin expression in human pancreatic tumours is affected by organ environment: the possible role of TGF-beta2. Br J Cancer 90:657–664

Coppelli FM, Grandis JR (2005) Oligonucleotides as anticancer agents: from the benchside to the clinic and beyond. Curr Pharm Des 11:2825–2840

Crooke ST (1999) Molecular mechanisms of action of antisense drugs. Biochim Biophys Acta 1489:31–44

Crookston KP, Webb DJ, Wolf BB, Gonias SL (1994) Classification of alpha 2-macroglobulin-cytokine interactions based on affinity of noncovalent association in solution under apparent equilibrium conditions. J Biol Chem 269:1533–1540

Danielpour D, Sporn MB (1990) Differential inhibition of transforming growth factor beta 1 and beta 2 activity by alpha 2-macroglobulin. J Biol Chem 265:6973–6977

Dean NM, Bennett CF (2003) Antisense oligonucleotide-based therapeutics for cancer. Oncogene 22:9087–9096

Derynck R, Zhang YE (2003) Smad-dependent and Smad-independent pathways in TGF-beta family signalling. Nature 425:577–584

Dumont N, Arteaga CL (2000) Transforming growth factor-beta and breast cancer: tumor promoting effects of transforming growth factor-beta. Breast Cancer Res 2:125–132

Eckstein F (1983) Phosphorothioate analogues of nucleotides—tools for the investigation of biochemical processes. Angew Chem Int Ed Engl 22:423–506

Frankel B, Longo SL, Ryken TC (1999) Human astrocytomas co-expressing Fas and Fas ligand also produce TGFbeta2 and Bcl-2. J Neurooncol 44:205–212

Friess H, Yamanaka Y, Buchler M, Ebert M, Beger HG, Gold LI, Korc M (1993) Enhanced expression of transforming growth factor beta isoforms in pancreatic cancer correlates with decreased survival. Gastroenterology 105:1846–1856

Gardlik R, Palffy R, Hodosy J, Lukacs J, Turna J, Celec P (2005) Vectors and delivery systems in gene therapy. Med Sci Monit 11:RA110–RA121

Geary RS, Yu RZ, Levin AA (2001) Pharmacokinetics of phosphorothioate antisense oligodeoxynucleotides. Curr Opin Investig Drugs 2:562–573

Gorelik L, Flavell RA (2001) Immune-mediated eradication of tumors through the blockade of transforming growth factor-beta signaling in T cells. Nat Med 7:1118–1122

Hau P, Stockhammer G, Kunst M, Mahapatra AK, Sastry KVR, Parfenov V, Leshinsky V, Jachimczak P, Bogdahn U, Schlingensiepen K-H (2006) Results of G004, a phase IIb actively controlled clinical trial with the TGF-b2 targeted compound AP 12009 for recurrent anaplastic astrocytoma. J Clin Oncol, ASCO Annual Meeting Proceedings 24:1566

Henry SP, Bolte H, Auletta C, Kornbrust DJ (1997) Evaluation of the toxicity of ISIS 2302, a phosphorothioate oligonucleotide, in a four-week study in cynomolgus monkeys. Toxicology 120:145–155

Jachimczak P, Bogdahn U, Schneider J, Behl C, Meixensberger J, Apfel R, Dorries R, Schlingensiepen KH, Brysch W (1993) The effect of transforming growth factor-beta 2-specific phosphorothioate-anti-sense oligodeoxynucleotides in reversing cellular immunosuppression in malignant glioma. J Neurosurg 78:944–951

Jachimczak P, Hessdorfer B, Fabel-Schulte K, Wismeth C, Brysch W, Schlingensiepen KH, Bauer A, Blesch A, Bogdahn U (1996) Transforming growth factor-beta-mediated autocrine growth regulation of gliomas as detected with phosphorothioate antisense oligonucleotides. Int J Cancer 65:332–337

Janji B, Melchior C, Gouon V, Vallar L, Kieffer N (1999) Autocrine TGF-beta-regulated expression of adhesion receptors and integrin-linked kinase in HT-144 melanoma cells correlates with their metastatic phenotype. Int J Cancer 83:255–262

Jemal A, Murray T, Ward E, Samuels A, Tiwari RC, Ghafoor A, Feuer EJ, Thun M (2005) Cancer statistics, 2005. CA Cancer J Clin 55:10–30

Jemal A, Siegel R, Ward E, Murray T, Xu J, Smigal C, Thun MJ (2006) Cancer statistics, 2006. CA Cancer J Clin 56:106–130

Kjellman C, Olofsson SP, Hansson O, Von Schantz T, Lindvall M, Nilsson I, Salford LG, Sjogren HO, Widegren B (2000) Expression of TGF-beta isoforms, TGF-beta receptors, and SMAD molecules at different stages of human glioma. Int J Cancer 89:251–258

Krieg AM (2002) CpG motifs in bacterial DNA and their immune effects. Annu Rev Immunol 20:709–760

Kurreck J (2003) Antisense technologies. Improvement through novel chemical modifications. Eur J Biochem 270:1628–1644

Lahn M, Kloeker S, Berry BS (2005) TGF-beta inhibitors for the treatment of cancer. Expert Opin Investig Drugs 14:629–643

Lee Y, Vassilakos A, Feng N, Jin H, Wang M, Xiong K, Wright J, Young A (2006) GTI-2501, an antisense agent targeting R1, the large subunit of human ribonucleotide reductase, shows potent anti-tumor activity against a variety of tumors. Int J Oncol 28:469–478

Levin AA (1999) A review of the issues in the pharmacokinetics and toxicology of phosphorothioate antisense oligonucleotides. Biochim Biophys Acta 1489:69–84

Levin AA, Monteith DK, Leeds JM, Nicklin PL, Geary RS, Butler M, Templin MV, Henry SP (1998) Toxicity of oligonucleotide therapeutic agents. In: Crooke ST (ed) Antisense research and application. Springer, Berlin Heidelberg New York, pp 169–215

Li D, Xie K, Wolff R, Abbruzzese JL (2004) Pancreatic cancer. Lancet 363:1049–1057

Li MO, Wan YY, Sanjabi S, Robertson AK, Flavell RA (2006) Transforming growth factor-beta regulation of immune responses. Annu Rev Immunol 24:99–146

Lieberman DM, Laske DW, Morrison PF, Bankiewicz KS, Oldfield EH (1995) Convection-enhanced distribution of large molecules in gray matter during interstitial drug infusion. J Neurosurg 82:1021–1029

Liu Q, Ling TY, Shieh HS, Johnson FE, Huang JS, Huang SS (2001) Identification of the high affinity binding site in transforming growth factor-beta involved in complex formation with alpha 2-macroglobulin. Implications regarding the molecular mechanisms of complex formation between alpha 2-macroglobulin and growth factors, cytokines, and hormones. J Biol Chem 276:46212–46218

Lowenfels AB, Maisonneuve P (2006) Epidemiology and risk factors for pancreatic cancer. Best Pract Res Clin Gastroenterol 20:197–209

Lysik MA, Wu-Pong S (2003) Innovations in oligonucleotide drug delivery. J Pharm Sci 92:1559–1573

Mahato RI (2005) Biomaterials for delivery and targeting of proteins and nucleic acids. CRC Press, Boca Raton

Mahato RI, Ye Z, Guntaka RV (2005) Antisense and antigene oligonucleotides: structure, stability and delivery. In: Mahato RI (ed) Biomaterials for delivering and targeting of proteins and nucleic acids. CRC Press, Boca Raton, pp 569–600

Maxwell M, Galanopoulos T, Neville-Golden J, Antoniades HN (1992) Effect of the expression of transforming growth factor-beta 2 in primary human glioblastomas on immunosuppression and loss of immune surveillance. J Neurosurg 76:799–804

Miller PS, McParland KB, Jayaraman K, Ts'o PO (1981) Biochemical and biological effects of nonionic nucleic acid methylphosphonates. Biochemistry 20:1874–1880

Moore MJ, Goldstein D, Hamm J, Figer A, Hecht J, Gallinger S, Au H, Ding J, Christy-Bittel J, Parulekar W (2005) Erlotinib plus gemcitabine compared to gemcitabine alone in patients with advanced pancreatic cancer. A phase III trial of the National Cancer Institute of Canada Clinical Trials Group [NCIC-CTG]. J Clin Oncol, 2005 ASCO Annual Meeting Proceedings 23:16S

Moustakas A, Pardali K, Gaal A, Heldin CH (2002) Mechanisms of TGF-beta signaling in regulation of cell growth and differentiation. Immunol Lett 82:85–91

Murphy-Ullrich JE, Poczatek M (2000) Activation of latent TGF-beta by thrombospondin-1: mechanisms and physiology. Cytokine Growth Factor Rev 11:59–69

Nygaard SJ, Haugland HK, Laerum OD, Lund-Johansen M, Bjerkvig R, Tysnes OB (1998) Dynamic determination of human glioma invasion in vitro. J Neurosurg 89:441–447

O'Connor-McCourt MD, Wakefield LM (1987) Latent transforming growth factor-beta in serum. A specific complex with alpha 2-macroglobulin. J Biol Chem 262:14090–14099

Oeklue R, Hesketh R (2000) The latent transforming growth factor beta binding protein (LTBP) family. Biochem J 352:601–610

Oft M, Heider KH, Beug H (1998) TGFbeta signaling is necessary for carcinoma cell invasiveness and metastasis. Curr Biol 8:1243–1252

Piek E, Heldin CH, Ten Dijke P (1999) Specificity, diversity, and regulation in TGF-beta superfamily signaling. FASEB J 13:2105–2124

Plank C, Mechtler K, Szoka FC Jr, Wagner E (1996) Activation of the complement system by synthetic DNA complexes: a potential barrier for intravenous gene delivery. Hum Gene Ther 7:1437–1446

Roberts AB (1998) Molecular and cell biology of TGF-beta. Miner Electrolyte Metab 24:111–119

Roehr B (1998) Fomivirsen approved for CMV retinitis. J Int Assoc Physicians AIDS Care 4:14–16

Schlingensiepen KH, Schlingensiepen R, Kunst M, Klinger I, Gerdes W, Seifert W, Brysch W (1993) Opposite functions of jun-B and c-jun in growth regulation and neuronal differentiation. Dev Genet 14:305–312

Schlingensiepen KH, Schlingensiepen R, Steinbrecher A, Hau P, Bogdahn U, Fischer-Blass B, Jachimczak P (2006) Targeted tumor therapy with the TGF-b2 antisense compound AP 12009. Cytokine Growth Factor Rev 17:129–139

Schlingensiepen R, Brysch W, Schlingensiepen KH (1997) Antisense: from technology to therapy: lab manual and textbook. Blackwell Science, Berlin

Schlingensiepen R, Goldbrunner M, Szyrach MN, Stauder G, Jachimczak P, Bogdahn U, Schulmeyer F, Hau P, Schlingensiepen KH (2005) Intracerebral and intrathecal infusion of the TGF-beta2-specific antisense phosphorothioate oligonucleotide AP 12009 in rabbits and primates: toxicology and safety. Oligonucleotides 15:94–104

Shaw JP, Kent K, Bird J, Fishback J, Froehler B (1991) Modified deoxyoligonucleotides stable to exonuclease degradation in serum. Nucleic Acids Res 19:747–750

Shen ZJ, Kim SK, Lee YS, Lee JW, Moon BJ (1999) Inhibition of transforming growth factor-beta 2 expression with phosphorothioate antisense oligonucleotides in U937 cells. Bioorg Med Chem Lett 9:13–18

Siech M, Schlosser W, Beger HG (2001) Modern techniques for operation for chronic pancreatitis and pancreatic carcinoma and postoperative consequences. Pancreatology 1:1–8

Stein CA, Tonkinson JL, Zhang LM, Yakubov L, Gervasoni J, Taub R, Rotenberg SA (1993) Dynamics of the internalization of phosphodiester oligodeoxynucleotides in HL60 cells. Biochemistry 32:4855–4861

Stupp R, Mason WP, van den Bent MJ, Weller M, Fisher B, Taphoorn MJ, Belanger K, Brandes AA, Marosi C, Bogdahn U, Curschmann J, Janzer RC, Ludwin SK, Gorlia T, Allgeier A, Lacombe D, Cairncross JG, Eisenhauer E, Mirimanoff RO (2005) Radiotherapy plus concomitant and adjuvant temozolomide for glioblastoma. N Engl J Med 352:987–996

Sung RS, Qin L, Bromberg JS (2001) TNFalpha and IFNgamma induced by innate anti-adenoviral immune responses inhibit adenovirus-mediated transgene expression. Mol Ther 3:757–767

Tari AM, Lopez-Berestein G (2001) Cellular uptake of antisense oligonucleotides. Curr Opin Investig Drugs 2:1450–1453

Theodosopoulos PV, Lamborn KR, Malec M, et al. (2001) Temozolomide in the treatment of recurrent malignant glioma. Proc ASCO, San Francisco

Tidd DM, Warenius HM (1989) Partial protection of oncogene, anti-sense oligodeoxynucleotides against serum nuclease degradation using terminal methylphosphonate groups. Br J Cancer 60:343–350

Wakefield LM, Roberts AB (2002) TGF-beta signaling: positive and negative effects on tumorigenesis. Curr Opin Genet Dev 12:22–29

Weller M, Fontana A (1995) The failure of current immunotherapy for malignant glioma. Tumor-derived TGF-beta, T-cell apoptosis, and the immune privilege of the brain. Brain Res Brain Res Rev 21:128–151

Wickstrom E (1986) Oligodeoxynucleotide stability in subcellular extracts and culture media. J Biochem Biophys Methods 13:97–102

Yang Y, Wilson JM (1995) Clearance of adenovirus-infected hepatocytes by MHC class I-restricted CD4+ CTLs in vivo. J Immunol 155:2564–2570

Yaswen P, Stampfer MR, Ghosh K, Cohen JS (1993) Effects of sequence of thioated oligonucleotides on cultured human mammary epithelial cells. Antisense Res Dev 3:67–77

Yingling JM, Blanchard KL, Sawyer JS (2004) Development of TGF-beta signalling inhibitors for cancer therapy. Nat Rev Drug Discov 3:1011–1022

Yung WK (2000) Temozolomide in malignant gliomas. Semin Oncol 27:27–34

Yung WK, Albright RE, Olson J, Fredericks R, Fink K, Prados MD, Brada M, Spence A, Hohl RJ, Shapiro W, Glantz M, Greenberg H, Selker RG, Vick NA, Rampling R, Friedman H, Phillips P, Bruner J, Yue N, Osoba D, Zaknoen S, Levin VA (2000) A phase II study of temozolomide vs. procarbazine in patients with glioblastoma multiforme at first relapse. Br J Cancer 83:588–593

Zamecnik P, Aghajanian J, Zamecnik M, Goodchild J, Witman G (1994) Electron micrographic studies of transport of oligodeoxynucleotides across eukaryotic cell membranes. Proc Natl Acad Sci U S A 91:3156–3160

Zamecnik PC, Stephenson ML (1978) Inhibition of Rous sarcoma virus replication and cell transformation by a specific oligodeoxynucleotide. Proc Natl Acad Sci U S A 75:280–284

17 NF-κB as a Molecular Target in the Therapy of Pancreatic Carcinoma

S. Sebens, A. Arlt, H. Schäfer

Recent Results in Cancer Research, Vol. 177

Abstract

The constitutive activation of the transcription factor nuclear-factor kappa B (NF-κB) is a hallmark of many highly malignant tumours such as the pancreatic ductal adenocarcinoma and accounts for profound chemoresistance. Inhibition of NF-κB activation has been shown to be a useful strategy for increasing the sensitivity towards cytostatic drug treatment in vitro and in vivo. Moreover, various pharmacological substances (e.g. thalidomide, bortezomib, sulphasalazine) have already entered clinical studies partially showing promising results for certain types of cancer. Further studies will be needed, in particular for pancreatic ductal adenocarcinoma, to evaluate the therapeutic efficacy of appropriate combinations of a NF-κB inhibitor and cytostatic drugs.

17.1 Introduction

The conservative treatment of pancreatic cancer still proves to be quite difficult and poorly effective due to the broad resistance of this carcinoma to any kind of cytostatic drug therapy. One factor which has gained much attention during the last couple of years is the transcription factor nuclear factor kappa B (NF-κB) which has been recognized as a central determinant in the induction and manifestation of chemoresistance in pancreatic carcinoma cells. Accordingly, the pharmacological inhibition of NF-κB represents a plausible strategy to efficiently sensitize chemoresistant tumour cells towards cytostatic drug treatment.

17.2 Regulation and Function of NF-κB

The ubiquitous transcription factor NF-κB comprises hetero- and homodimeric protein complexes composed of members of the Rel/NF-κB protein family: RelA/p65, c-Rel, RelB, p50/NF-κB1 and p52/NF-κB2. Most abundant are the heterodimer RelA/NF-κB1 (p65/p50) and the homodimer NF-κB1/NF-κB1 (p50/p50), the former being transcriptionally active in many cell types. In non-stimulated cells, NF-κB is retained in the cytoplasm by inhibitory proteins of the inhibitor of NF-κB (IκB) family thereby masking the NF-κB nuclear localization domain and inhibiting its DNA binding activity (Fig. 17.1). Upon the canonical ("classical") activation by a great variety of cellular stimuli, i.e. cytokines, growth factors or viral proteins, the IκB kinase (IKK) complex– composed of the catalytic subunits IKK-α and IKK-β and the regulatory subunit IKK-γ/NF-κB essential modulator (NEMO)—becomes activated and subsequently phosphorylates IκB proteins. Then IκB proteins are subject to rapid polyubiquitination, followed by degradation by the 26S-proteasome. Thereby, NF-κB becomes released from IκB and translocates into the nucleus where it exerts its action as a transcription factor and, possibly, other yet-to-be-defined functions [1]. One the one hand, activation of NF-κB can be induced by different stimuli, and on the other hand, it is involved in the regulation of a multitude of genes amongst them those encoding for cytokines, growth factors, and anti- and proapoptotic proteins [1, 2]. Thus, NF-κB is an important regulator of cellular processes such as proliferation, apoptosis, cell growth and differentiation. Therefore, under

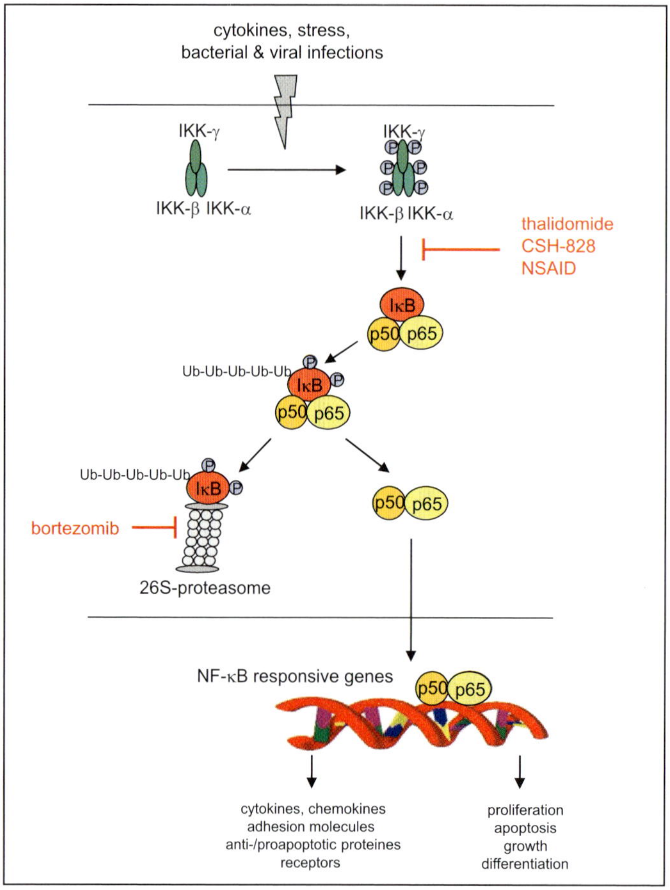

Fig. 17.1 Activation and inhibition of NF-κB. In non-stimulated cells, NF-κB (here represented as the heterodimer p50/p65) is inactive and sequestered in the cytoplasm by its inhibitor IκB. Cytokines, cellular stress, and bacterial and viral infections lead to the phosphorylation and, thereby, to the activation of the IKK complex (IKK-α, IKK-β, IKK-γ), which in turn phosphorylates IκB proteins. After additional polyubiquitination, IκB becomes degraded by the 26S-proteasome. Thus, NF-κB, released from IκB, is able to translocate into the nucleus leading to the expression of NF-κB responsive genes. Since many different genes are regulated by NF-κB, this transcription factor is essential for the control of cellular processes such as proliferation, apoptosis, cell growth and differentiation under physiological as well as under pathological conditions. NF-κB inhibitors being under clinical investigation, they either block IKK activity (thalidomide, CSH-828, non-steroidal anti-inflammatory drugs, NSAIDs) or the 26S-proteasome (bortezomib)

physiological conditions induction and activation of NF-κB is of vital importance in immune and inflammatory responses as well as in cellular homeostasis and organogenesis [3].

17.3 Constitutive Activation of NF-κB and Its Role in Carcinogenesis

Besides its fundamental role in many physiological conditions, NF-κB is also involved in pathological conditions such as chronic inflammation and carcinogenesis [4, 5]. Constitutive activation of NF-κB has been observed in haematological tumour diseases [6] as well as in various solid tumours, e.g. in melanoma [7] and carcinoma of the mamma [8], the colon [9], the prostate [10] and the pancreas [11, 12]. Aetiologically, constitutive activation of NF-κB in tumours can occur due to various conditions and factors. First of all, chronic bacterial or viral infections being major risk factors for various types of cancer, they can induce permanent NF-κB activation [1]. Furthermore, pro-inflammatory cytokines such as interleukin (IL)-1β [13], IL-1α [14] and tumour necrosis factor (TNF)-α [15] either released by immune cells or by other adjacent stromal cells might lead to constitutive nuclear translocation and DNA binding activity of NF-κB. Since some of these “inducer” cytokines are NF-κB target genes at the same time, an autocrine or paracrine amplification loop emerges leading to the constitutive cytokine-driven NF-κB activation, e.g. in pancreatic carcinoma cells [13]. Point mutation of the k-ras oncogene, which is a common and early event in the carcinogenesis of pancreatic cancer, might also result in an enduring activation of NF-κB [11, 16]. In addition, overexpression and activation of the epidermal growth factor (EGF) receptor might contribute to tumour progression and an invasive phenotype of pancreatic cancer by permanent activation of NF-κB [17, 18]. Finally, chromosomal aberrations, e.g. in the genes *c-rel*, *rela*, *nfκb1*, *nfκb2* or *iκbα* have been found in haematological as well as in solid tumours, affecting expression or function of NF-κB directly or indirectly via alterations of IκB [19].

This constitutive NF-κB nuclear translocation results in the activation of a number of different genes leading to a permanently increased expression of pro-inflammatory and pro-oncogenic proteins such as inducible nitric oxide synthetase (iNOS), IL-1β, IL-8 or cyclin D1 [1, 4, 20]. Overexpression of the latter protein has been shown to promote cell survival and cell growth. Furthermore, constitutive NF-κB activation also contributes to tumour growth and tumour aggressiveness by increasing the angiogenic and invasive potential of tumour cells via increased expression of proangiogenic factors such as vascular endothelial growth factor (VEGF) and IL-8 [2, 10]. However, the most important tumourigenic mechanism by which NF-κB promotes tumour cell growth and carcinogenesis is the inhibition of programmed cell death (apoptosis) thus enabling propagation of genetically altered cells. The efficient prevention of apoptosis provided by NF-κB activity also implicates the most effective mechanism of tumour cells to gain protection from cytostatic drug treatment.

17.4 NF-κB as Determinant of Chemoresistance

While there are some reports indicating a rather apoptosis-promoting role for NF-κB [21–23], the majority of studies demonstrate NF-κB as a potent apoptosis suppressor. Although the crucial role of NF-κB in the protection notably from TNF-α and chemotherapeutic drug-induced apoptosis is widely proved, the exact mechanisms by which apoptosis prevention occurs is only now beginning to emerge. Several genes that certainly play a role in apoptosis inhibition, and whose expression is regulated by NF-κB, have been already identified. Thus, activation of NF-κB leads either to the up-regulation of anti-apoptotic genes or to the down-regulation of apoptotic genes. A prevalent mechanism by which activated NF-κB induces chemoresistance is the increased expression of cellular inhibitors of apoptosis (cIAP1, cIAP2, TRAF1, TRAF2, survivin) or the increased expression of the pro-survival bcl-2 homologue Bfl-1/A1 or of bcl-x(L) [24–27]. Increased expression of either apoptosis inhibitor that has been found in several tumour entities, e.g. in pancreatic carcinoma, leads to the disruption of caspase activation and thereby to the failure of apoptosis execution. Another mechanism by which activated NF-κB mediates resistance to chemotherapeutic drugs in pancreatic carcinoma cells represents the direct inactivation of caspases [28]. As a result of an IL-1β-driven constitutive activation of NF-κB, expression of inducible NOS (iNOS) and subsequently the release of nitric oxide (NO) are enhanced, leading to the inactivation of a broad spectrum of caspases. This efficient NO-mediated caspase inhibition obviously occurs via nitrosylation of certain cystein residues in the active site of the caspases [28]. In conclusion, NF-κB-mediated chemoresistance can be induced either by intrinsic mechanisms—e.g. by chromosomal aberrations or by interactions of tumour cells with adjacent stromal cells (fibroblasts, endothelial or immune cells)—or by extrinsic mechanisms, e.g. during a course of chemotherapy. Thus, constitutive activation of NF-κB significantly accounts for the pre-existing as well as for the acquired chemoresistance of pancreatic carcinoma cells [28, 29].

17.5 Inhibition of NF-κB as Strategy for Chemosensitization

In 1996 already, Wang et al. reported on the potential of NF-κB inhibition for improving the efficacy of cancer therapies [15]. Since chemoresistance of various tumours depends on the constitutive activation of NF-κB, a multitude of strategies has been developed and verified to prevent the activation or transcriptional activity of NF-κB, thereby enhancing chemosensitivity.

Three main strategies exist to inhibit NF-κB activation and function:

1. Inhibition of NF-κB protein expression
2. Interference with DNA binding of NF-κB
3. Inhibition of NF-κB activation

17.5.1 Inhibition of NF-κB Protein Expression

Guo et al. demonstrated that NF-κB protein expression blocking can be effectively achieved by delivery of p65-specific small interfering RNA (siRNA) to tumour cells in vivo indicating that inhibition of NF-κB activity by siRNA may have therapeutic potential [30]. Despite these promising findings, this technology requires significant improvement with respect to efficiency of delivery, duration of action and improved specificity and safety, before clinical application can be considered [31, 32].

17.5.2 Interference with DNA Binding of NF-κB

Some inhibitors such as Evans blue, Gallic acid and coumarin, and the novel quinone derivative E3330 have been shown to inhibit binding of the NF-κB subunit p50 to the DNA [33], but the exact mechanism of action remains to be elucidated. Further approaches may be the development and the design of ligands binding either to the κB site of the DNA or directly to the DNA binding sequence of the NF-κB protein. Although this can be accomplished by use of decoy κB sites or their analogues, such molecules might be quite large and polar, thus hampering their cellular uptake and bioavailability [34].

17.5.3 Inhibition of NF-κB Activation

The third and most advanced strategy of NF-κB inhibition—interference with its activation at different points of the activation signalling cascade—has already proved to be feasible and, most notably, to overcome chemoresistance in various tumour entities [34]. First of all, inhibitors of the 26S-proteasome (Fig. 17.1) have been shown to prevent NF-κB nuclear translocation and activity by inhibiting IκB degradation [35, 36]. To date, one proteasome inhibitor [PS-341, bortezomib, Velcade (Janssen-Cilag International, Beerse, Belgium)] has entered clinical application and will be discussed below in more detail. However, therapeutic effects seen after treatment with a proteasome inhibitor cannot only be attributed to inhibition of IκB degradation (and NF-κB activation) but also to the inhibited degradation of other proteins. Beside the low specificity of proteasome inhibitors, it has to take into consideration that abrogation of proteasomal degradation might also lead to the accumulation of proteins such as β-catenin, which can rather promote than suppress carcinogenesis [37].

Beside three recent publications describing IKK activity in a NF-κB-independent manner in Drosophila [38–40], there is little evidence that either IKKα or IKKβ phosphorylate proteins that are not involved in NF-κB signalling. Thus, the most effective and selective approach for blocking NF-κB activation might be given by inhibition of the IKKs (Fig. 17.1). So far, three main groups of agents exist that specifically inhibit IKK activity: immunomodulatory drugs (e.g. thalidomide and its derivates, flavonoids and cyclopentenone prostaglandins), the non-steroidal anti-inflammatory drugs (NSAID) including aspirin and salicylates, sulindac and its analogues, sulphasalazine and its metabolites and newly developed selective IKK inhibitors (e.g. CHS-828) [34]. Since thalidomide, sulphasalazine and CHS-828 have already been applied in preclinical as well as in clinical studies, the therapeutic potential of these substances in the treatment of chemoresistant tumour diseases can be evaluated soonest and is therefore described in more detail below.

17.5.3.1 Inhibition of NF-κB Activation by Blocking Proteasome Activity

Bortezomib

The therapeutic efficacy of the proteasome inhibitor bortezomib was broadly investigated in vitro and in vivo in different experimental settings using cells of prostate carcinoma [41], colorectal carcinoma [42], melanoma [43] or non-small cell lung carcinoma [44]. Bortezomib sensitizes tumour cells to apoptosis induced by camptothecin CPT-11, gemcitabine or temozolomide [42–44]. Moreover, treatment with bortezomib alone already induces growth arrest and apoptosis which can be potentiated by co-treatment with chemotherapeutic drugs [41]. Fahy et al. demonstrated that bortezomib increases sensitivity to apoptosis-inducing agents by down-regulation of bcl-2 [45]. In androgen-dependent human prostate LNCaP cancer cells, bortezomib-induced growth arrest and apoptosis is accompanied by markedly elevated levels of p21(waf1) and p53 [41]. Most studies were performed in models of multiple myeloma showing that bortezomib decreases the apoptotic threshold to chemotherapeutic drugs such as doxorubicin and melphalan in multiple myeloma cell lines or even reverses chemoresistance in cells from multiple myeloma patients [46, 47]. As shown by gene expression profiling, bortezomib treatment results in the down-regulation of several effectors mediating a protective cellular response to genotoxic stress (e.g. topoisomerase II beta, RAD1, Ku autoantigen). Several encouraging results were also obtained in models of pancreatic carcinoma. Nawrocki et al. showed that bortezomib alone as well as in combination with docetaxel reduces tumour growth of orthotopic human pancreatic tumour xenografts [48, 49]. This significant tumour reduction can be attributed to an inhibited proliferation, increased apoptosis and reduced microvessel density. These data indicate that bortezomib inhibits growth of pancreatic tumours via direct effects on tumour cells and indirect effects on the tumour microenvironment. Furthermore, these results are supported by similar findings achieved in a xenotransplant model with human pancreatic carcinoma cells using the combination of the proteasome inhibitor MG132 and etoposide [50].

17.5.3.2 Inhibition of NF-κB Activation by Interfering with the IKK Complex

Thalidomide

Thalidomide was originally developed in the 1950s as a sedative and anti-nausea drug but was rapidly withdrawn due to teratogenicity. Meanwhile, thalidomide and its derivates (Actimid, Revlimid) have been proved to possess potent anti-tumour activity which is mainly based on the abrogation of NF-κB activation by inhibition of the IKKβ activity. Thalidomide has been shown to increase chemosensitivity in tumour models with melanoma [51] and glioblastoma [52]. Most intensively, the anti-tumour activity of thalidomide was investigated in experimental settings of multiple myeloma. Beside its potent anti-angiogenic activity (which is partially also mediated by NF-κB inhibition), thalidomide has shown several other anti-tumour activities in multiple myeloma cells: direct induction of apoptosis, growth arrest and inhibition of cytokine and growth factor secretion [53–55]. Mitsiades et al. could show that thalidomide treatment of multiple myeloma cell lines and cells from multiple myeloma patients increases sensitivity to apoptosis induced by Fas, Trail or dexamethasone [56]. Furthermore, thalidomide-treated cells exhibit a clearly reduced NF-κB activity, reduced expression of cIAP2 and FLICE inhibitory protein (FLIP) as well as an increased activation of caspase 8. Marriott et al. evaluated the anti-tumour activity of thalidomide and certain analogues in the treatment of different solid tumour cell lines (colorectal, pancreatic, prostate) in vitro and in vivo [57]. The thalidomide analogue phosphodiesterase type IV inhibitor effectively reduces tumour cell viability, thereby leading to inhibition of tumour growth in vivo. This effect appears to be mediated by decreased expression levels of bcl-2 and an increased induction of caspase 3.

CHS-828

CHS-828 (N-(6-(4-chlorophenoxy)hexyl)-N′-cyano-N″-4-pyridylguanidine) belongs to a new group of anti-tumoural substances, the pyridyl cyanoguanidines, and inhibits NF-κB activation by blocking IKK activity [58]. Hjarnaa et al. demonstrated that CHS-828 exerts significant cytotoxic effects on human breast and lung cancer cell lines that were not seen on normal fibroblasts and endothelial cells [59]. In nude mice bearing human tumour xenografts, CHS-828 reduces growth of MCF-7 breast cancer tumours and leads to the regression of small-cell lung cancer tumours. Aleskog et al. observed significant cytotoxic activity of CHS-828 in haematological as well as in solid tumour cells, although haematological tumour cells appear to be more responsive than those of solid tumours [60]. Furthermore, CHS-828 induces significant cytotoxic effects in myeloma cell lines in vitro and in vivo [61]. A recent publication of Johanson et al. demonstrated anti-tumoural activity of CHS-828 against different neuroendocrine tumours [62]. One study has reported on the treatment of U-937 GTB lymphoma cells with a combination of CHS-828 and etoposide [63]. Some promising synergistic cytotoxic effects could be observed, but the enhanced apoptosis induction by etoposide apparently depends on the duration of exposure to CHS-828. Thus, further studies evaluating the therapeutic efficacy of CHS-828 in combination with etoposide or other chemotherapeutic drugs seem to be warranted.

Sulphasalazine

Sulphasalazine is an anti-inflammatory drug that has been used for a long time in the treatment of inflammatory bowel disease or of rheumatoid arthritis. It is metabolically cleaved following oral administration to 5-amino-salicylic acid (5-Asa) and sulphapyridine. Its mode of action has been linked to the ability to inhibit IKK kinase activity and hence the activation of NF-κB [34, 64, 65]. Sulphasalazine has been shown to inhibit proliferation of human mammary carcinoma cells [66] and lymphoma cells [67] in vitro. Robe et al. observed growth inhibitory properties of sulphasalazine in human glioblastoma cells in vitro and in vivo [68]. In addition, sulphasalazine is able to efficiently induce apoptosis in glioblastoma cells as determined by DNA fragmentation and caspase cleavage. Thus, decreased proliferation and increased apoptosis account for significant remission of experimental U87 tumours in the brain of nude mice after sulphasalazine treatment. Arlt et al. intensively evaluated the NF-κB blocking activity of sulphasalazine in the sensitization of pancreatic carcinoma cells in vitro [13, 69, 70]. Pre-treatment of chemoresistant pancreatic carcinoma cells with sulphasalazine clearly increases the apoptotic response towards cytostatic drugs such as etoposide, doxorubicin, gemcitabine or 5-fluorouracil. Moreover, combined treatment of severe combined immunodeficiency (SCID) mice bearing human pancreatic tumour xenografts with sulphasalazine and either etoposide or gemcitabine significantly reduces tumour outgrowth [50]. Immunohistochemical analysis revealed that tumours of combined treated animals exhibit a significantly increased number of apoptotic cells, a markedly reduced number of proliferating tumour cells and a decreased microvessel density, effects similarly seen with combined treatment of cytostatic drugs and the proteasome inhibitors MG132 [50] or bortezomib [48, 49].

17.6 NF-κB Inhibitors in Clinical Trials

17.6.1 Bortezomib

The proteasome inhibitor bortezomib has already applied in a variety of clinical studies to improve the therapy of different malignancies, a fact which is reflected by 196 entries in Medline if searching for the terms "bortezomib" and "clinical trial". The vast majority of studies were conducted with patients suffering from multiple myeloma [71–73]. Richardson et al. had 669 patients in their study comparing the therapeutic efficacy of bortezomib with high-dose dexamethasone in terms of tumour response, progression time and time of survival [73]. All patients displayed an advanced relapsed tumour stage and had received one to three previous therapies before entering the study. Patients that were treated with bortezomib showed a higher tumour response rate compared to patients treated with dexamethasone. The combined complete and partial response rates were 38% for the bortezomib group and 18% for the dexamethasone group ($p<0.001$). Moreover, median times to progression were 189 days for patients after bortezomib and 106 days for patients after dexamethasone treatment, respectively ($p<0.001$). The 1-year survival rate was 80% for patients receiving bortezomib and 66% for patients taking dexamethasone ($p<0.003$). Most studies indicate that bortezomib is well tolerated. However, the most common grade 3 and 4 toxicities of bortezomib were thrombocytopenia, lymphopenia and peripheral neuropathy, the latter also being reversible after dose reduction or discontinuation [74]. Furthermore, bortezomib showed remarkable single-agent activity in patients with other lymphomas such as non-Hodgkin's lymphoma or mantle cell lymphomas [75, 76].

In contrast, monotherapy with bortezomib exhibited no or only minimal activity in various advanced solid tumours such as metastatic sarcomas [77], metastatic colorectal carcinoma [78], metastatic malignant melanoma [79] or metastatic neuroendocrine tumours [80]. Thus, for further studies of solid malignancies, the authors univocally recommend the use of bortezomib in combination with cytostatic drugs. Aghajanian et al. determined in a single-arm phase I study the maximal-tolerated dose and safety of a combination of bortezomib and carboplatin in recurrent ovarian cancer [81]. Besides assessment of the recommended dose of bortezomib, the overall response rate was 47%, including five partial and two complete responses, one of the latter occurring in a patient with platinum-resistant disease.

So far, only one study has been performed evaluating the therapeutic efficacy of bortezomib in the treatment of metastatic pancreatic carcinoma [82]. There were 44 patients enrolled for treatment with bortezomib alone and 43 patients for combined treatment with bortezomib and gemcitabine. Response rates were 0% and 10%, the median times to progression were 1.2 and 2.4 months and median survival times were 2.5 and 4.8 months, respectively. Thus, bortezomib alone or a combination of this drug with gemcitabine did not yield better results in the treatment of metastatic pancreatic carcinoma than expected for gemcitabine alone. It has to be critically noted that treatment with gemcitabine alone was not the subject of this study, thus it does not allow for proper direct comparison. Furthermore, patients progressing upon bortezomib monotherapy were allowed to receive bortezomib with gemcitabine, hence attenuating the assessable effect of the combined treatment. Further studies—in particular for the treatment of solid tumour diseases—should be aspire towards combinations of bortezomib and cytostatic drugs to better exploit the benefit of proteasome-dependent NF-κB inhibition for chemosensitization.

17.6.2 Thalidomide

The first study showing anti-tumour activity of thalidomide in the therapy of refractory multiple myeloma was published in 1999 by Singhal et al. [83]. Since then, several clinical studies have been undertaken to prove therapeutic efficacy of thalidomide in the treatment of haematological as well as of solid tumours. Many encouraging results were obtained in phase II and III studies with advanced multiple myeloma [84–87]. Rajkumar et al. enrolled 207 patients with newly diagnosed multiple myeloma in a phase III study comparing the combination of thalidomide and dexamethasone (103 patients) with dexamethasone alone (104 patients) [84]. The combined treatment showed a significant better response rate compared to dexamethasone monotherapy (63% versus 41%, $p<0.002$). Albeit this convincing anti-tumour activity was achieved by additional thalidomide treatment, a significant higher incidence of grade 4 and 5 toxicities (e.g. peripheral neuropathy) was observed in patients receiving combined treatment compared to patients treated with dexamethasone alone (45% versus 21%, $p<0.001$). However, Kyriakou et al. described a combination of cyclophosphamide and dexamethasone with low-dose thalidomide as a well-tolerated and effective therapeutic regimen for patients with relapsed or refractory multiple myeloma [87]. Therefore, efforts still have to be undertaken to optimally balance maximal anti-tumour activity with the adverse effects of thalidomide.

Up to now, monotherapy with thalidomide hardly induced any objective response rates against solid tumours, e.g. of advanced melanoma, renal cell, ovarian or breast cancer [88, 89]. This holds true for the combination of thalidomide and capecitabine in the therapy of patients with metastatic colorectal carcinoma who were refractory to previous therapies [90]. Interesting results were obtained in a phase II trial treating patients with metastatic neuroendocrine tumours with a combination of thalidomide and temozolomide [91]. In this single-arm study, 40% and 29% of 29 patients showed an objective biochemical and radiologic response, respectively. The median duration of response was 13.5 months, the 1-year survival rate was 79% and the 2-year survival rate was 61%.

Gordon et al. evaluated in a radomized placebo-controlled trial the efficacy of thalidomide in the attenuation of tumour cachexia in 50 patients with advanced pancreatic carcinoma [92]. Tumour cachexia, which mainly depends on NF-κB activity and the release of pro-inflammatory cytokines [93], represents a common problem in approximately 80% of patients with pancreatic carcinoma and is associated with a much worse clinical outcome. In this study, 33 patients (16 placebo, 17 thalidomide) were evaluated after 4 weeks of treatment showing that patients receiving thalidomide had gained weight by an average of 0.37 kg compared with a median weight loss of 2.21 kg in the placebo group ($p=0.005$). Moreover, evaluation of 20 patients (8 placebo, 12 thalidomide) after 8 weeks revealed a median weight loss of 0.06 kg in patients treated with thalidomide compared with a loss of 3.62 kg in the control group ($p=0.034$). In conclusion, thalidomide was well tolerated and effectively diminished weight loss in patients suffering from advanced pancreatic carcinoma. It would be of great value to further investigate its anti-tumour activity, particularly in combination with cytostatic drugs in the therapy of pancreatic carcinoma.

17.6.3 CSH-828

Until now, two phase I studies have been conducted evaluating the maximal tolerated dose (MTD), the recommended dose and the toxicity of CHS-828 [94, 95]. Sixteen and 27 patients, respectively, with different histologically proved solid malignancies were included in these studies. Most patients had already received previous treatments with chemotherapy, radiotherapy, surgery, and/or hormonal therapy. For further studies, Hovstadius et al. recommended a dose of 20 mg CHS-828 once daily for 5 days in cycles of 28-days duration [94]. Haematological toxicity (thrombocytopenia, lymphocytopenia) was generally mild. Other side-effects were most frequently nausea, vomiting, diarrhoea, fatigue and localized genital mucositis. No objective tumour responses could be noted, although seven patients showed stable disease after two courses of therapy. Ravaud et al. concluded that a dose of 420 mg of CHS-828 administered every 3 weeks is recommended for further studies, while 500 mg is the MTD [95]. Haematological toxicities such as anaemia and thrombocytopenia as well as gastrointestinal side-effects (pain, nausea, vomiting, diarrhoea) were frequent. In both studies there was a large variation in pharmacokinetics of CHS-828 both between and within patients. To overcome this problem, a series of improved pro-drugs of CHS-828 was synthesized. The best compound was EB1627 showing improved solubility and potent anti-tumour activity alone or in combination with cytostatic drugs in animal models [96]. For further studies it will be worthwhile to evaluate whether combinations of CHS-828 or of the improved pro-drug EB1627 with other drugs might be more potent in the treatment of solid tumour diseases.

17.6.4 Sulphasalazine

Since Sulphasalazine has already been used for decades to treat inflammatory diseases and its administration has been proved to be safe and well tolerable, this drug seems particularly qualified for NF-κB inhibition in cancer treatment. Currently, a prospective, double-blind, randomized phase 1–2 study is being conducted to prove the safety and efficacy of sulphasalazine for the therapy of advanced malignant gliomas [97]. The primary study objectives are the evaluation of the maximal daily oral dose of sulphasalazine and the assessment of any clinical and radiological tumour responses. Determination of overall and progression-free survival will be secondary objectives. Overall, 20 patients will be enrolled in the study.

Based on our own comprehensive experimental and preclinical investigations [13, 50, 69, 70, 98], the University Hospital Schleswig-Holstein Campus Kiel will launch a pilot study applying sulphasalzine as a chemosensitizer for the treatment of pancreatic carcinoma. Overall, 20 patients with an advanced inoperable pancreatic adenocarcinoma will be enclosed in a prospective, single-arm, multi-centre study to explore the compatibility and efficacy of the combination of sulphasalazine and gemcitabine.

17.7 Concluding Remarks

Since inflammation, a crucial risk factor for tumour development and progression, and chemoresistance both broadly depend on activation of NF-κB, this signalling molecule represents an attractive target for cancer prevention and therapy. However, NF-κB in immune cells is an important mediator and regulator of immune function so that its permanent inhibition might lead to severe immunosuppression. Thus, prolonged inhibition of NF-κB seems not to be applicable for tumour prevention. In contrast, suppression of NF-κB activity might be more useful in the therapy of already existing tumours, thus implying NF-κB inhibitor administration will be of shorter durations. Although it must be kept in mind that under certain circumstances NF-κB inhibition might also contribute to tumour progression, the most likely outcome of this interference in existing tumours will be impairment of the tumour microenvironment (e.g. by reducing tumour vascularization) and increased tumour cell apoptosis. Since, in particular, solid tumours apparently exhibit comprehensive protection from apoptosis induction, the mere inhibition of NF-κB appears to be insufficient for a pronounced anti-tumour effect. Thus, it is reasonable to use NF-κB inhibitors as chemosensitizing adjuvants in combination with cytostatic drugs.

Several preclinical and clinical studies have revealed that the transcription factor NF-κB is a promising molecular target that can be used for sensitization of a variety of tumours to chemotherapeutic drugs. NF-κB inhibitors, such as bortezomib, thalidomide or sulphasalazine, that have been already employed in clinical studies should be further evaluated in combination with cytostatic drugs, particularly in the therapy of profoundly chemoresistant tumours (e.g. pancreatic carcinoma). One focus of recent research is the design and development of more specific IKK inhibitors; they will enter clinical application within the next few years. These improved NF-κB inhibitors will presumably have fewer side-effects with respect to immunosuppression and are likely to be more potent in anti-cancer therapy.

References

1. Karin M (2006) Nuclear factor-kappaB in cancer development and progression. Nature 441:431–436
2. Takada Y, Kobayashi Y, Aggarwal BB (2005) Evodiamine abolishes constitutive and inducible NF-kappaB activation by inhibiting IkappaBalpha kinase activation, thereby suppressing NF-kappaB-regulated antiapoptotic and metastatic gene expression, up-regulating apoptosis, and inhibiting invasion. J Biol Chem 280:17203–17212
3. Ghosh S, May MJ, Kopp EB (1998) NF-kappaB and Rel proteins: evolutionarily conserved mediators of immune responses. Annu Rev Immunol 16:225–260
4. Garcea G, Dennison AR, Steward WP, Berry DP (2005) Role of inflammation in pancreatic carcinogenesis and the implications for future therapy. Pancreatology 5:514–529
5. Farrow B, Evers BM (2002) Inflammation and the development of pancreatic cancer. Surg Oncol 10:153–169
6. Reuther JY, Reuther GW, Cortez D, Pendergast AM, Baldwin AS Jr (1998) A requirement for NF-kappaB activation in Bcr-Abl-mediated transformation. Genes Dev 12:968–981
7. Ghiorzo P, Mantelli M, Gargiulo S, Gramigni C, Pastorino L, Banelli B, Villaggio B, Coccia MC, Sementa AR, Garre C, Bianchi-Scarra G (2004) Inverse correlation between p16INK4A expression and NF-kappaB activation in melanoma progression. Hum Pathol 35:1029–1037
8. Sovak MA, Arsura M, Zanieski G, Kavanagh KT, Sonenshein GE (1999) The inhibitory effects of transforming growth factor beta1 on breast cancer cell proliferation are mediated through regulation of aberrant nuclear factor-kappaB/Rel expression. Cell Growth Differ 10:537–544
9. Dejardin E, Deregowski V, Chapelier M, Jacobs N, Gielen J, Merville MP, Bours V (1999) Regulation of NF-kappaB activity by I kappaB-related proteins in adenocarcinoma cells. Oncogene 18:2567–2577
10. Uzzo RG, Crispen PL, Golovine K, Makhov P, Horwitz EM, Kolenko VM (2006) Diverse effects of zinc on NF-kappaB and AP-1 transcription factors: implications for prostate cancer progression. Carcinogenesis 27:1980–1990

11. Wang W, Abbruzzese JL, Evans DB, Larry L, Cleary KR, Chiao PJ (1999) The nuclear factor-kappa B RelA transcription factor is constitutively activated in human pancreatic adenocarcinoma cells. Clin Cancer Res 5:119–127
12. Muerkoster S, Arlt A, Sipos B, Witt M, Grossmann M, Kloppel G, Kalthoff H, Folsch UR, Schafer H (2005) Increased expression of the E3-ubiquitin ligase receptor subunit betaTRCP1 relates to constitutive nuclear factor-kappaB activation and chemoresistance in pancreatic carcinoma cells. Cancer Res 65:1316–1324
13. Arlt A, Vorndamm J, Muerkoster S, Yu H, Schmidt WE, Folsch UR, Schafer H (2002) Autocrine production of interleukin 1beta confers constitutive nuclear factor kappaB activity and chemoresistance in pancreatic carcinoma cell lines. Cancer Res 62:910–916
14. Niu J, Li Z, Peng B, Chiao PJ (2004) Identification of an autoregulatory feedback pathway involving interleukin-1alpha in induction of constitutive NF-kappaB activation in pancreatic cancer cells. J Biol Chem 279:16452–16462
15. Wang CY, Mayo MW, Baldwin AS Jr (1996) TNF- and cancer therapy-induced apoptosis: potentiation by inhibition of NF-kappaB. Science 274:784–787
16. Hu L, Shi Y, Hsu JH, Gera J, Van Ness B, Lichtenstein A (2003) Downstream effectors of oncogenic ras in multiple myeloma cells. Blood 101:3126–3135
17. Zhang H, Ma G, Dong M, Zhao M, Shen X, Ma Z, Guo K (2006) Epidermal growth factor promotes invasiveness of pancreatic cancer cells through NF-kappaB-mediated proteinase productions. Pancreas 32:101–109
18. Liptay S, Weber CK, Ludwig L, Wagner M, Adler G, Schmid RM (2003) Mitogenic and antiapoptotic role of constitutive NF-kappaB/Rel activity in pancreatic cancer. Int J Cancer 105:735–746
19. Rayet B, Gelinas C (1999) Aberrant rel/nfkb genes and activity in human cancer. Oncogene 18:6938–6947
20. Shishodia S, Aggarwal BB (2002) Nuclear factor-kappaB activation: a question of life or death. J Biochem Mol Biol 35:28–40
21. Packham G, Lahti JM, Fee BE, Gawn JM, Coustan-Smith E, Campana D, Douglas I, Kidd VJ, Ghosh S, Cleveland JL (1997) Fas activates NF-kappaB and induces apoptosis in T-cell lines by signaling pathways distinct from those induced by TNF-alpha. Cell Death Differ 4:130–139
22. Ivanov VN, Ronai Z (2000) p38 protects human melanoma cells from UV-induced apoptosis through down-regulation of NF-kappaB activity and Fas expression. Oncogene 19:3003–3012
23. Gupta RA, Polk DB, Krishna U, Israel DA, Yan F, DuBois RN, Peek RM Jr (2001) Activation of peroxisome proliferator-activated receptor gamma suppresses nuclear factor kappa B-mediated apoptosis induced by Helicobacter pylori in gastric epithelial cells. J Biol Chem 276:31059–31066
24. Chu ZL, McKinsey TA, Liu L, Gentry JJ, Malim MH, Ballard DW (1997) Suppression of tumour necrosis factor-induced cell death by inhibitor of apoptosis c-IAP2 is under NF-kappaB control. Proc Natl Acad Sci U S A 94:10057–10062
25. Greten FR, Weber CK, Greten TF, Schneider G, Wagner M, Adler G, Schmid RM (2002) Stat3 and NF-kappaB activation prevents apoptosis in pancreatic carcinogenesis. Gastroenterology 123:2052–2063
26. Stehlik C, de Martin R, Kumabashiri I, Schmid JA, Binder BR, Lipp J (1998) Nuclear factor (NF)-kappaB-regulated X-chromosome-linked iap gene expression protects endothelial cells from tumour necrosis factor alpha-induced apoptosis. J Exp Med 188:211–216
27. Wang CY, Mayo MW, Korneluk RG, Goeddel DV, Baldwin AS Jr (1998) NF-kappaB antiapoptosis: induction of TRAF1 and TRAF2 and c-IAP1 and c-IAP2 to suppress caspase-8 activation. Science 281:1680–1683
28. Sebens Muerkoster S, Lust J, Arlt A, Hasler R, Witt M, Sebens T, Schreiber S, Folsch UR, Schafer H (2006) Acquired chemoresistance in pancreatic carcinoma cells: induced secretion of IL-1beta and NO lead to inactivation of caspases. Oncogene 25:4628
29. Muerkoster S, Wegehenkel K, Arlt A, Witt M, Sipos B, Kruse ML, Sebens T, Kloppel G, Kalthoff H, Folsch UR, Schafer H (2004) Tumour stroma interactions induce chemoresistance in pancreatic ductal carcinoma cells involving increased secretion and paracrine effects of nitric oxide and interleukin-1beta. Cancer Res 64:1331–1337
30. Guo J, Verma UN, Gaynor RB, Frenkel EP, Becerra CR (2004) Enhanced chemosensitivity to irinotecan by RNA interference-mediated down-regulation of the nuclear factor-kappaB p65 subunit. Clin Cancer Res 10:3333–3341
31. Kalota A, Shetzline SE, Gewirtz AM (2004) Progress in the development of nucleic acid therapeutics for cancer. Cancer Biol Ther 3:4–12

32. Wall NR, Shi Y (2003) Small RNA: can RNA interference be exploited for therapy? Lancet 362:1401–1403
33. Pande V, Ramos MJ (2005) NF-kappaB in human disease: current inhibitors and prospects for de novo structure based design of inhibitors. Curr Med Chem 12:357–374
34. Karin M, Yamamoto Y, Wang QM (2004) The IKK NF-kappa B system: a treasure trove for drug development. Nat Rev Drug Discov 3:17–26
35. Zavrski I, Jakob C, Schmid P, Krebbel H, Kaiser M, Fleissner C, Rosche M, Possinger K, Sezer O (2005) Proteasome: an emerging target for cancer therapy. Anticancer Drugs 16:475–481
36. Al-Aynati MM, Radulovich N, Riddell RH, Tsao MS (2004) Epithelial-cadherin and beta-catenin expression changes in pancreatic intraepithelial neoplasia. Clin Cancer Res 10:1235–1240
37. Koenig A, Mueller C, Hasel C, Adler G, Menke A (2006) Collagen type I induces disruption of E-cadherin-mediated cell-cell contacts and promotes proliferation of pancreatic carcinoma cells. Cancer Res 66:4662–4671
38. Shapiro RS, Anderson KV (2006) Drosophila Ik2, a member of the I kappa B kinase family, is required for mRNA localization during oogenesis. Development 133:1467–1475
39. Kuranaga E, Kanuka H, Tonoki A, Takemoto K, Tomioka T, Kobayashi M, Hayashi S, Miura M (2006) Drosophila IKK-related kinase regulates nonapoptotic function of caspases via degradation of IAPs. Cell 126:583–596
40. Oshima K, Takeda M, Kuranaga E, Ueda R, Aigaki T, Miura M, Hayashi S (2006) IKKvarepsilon regulates F actin assembly and interacts with Drosophila IAP1 in cellular morphogenesis. Curr Biol 16:1531–1537
41. Ikezoe T, Yang Y, Saito T, Koeffler HP, Taguchi H (2004) Proteasome inhibitor PS-341 down-regulates prostate-specific antigen (PSA) and induces growth arrest and apoptosis of androgen-dependent human prostate cancer LNCaP cells. Cancer Sci 95:271–275
42. Cusack JC Jr, Liu R, Houston M, Abendroth K, Elliott PJ, Adams J, Baldwin AS Jr (2001) Enhanced chemosensitivity to CPT-11 with proteasome inhibitor PS-341: implications for systemic nuclear factor-kappaB inhibition. Cancer Res 61:3535–3540
43. Amiri KI, Horton LW, LaFleur BJ, Sosman JA, Richmond A (2004) Augmenting chemosensitivity of malignant melanoma tumours via proteasome inhibition: implication for bortezomib (VELCADE, PS-341) as a therapeutic agent for malignant melanoma. Cancer Res 64:4912–4918
44. Denlinger CE, Rundall BK, Keller MD, Jones DR (2004) Proteasome inhibition sensitizes non-small-cell lung cancer to gemcitabine-induced apoptosis. Ann Thorac Surg 78:1207–1214
45. Fahy BN, Schlieman MG, Mortenson MM, Virudachalam S, Bold RJ (2005) Targeting BCL-2 overexpression in various human malignancies through NF-kappaB inhibition by the proteasome inhibitor bortezomib. Cancer Chemother Pharmacol 56:46–54
46. Ma MH, Yang HH, Parker K, Manyak S, Friedman JM, Altamirano C, Wu ZQ, Borad MJ, Frantzen M, Roussos E, Neeser J, Mikail A, Adams J, Sjak-Shie N, Vescio RA, Berenson JR (2003) The proteasome inhibitor PS-341 markedly enhances sensitivity of multiple myeloma tumour cells to chemotherapeutic agents. Clin Cancer Res 9:1136–1144
47. Mitsiades N, Mitsiades CS, Richardson PG, Poulaki V, Tai YT, Chauhan D, Fanourakis G, Gu X, Bailey C, Joseph M, Libermann TA, Schlossman R, Munshi NC, Hideshima T, Anderson KC (2003) The proteasome inhibitor PS-341 potentiates sensitivity of multiple myeloma cells to conventional chemotherapeutic agents: therapeutic applications. Blood 101:2377–2380
48. Nawrocki ST, Bruns CJ, Harbison MT, Bold RJ, Gotsch BS, Abbruzzese JL, Elliott P, Adams J, McConkey DJ (2002) Effects of the proteasome inhibitor PS-341 on apoptosis and angiogenesis in orthotopic human pancreatic tumour xenografts. Mol Cancer Ther 1:1243–1253
49. Nawrocki ST, Sweeney-Gotsch B, Takamori R, McConkey DJ (2004) The proteasome inhibitor bortezomib enhances the activity of docetaxel in orthotopic human pancreatic tumour xenografts. Mol Cancer Ther 3:59–70
50. Muerkoster S, Arlt A, Witt M, Gehrz A, Haye S, March C, Grohmann F, Wegehenkel K, Kalthoff H, Folsch UR, Schafer H (2003) Usage of the NF-kappaB inhibitor sulfasalazine as sensitizing agent in combined chemotherapy of pancreatic cancer. Int J Cancer 104:469–476

51. Heere-Ress E, Boehm J, Thallinger C, Hoeller C, Wacheck V, Birner P, Wolff K, Pehamberger H, Jansen B (2005) Thalidomide enhances the antitumour activity of standard chemotherapy in a human melanoma xenotransplantation model. J Invest Dermatol 125:201–206
52. Son MJ, Kim JS, Kim MH, Song HS, Kim JT, Kim H, Shin T, Jeon HJ, Lee DS, Park SY, Kim YJ, Kim JH, Nam DH (2006) Combination treatment with temozolomide and thalidomide inhibits tumour growth and angiogenesis in an orthotopic glioma model. Int J Oncol 28:53–59
53. D'Amato RJ, Loughnan MS, Flynn E, Folkman J (1994) Thalidomide is an inhibitor of angiogenesis. Proc Natl Acad Sci U S A 91:4082–4085
54. Gupta D, Treon SP, Shima Y, Hideshima T, Podar K, Tai YT, Lin B, Lentzsch S, Davies FE, Chauhan D, Schlossman RL, Richardson P, Ralph P, Wu L, Payvandi F, Muller G, Stirling DI, Anderson KC (2001) Adherence of multiple myeloma cells to bone marrow stromal cells upregulates vascular endothelial growth factor secretion: therapeutic applications. Leukemia 15:1950–1961
55. Hideshima T, Chauhan D, Shima Y, Raje N, Davies FE, Tai YT, Treon SP, Lin B, Schlossman RL, Richardson P, Muller G, Stirling DI, Anderson KC (2000) Thalidomide and its analogs overcome drug resistance of human multiple myeloma cells to conventional therapy. Blood 96:2943–2950
56. Mitsiades N, Mitsiades CS, Poulaki V, Chauhan D, Richardson PG, Hideshima T, Munshi NC, Treon SP, Anderson KC (2002) Apoptotic signaling induced by immunomodulatory thalidomide analogs in human multiple myeloma cells: therapeutic implications. Blood 99:4525–4530
57. Marriott JB, Clarke IA, Czajka A, Dredge K, Childs K, Man HW, Schafer P, Govinda S, Muller GW, Stirling DI, Dalgleish AG (2003) A novel subclass of thalidomide analogue with anti-solid tumour activity in which caspase-dependent apoptosis is associated with altered expression of bcl-2 family proteins. Cancer Res 63:593–599
58. Olsen LS, Hjarnaa PJ, Latini S, Holm PK, Larsson R, Bramm E, Binderup L, Madsen MW (2004) Anticancer agent CHS 828 suppresses nuclear factor-kappa B activity in cancer cells through downregulation of IKK activity. Int J Cancer 111:198–205
59. Hjarnaa PJ, Jonsson E, Latini S, Dhar S, Larsson R, Bramm E, Skov T, Binderup L (1999) CHS 828, a novel pyridyl cyanoguanidine with potent antitumour activity in vitro and in vivo. Cancer Res 59:5751–5757
60. Aleskog A, Bashir-Hassan S, Hovstadius P, Kristensen J, Hoglund M, Tholander B, Binderup L, Larsson R, Jonsson E (2001) Activity of CHS 828 in primary cultures of human hematological and solid tumours in vitro. Anticancer Drugs 12:821–827
61. Hovstadius P, Lindhagen E, Hassan S, Nilsson K, Jernberg-Wiklund H, Nygren P, Binderup L, Larsson R (2004) Cytotoxic effect in vivo and in vitro of CHS 828 on human myeloma cell lines. Anticancer Drugs 15:63–70
62. Johanson V, Arvidsson Y, Kolby L, Bernhardt P, Sward C, Nilsson O, Ahlman H (2005) Antitumoural effects of the pyridyl cyanoguanidine CHS 828 on three different types of neuroendocrine tumours xenografted to nude mice. Neuroendocrinology 82:171–176
63. Martinsson P, Ekelund S, Nygren P, Larsson R (2002) The combination of the antitumoural pyridyl cyanoguanidine CHS 828 and etoposide in vitro—from cytotoxic synergy to complete inhibition of apoptosis. Br J Pharmacol 137:568–573
64. Wahl C, Liptay S, Adler G, Schmid RM (1998) Sulfasalazine: a potent and specific inhibitor of nuclear factor kappa B. J Clin Invest 101:1163–1174
65. Kopp E, Ghosh S (1994) Inhibition of NF-kappa B by sodium salicylate and aspirin. Science 265:956–959
66. Narang VS, Pauletti GM, Gout PW, Buckley DJ, Buckley AR (2003) Suppression of cystine uptake by sulfasalazine inhibits proliferation of human mammary carcinoma cells. Anticancer Res 23:4571–4579
67. Gout PW, Simms CR, Robertson MC (2003) In vitro studies on the lymphoma growth-inhibitory activity of sulfasalazine. Anticancer Drugs 14:21–29
68. Robe PA, Bentires-Alj M, Bonif M, Rogister B, Deprez M, Haddada H, Khac MT, Jolois O, Erkmen K, Merville MP, Black PM, Bours V (2004) In vitro and in vivo activity of the nuclear factor-kappaB inhibitor sulfasalazine in human glioblastomas. Clin Cancer Res 10:5595–5603
69. Arlt A, Vorndamm J, Breitenbroich M, Folsch UR, Kalthoff H, Schmidt WE, Schafer H (2001) Inhibition of NF-kappaB sensitizes human pancreatic carcinoma cells to apoptosis induced by etoposide (VP16) or doxorubicin. Oncogene 20:859–868
70. Arlt A, Gehrz A, Muerkoster S, Vorndamm J, Kruse ML, Folsch UR, Schafer H (2003) Role of NF-kappaB and Akt/PI3 K in the resistance of pancreatic carcinoma cell lines against gemcitabine-induced cell death. Oncogene 22:3243–3251

71. Jagannath S, Barlogie B, Berenson J, Siegel D, Irwin D, Richardson PG, Niesvizky R, Alexanian R, Limentani SA, Alsina M, Adams J, Kauffman M, Esseltine DL, Schenkein DP, Anderson KC (2004) A phase 2 study of two doses of bortezomib in relapsed or refractory myeloma. Br J Haematol 127:165–172
72. Oakervee HE, Popat R, Curry N, Smith P, Morris C, Drake M, Agrawal S, Stec J, Schenkein D, Esseltine DL, Cavenagh JD (2005) PAD combination therapy (PS-341/bortezomib, doxorubicin and dexamethasone) for previously untreated patients with multiple myeloma. Br J Haematol 129:755–762
73. Richardson PG, Sonneveld P, Schuster MW, Irwin D, Stadtmauer EA, Facon T, Harousseau JL, Ben-Yehuda D, Lonial S, Goldschmidt H, Reece D, San-Miguel JF, Blade J, Boccadoro M, Cavenagh J, Dalton WS, Boral AL, Esseltine DL, Porter JB, Schenkein D, Anderson KC (2005) Bortezomib or high-dose dexamethasone for relapsed multiple myeloma. N Engl J Med 352:2487–2498
74. Richardson PG, Briemberg H, Jagannath S, Wen PY, Barlogie B, Berenson J, Singhal S, Siegel DS, Irwin D, Schuster M, Srkalovic G, Alexanian R, Rajkumar SV, Limentani S, Alsina M, Orlowski RZ, Najarian K, Esseltine D, Anderson KC, Amato AA (2006) Frequency, characteristics, and reversibility of peripheral neuropathy during treatment of advanced multiple myeloma with bortezomib. J Clin Oncol 24:3113–3120
75. Goy A, Younes A, McLaughlin P, Pro B, Romaguera JE, Hagemeister F, Fayad L, Dang NH, Samaniego F, Wang M, Broglio K, Samuels B, Gilles F, Sarris AH, Hart S, Trehu E, Schenkein D, Cabanillas F, Rodriguez AM (2005) Phase II study of proteasome inhibitor bortezomib in relapsed or refractory B-cell non-Hodgkin's lymphoma. J Clin Oncol 23:667–675
76. O'Connor OA, Wright J, Moskowitz C, Muzzy J, MacGregor-Cortelli B, Stubblefield M, Straus D, Portlock C, Hamlin P, Choi E, Dumetrescu O, Esseltine D, Trehu E, Adams J, Schenkein D, Zelenetz AD (2005) Phase II clinical experience with the novel proteasome inhibitor bortezomib in patients with indolent non-Hodgkin's lymphoma and mantle cell lymphoma. J Clin Oncol 23:676–684
77. Maki RG, Kraft AS, Scheu K, Yamada J, Wadler S, Antonescu CR, Wright JJ, Schwartz GK (2005) A multicenter Phase II study of bortezomib in recurrent or metastatic sarcomas. Cancer 103:1431–1438
78. Mackay H, Hedley D, Major P, Townsley C, Mackenzie M, Vincent M, Degendorfer P, Tsao MS, Nicklee T, Birle D, Wright J, Siu L, Moore M, Oza A (2005) A phase II trial with pharmacodynamic endpoints of the proteasome inhibitor bortezomib in patients with metastatic colorectal cancer. Clin Cancer Res 11:5526–5533
79. Markovic SN, Geyer SM, Dawkins F, Sharfman W, Albertini M, Maples W, Fracasso PM, Fitch T, Lorusso P, Adjei AA, Erlichman C (2005) A phase II study of bortezomib in the treatment of metastatic malignant melanoma. Cancer 103:2584–2589
80. Shah MH, Young D, Kindler HL, Webb I, Kleiber B, Wright J, Grever M (2004) Phase II study of the proteasome inhibitor bortezomib (PS-341) in patients with metastatic neuroendocrine tumours. Clin Cancer Res 10:6111–6118
81. Aghajanian C, Dizon DS, Sabbatini P, Raizer JJ, Dupont J, Spriggs DR (2005) Phase I trial of bortezomib and carboplatin in recurrent ovarian or primary peritoneal cancer. J Clin Oncol 23:5943–5949
82. Alberts SR, Foster NR, Morton RF, Kugler J, Schaefer P, Wiesenfeld M, Fitch TR, Steen P, Kim GP, Gill S (2005) PS-341 and gemcitabine in patients with metastatic pancreatic adenocarcinoma: a North Central Cancer Treatment Group (NCCTG) randomized phase II study. Ann Oncol 16:1654–1661
83. Singhal S, Mehta J, Desikan R, Ayers D, Roberson P, Eddlemon P, Munshi N, Anaissie E, Wilson C, Dhodapkar M, Zeddis J, Barlogie B (1999) Antitumour activity of thalidomide in refractory multiple myeloma. N Engl J Med 341:1565–1571
84. Rajkumar SV, Blood E, Vesole D, Fonseca R, Greipp PR (2006) Phase III clinical trial of thalidomide plus dexamethasone compared with dexamethasone alone in newly diagnosed multiple myeloma: a clinical trial coordinated by the Eastern Cooperative Oncology Group. J Clin Oncol 24:431–436
85. Wang M, Weber DM, Delasalle K, Alexanian R (2005) Thalidomide-dexamethasone as primary therapy for advanced multiple myeloma. Am J Hematol 79:194–197
86. Badros AZ, Goloubeva O, Rapoport AP, Ratterree B, Gahres N, Meisenberg B, Takebe N, Heyman M, Zwiebel J, Streicher H, Gocke CD, Tomic D, Flaws JA, Zhang B, Fenton RG (2005) Phase II study of G3139, a Bcl-2 antisense oligonucleotide, in combination with dexamethasone and thalidomide in relapsed multiple myeloma patients. J Clin Oncol 23:4089–4099

87. Kyriakou C, Thomson K, D'Sa S, Flory A, Hanslip J, Goldstone AH, Yong KL (2005) Low-dose thalidomide in combination with oral weekly cyclophosphamide and pulsed dexamethasone is a well tolerated and effective regimen in patients with relapsed and refractory multiple myeloma. Br J Haematol 129:763–770
88. Eisen T, Boshoff C, Mak I, Sapunar F, Vaughan MM, Pyle L, Johnston SR, Ahern R, Smith IE, Gore ME (2000) Continuous low dose thalidomide: a phase II study in advanced melanoma, renal cell, ovarian and breast cancer. Br J Cancer 82:812–817
89. Reiriz AB, Richter MF, Fernandes S, Cancela AI, Costa TD, Di Leone LP, Schwartsmann G (2004) Phase II study of thalidomide in patients with metastatic malignant melanoma. Melanoma Res 14:527–531
90. McCollum AD, Wu B, Clark JW, Kulke MH, Enzinger PC, Ryan DP, Earle CC, Michelini A, Fuchs CS (2006) The combination of capecitabine and thalidomide in previously treated, refractory metastatic colorectal cancer. Am J Clin Oncol 29:40–44
91. Kulke MH, Stuart K, Enzinger PC, Ryan DP, Clark JW, Muzikansky A, Vincitore M, Michelini A, Fuchs CS (2006) Phase II study of temozolomide and thalidomide in patients with metastatic neuroendocrine tumours. J Clin Oncol 24:401–406
92. Gordon JN, Trebble TM, Ellis RD, Duncan HD, Johns T, Goggin PM (2005) Thalidomide in the treatment of cancer cachexia: a randomised placebo controlled trial. Gut 54:540–545
93. Zhou W, Jiang ZW, Jiang J, Li N, Li JS (2004) Role of NF-kappa B in cancer cachexia [in Chinese]. Zhonghua Wai Ke Za Zhi 42:683–686
94. Hovstadius P, Larsson R, Jonsson E, Skov T, Kissmeyer AM, Krasilnikoff K, Bergh J, Karlsson MO, Lonnebo A, Ahlgren J (2002) A Phase I study of CHS 828 in patients with solid tumour malignancy. Clin Cancer Res 8:2843–2850
95. Ravaud A, Cerny T, Terret C, Wanders J, Bui BN, Hess D, Droz JP, Fumoleau P, Twelves C (2005) Phase I study and pharmacokinetic of CHS-828, a guanidino-containing compound, administered orally as a single dose every 3 weeks in solid tumours: an ECSG/EORTC study. Eur J Cancer 41:702–707
96. Binderup E, Bjorkling F, Hjarnaa PV, Latini S, Baltzer B, Carlsen M, Binderup L (2005) EB1627: a soluble prodrug of the potent anticancer cyanoguanidine CHS828. Bioorg Med Chem Lett 15:2491–2494
97. Robe PA, Martin D, Albert A, Deprez M, Chariot A, Bours V (2006) A phase 1–2, prospective, double blind, randomized study of the safety and efficacy of Sulfasalazine for the treatment of progressing malignant gliomas: study protocol of [ISRCTN45828668]. BMC Cancer 6:29
98. Muerkoster S, Arlt A, Gehrz A, Vorndamm J, Witt M, Grohmann F, Folsch UR, Schafer H (2004) Autocrine IL-1beta secretion leads to NF-kappabeta-mediated chemoresistance in pancreatic carcinoma cells in vivo [in German]. Med Klin (Munich) 99:185–190

18 Immunotherapeutic Approaches in Pancreatic Cancer

J. Stieler

Recent Results in Cancer Research, Vol. 177

Abstract

With growing understanding of the regulation of immune responses, multiple new immunotherapeutic targets have evolved. This article gives a survey over the current approaches in pancreatic cancer therapy including peptide vaccinations, unspecific immunotherapy, allogene modified tumor cell vaccines, and vector-based vaccines. Although several trials have shown detectable immune responses, such as delayed-type hypersensitivity reactions and cytokine release in enzyme-linked immunosorbent spot (ELISPOTS) assays, and some have reported prolonged survival for immune responders, immunotherapy remains experimental. However, some approaches have made it into a phase III setting. In addition, the emerging concept of tumor stem cells may lead to a new focus on immunotherapy, since these often highly chemotherapy-resistant cells are thought to be the source of recurrences.

18.1 Natural Course of Pancreatic Cancer and Immune Responses Detected

Untreated metastatic pancreatic cancer patients have a median survival of only about 4 months; for locally advanced cancers patients the life expectancy is about 6–8 months. Even after resection, recurrence occurs in the majority of the patients, leading to a median survival of about 18 months after R0 resection. With conventional chemotherapy the aim of treatment is restricted to palliation.

In healthy human subjects malignant transformations occur every day, but the immune systems manages to eliminate the potential threats. For malignant melanoma patients, spontaneous remissions of cancer lesions have been described in numerous case reports [57]. However, reports of spontaneously regressing pancreatic cancer do not exist; this may be because pancreatic cancer is generally diagnosed in a late stage, when the tumor must have found ways to overcome the hosts immune response. For the fate of early lesions, little is known about what percentage of them spontaneously regress or proceed into invasive cancer. One the one hand, this shows the putative potential of immune therapies against these cancer cells, but on the other hand it shows the potential of tumors to overcome immune responses with several escape mechanisms, some of which have been already characterized.

In pancreatic cancer patients, tumor-specific T4 and T8 cells have been isolated from the bone marrow [61, 62]. Furthermore, antibodies against tumor-associated antigens such as MUC-1 or the cancer testis antigen SCP-1 have been described [77, 89], partly associated with a better prognosis [17]. These findings show the immunogenicity of pancreatic cancer.

18.2 Tumor Stem Cell Hypothesis

Tumor immune therapy may not necessarily compete with conventional chemotherapy. As chemotherapy is only active in proliferating cells and therefore will reduce the number of tumor cells, in most cases it does not cure the patient. Immune therapy may in the future have a role in eliminating the quiescent tumor (stem) cells [65]. The concept of tumor stem cells is based on the finding that every tumor is a functional heterogeneous population of cells that undergoes, at least to a certain degree, some proliferation and differentiation, which implies the existence of a small subsets of cells capable of unlimited self-renewal. These cells are supposed to be the source of metastasis, recurrence, and minimal residual disease. In some human malignancies such as brain tumors and breast cancer, these cells that are capable of giving rise to recurrence have been characterized more precisely by surface markers [1, 20, 68, 69]. As such cells may differ in their expression of tumor-specific antigens from the majority of the tumor tissue, specific markers for tumor stem cells may need to be developed. For pancreatic cancer, such cancer stem cells have been identified in a mouse model [35]; the identified cells were CD44-, CD24-, and ESA-positive, they formed about 0.2%–0.8% of the cancer cells, and they had a more than 100 times higher tumor-forming potential than other cells derived from the same tumor.

18.3 Mechanisms of Immune Escape

Pancreatic cancer cells have an arsenal of local and systemic mechanisms to escape immunological control. Secretion of transforming growth factor (TGF)-beta, interleukin (IL)-6 and IL-10 exerts a systemic and local immunosuppressive effect [88]; secreted vascular endothelial growth factor (VEGF) may prevent dendritic cell maturation [42]. Accumulation of immunosuppressive Treg cells [37, 38], expression of nonfunctional Fas-receptor, and the killing of lymphocytes by Fas-Ligand expression have been described for pancreatic cancer [13, 43, 74, 75]. Furthermore, decreased expression of HLA-class I molecules [55], a reduced expression of the transporter associated with antigen processing (TAP) and b2-microglobulin, a reduced expression of costimulatory molecules of the B7 family necessary for establishing a profound immune response, and an increased expression of coinhibitory molecules of B7-H1 and B7-H4 have all been found to be mechanisms of immune escape in solid tumors [24, 32]. A mechanical barrier for invading cells is formed by the desmoplastic reaction found in the majority of pancreatic cancers.

18.4 Tumor Response

The first obstacle to immunotherapy in cancer is to find antigens expressed only or at least mostly in malignant tissue and not in normal tissue, and the second is to evoke a strong immune reaction against these antigens.

In the immune response to tumor cells, antigen-presenting cells present processed tumor antigens to naive CD8+ T cells by cross-presentation leading to antigen-specific cytotoxic T lymphocytes. These cytotoxic T lymphocytes are thought to mediate most of the antitumor response. MHC-2 presentation of ingested tumor antigens may activate CD4+ T lymphocytes leading to antibody production by B lymphocytes and stimulation of CD8+ T lymphocytes by cytokines. Natural killer (NK) cells can be activated by loss of inhibitory MHC-1 molecules and antibody binding to tumor cells. Macrophages may also kill tumor cells by secretion of nitrous oxide, reactive oxygen intermediates, tumor necrosis factor (TNF), and lysosomal enzymes. How macrophages are activated is not completely clear yet.

To generate a profound immune reaction, an antigen needs to be presented in association with other stimuli such as costimulatory molecules. Otherwise, immune tolerance instead of an immune reaction may result.

18.5 Isolation of Tumor Antigens

Tumor-associated antigens, which means antigens expressed stronger by the malignant clones but also expressed on normal tissue, can be distinguished from tumor-specific antigens such as mutated proteins found only in tumor cells. To isolate immunogenic tumor antigens, several approaches are in use. The first one is the serial analysis of gene expression (SAGE). Gene expression in tumor cells and normal tissue is compared to identify genes more strongly expressed in tumors. From the given proteins, candidate proteins are determined and computer algorithms are used to predict HLA binding epitopes in these proteins. From patients vaccinated with whole cell tumor vaccines, CD8+ T cells are collected before and after vaccination, and these cells are exposed to antigen-presenting T2 cells that have been engineered to express the previously determined peptides. The effect of the isolated HLA-restricted peptides can thus be quantified and potential tumor antigens can be determined.

A similar possibility is to identify tumor cell MHC class I bound peptides by eluting them with acid treatment and fractioning them with reverse high-performance chromatography. Then, these fractions can be tested for their ability to provoke cell lysis in MHC matched nontumor cells cocultivated by tumor-specific cytotoxic T lymphocytes (CTLs). The peptides can subsequently be analyzed and compared to databases of protein sequences.

Another method is serological analysis of recombinant tumor cDNA expression libraries (SEREX). Genes from this library are then transfected into MHC class I+ cell lines, and these cells are tested in coculture with tumor-specific CTLs. Thus, genes leading to lysis of the transfected cell can be determined to be a potential target.

18.6 Does It Make Sense to Combine Immunotherapy with Chemotherapy?

As conventional chemotherapy affects bone marrow and renders the patient susceptible to infection, it seems on first sight contradictory to combine immunotherapy based on an intact immune system with chemotherapy. In fact, several trials have shown that chemotherapy may even enhance immune responses; low-dose cyclophosphamide has been known for many years to enhance vaccination effects and CD8+ T cell-mediated responses, an effect probably due to increased (augmented) freeing of type 1 interferons, decreased regulatory T cells, and an increase in the recruitment of myeloid dendritic cells [58]. Chemotherapy with other agents, or chemoradiation, may furthermore induce the death of tumor cells and so increase presentation of tumor-associated antigens by dendritic cells. For gemcitabine and combinations with cisplatin, several authors have shown that chemotherapy may in fact restore normal immune function by reducing myeloid suppressor cells, thereby even improving upon the antitumor immune activity [3, 10, 48, 72].

18.7 Passive Immunization

The most evolved and so far most effective way of immunotherapy in cancer patients has been monoclonal antibodies, which are directed against growth factors or their receptors. In pancreatic cancer, several antibodies have made their way into clinical testing. The epidermal growth factor receptor (EGFR) antibody cetuximab, which has proven efficacy in colorectal cancer, has been evaluated in a phase III trial in combination with gemcitabine. In the preceding phase II study, a time to progression of 3.8 months and a median overall survival of 7.1 months was reached, which compares slightly positively compared with historic controls of gemcitabine alone [84]. In the phase III trial, which was presented on ASCO 2007, the combination showed no significant benefit with an overall survival of 6 months for gemcitabine alone and 6.5 months for the combination, but subgroup analysis for the patients with higher grades of skin reactions have not yet been reported [90]. Further studies in combination with radiotherapy are underway [30]. The rationale for combining the antibody with radiotherapy is, above all, to attain a marked increase of efficacy in radiotherapy in head and neck cancer, where EGFR is involved in tissue regeneration after radiation. Another humanized EGFR antibody, matuzumab, is under evaluation in pancreatic cancer too [16].

Another antibody that has been quite successful in colorectal cancer in combination with chemotherapy is bevacizumab. This antibody binds to free VEGF and may therefore reduce VEGF receptor (VEGFR) activation and thus neovascularization, which is essential for growth of metastases. In pancreatic cancer, in combination with gemcitabine, a phase II study showed an encouraging 8.8-month median survival in metastasized patients [25]. However, the phase III study to evaluate the combination in comparison to gemcitabine has recently been closed prematurely due to lack of efficacy in an interim analysis [26].

The combination of this antibody with radiotherapy and capecitabine in a phase I trial has also been reported and showed some increased toxicity [9]. More trials evaluating combinations of bevacizumab and several chemotherapeutic combinations, some even including radiotherapy, are underway.

Epithelial cell adhesion molecule (EPCAM) is molecule expressed in several epithelial cancers including pancreatic cancer. Antibodies against this epitope have been under clinical evaluation [67] and have led to some minor responses [80]. Attempts to increase the efficacy of the first-generation murine antibodies by improving antigen affinity have led to more side effects such as pancreatitis, but another approach might be aimed toward improving affinity of the Fc part to its receptor [76].

Mesothelin, a cell surface glycoprotein, is another tumor antigen expressed by almost 100% of pancreatic adenocarcinomas, but not in normal pancreatic tissue [19]. Early trials with monoclonal antibodies against this target are also underway.

While antibodies will (1) suppress functioning of cell surface molecules, (2) mark tumor cells for complement-mediated lysis, or (3) act as immune effector cells, they can also be used to deliver drugs, radioactive isotopes, cytokines, or toxins to the tumor cell. Some early clinical trials using such approaches are underway in pancreatic cancer, but they have not yet proved their efficacy and tolerability in clinical settings (Table 18.1).

18.8 Peptide Vaccines

Several trials have addressed active immunization with peptides derived from tumor-associated antigens. In general, peptide vaccines are not immunogenic enough and are therefore combined with granulocyte-macrophage colony stimulating factor (GM-CSF) to attract dendritic cells, or they are given together with strong immunogenic stimuli, for example diphtheria toxin, to intensify the response. The largest trial so far has been one investigating the effect of a gastrin-derived peptide linked to diphtheria toxin to enhance immunogenicity and recruitment of dendritic cells. Gastrin has previously shown to be a growth factor for pancreatic cancer cells in vitro [23, 79], and a phase II study of the vaccine showed a significant advantage for antibody responders against nonresponders of 217 versus 121 days median survival [5]. In the succeeding placebo-controlled phase III trial of gemcitabine +/− G17DT no differences in response, time to progression, or survival could be shown, but there was a tendency toward prolonged survival in patients with higher antibody titers [66].

Other attempts have included vaccination with mutated ras-peptide, which is closely linked to pancreatic carcinogenesis. About 90% of pancreatic adenocarcinomas show *ras* mutations. Immune responses were measured by delayed-type hypersensitivity (DTH), mutated ras-specific IgG levels, and enzyme-linked immunosorbent spot (ELISPOT), and GM-CSF was given as an attractant for dendritic cells [7, 86, 87]. Immune responses were detectable in IgG levels, DTH, and in an increase of mutated-ras-specific CTLs, but it is still unclear if these immune responses transfer into clinical responses.

Other targets in peptide vaccination have been MUC-1, a mucopolysaccharide usually expressed in the apical area of ductal pancreatic cells whose expression is enforced in pancreatic adenocarcinoma. MUC-1 levels in the sera of patients may also be useful in making the distinction between benign and malignant pancreatic lesions [14, 73], and higher levels of MUC-1 IgG antibodes in pancreatic cancer patients have been found to be significantly associated with survival in some minor studies [17]. Vaccination trials with a MUC-1-derived peptide and Freund's adjuvants have passed phase I with good tolerability [51, 85].

Survivin, which is another tumor-associated antigen, is also under investigation as a vaccine, and in a case report, a complete remission of liver metastasis has been reported [18, 82].

Telomerase is an enzyme necessary for unlimited replicative potential of cells since every division of a cell leads to a small loss in the telomere repeat sequence of the chromosome. Telomerase repairs these losses. Telomerase is expressed in a variety of human tumors [15]; in pancreatic cancer it is expressed in 85%–90% of tumors. Telomerase-specific T cells are capable of killing pancreatic cancer cells in vitro and in vivo [60]. A peptide derived from the catalytic subunit of human telomerase (GV1001) has been shown to evoke, when given together with GM-CSF, noticeable responses as measured by ELISPOT

Table 18.1 Current immunotherapy-based approaches in pancreatic cancer according to the Clinical Trials Database (http://clinicaltrials.gov/)

No.	Phase	Drugs/radiation	Indication
NCT00307723	I/II	5-FU, oxaliplatin, bevacizumab, radiation, gemcitabine, bevacizumab	Loc. advanced
NCT00100815	II	Gemcitabine, capecitabine, bevacizumab	Metastatic/unresectable
NCT00350753	II	Erlotinib, bevacizumab	Upper GI cancer
NCT00305877	II	Bevacizumab or cetuximab plus gemcitabine, capecitabine and radiation	Completely resected pancreatic cancer
NCT00066677	II	Docetaxel +/− bevacizumab	Second line
NCT00101348	I/II	Erlotinib, cetuximab +/− bevacizumab	Several cancers including pancreatic cancer
NCT00260364	I/II	Gemcitabine, capecitabine, erlotinib, bevacizumab	Metastatic/unresectable
NCT00365144	II	Bevacizumab + erlotinib	Second line after Gemcitabine
NCT00091026	II	Bevacizumab + gemcitabine + cetuximab or erlotinib	Loc. advanced/metastatic
NCT00126633	II	Gemcitabine, cisplatin, bevacizumab	Metastatic
NCT00410774	I/II	Gemcitabine + bevacizumab	Completely resected
NCT00366457	II	Gemcitabine, erlotinib, bevacizumab	Metastatic/unresectable
NCT00222469	II	Gemcitabine, oxaliplatin, bevacizumab	Metastatic/unresectable
NCT00336648	II	Gemcitabine, bevacizumab, radiation	Neoadjuvant
NCT00326911	II	Cetuximab, bevacizumab +/− gemcitabine	Metastatic/unresectable
NCT00325494	I	MORAb-009 (mesothelin-antibody)	≥ Second line, mesothelin expressing tumors
NCT00002475	II	Cyclophosphamide plus interferon-treated, irradiated tumor cell vaccine (autologous or allogeneic) plus GM-CSF	Various tumors
NCT00108875	I/II	Survivin peptide	Different tumors, Second line
NCT00364364	I	Radiolabeled mesothelin-antibody	Pancreatic cancer
NCT00352131	I	HuC242-DM4, toxin-linked monoclonal AB against CanAg	CanAg expressing pancreatic and colon cancers, failed standard therapy
NCT00305760	II	Cyclophosphamide, GM-CSF transfected allogeneic tumor cells, cetuximab	Refractory to standard therapy or refusing standard therapy pancreatic cancer patients
NCT00112580	II	Ipilimumab (CTLA-4 antibody)	Stage IV irresectable pancreatic cancer
NCT00401570	II	Volociximab (anti-alpha5beta1-integrin-antibody) plus gemcitabine	Inoperable first line
NCT00010270	I	LMB-9 immunotoxin	Different tumors refractory to standard therapy, Lewis-Y antigen overexpression
NCT00098592	I	Sorafenib and bevacizumab	Solid tumors refractory to standard therapy
NCT00024674 (terminated)	I	Toxin-linked mesothelin antibody	Different tumors, recurrence after appropriate first line therapy

CTLA, cytotoxic T lymphocyte-associated protein; GM-CSF, granulocyte-macrophage colony stimulating factor and DTH in up to 75% of the patients. In the phase I/II study, patients reached a median survival of 8.6 months [4]. Consequently, this vaccine is currently being evaluated in a phase III setting in combination with gemcitabine and capecitabine (Telovax trial) comparing chemotherapy alone with either sequential or parallel administration of the vaccinations.

18.9 Nonspecific Immune Stimulation

Another approach of immunotherapy is nonspecific immune stimulation. This approach has attracted new interest after the amazing results of a phase II adjuvant chemoradiation trial that used cisplatin, 5-fluorouracil (5-FU), and interferon-alpha in a high-risk collective and reached a median survival of 46 months [47]. Consequently, confirming phase III trials have been initiated, and one of these was accompanied by immune surveillance programs [59]. Increased MUC-1 and CA 19-9-dependent granzyme B release, a time-dependent increase of IL-12 and TNF-alpha levels, increased spontaneous cytotoxicity, and increased peripheral dendritic cells, macrophages, central and effector memory T cells, CD8+ cells and CD40+ cells were all observed after a dose of interferon alpha [59]. These changes were not observed in the 5-FU (alone) arm. This phase III trial is still recruiting; therefore no survival or response data are available [27].

18.10 Tumor Cell Vaccine

Tumor cells can also be modified in vitro to secrete GM-CSF and be given back to the patient after irradiation of these cells [31]. GM-CSF is used to enhance dendritic cell accrual. Autologous or allogenic tumor cells may be used [22, 70], and immunological responses have been reported. The theoretical advantage in using whole cell vaccines is that a broad spectrum of possible antigen is presented; however, cell vaccines, such as in vitro-modified dendritic cells, need an enormous logistical background that limits their use. In a trial using GM-CSF-transfected and irradiated allogenic pancreatic cancer cells, resected pancreatic cancer patients who received adjuvant chemoradiation as well experienced vaccine reactions; a promising 1- and 2-year survival of 88% and 76% was reached [33].

18.11 Pulsed Dendritic Cells

Another approach of immunotherapy is to load dendritic cells in vitro directly with tumor-derived antigens and to give these cells back to the patient. This can be done by pulsing them with tumor-derived peptides or by transfection with the DNA or RNA of target molecules [53].

Vaccination with peptide-pulsed mononuclear cells derived from peripheral blood with mutated p53 or kras-derived peptides in patients previously shown to harbor the given mutations has been used to augment immune responses. In 28% of patients a CTL response and in 42% a positive IFN-gamma response was shown in various tumor patients including pancreatic cancer patients. Responders had a significantly prolonged survival (393 versus 98 days for CTL responders and 470 versus 88 days for IFN gamma responders [6].

Muc-1, which has already been used as a peptide vaccine as well, can also be pulsed on dendritic cells [8, 29, 81] and is capable of increasing antigen-specific interferon release by CD8+ T cells up to tenfold in 4 out of 10 patients [44], but it is still unclear if this also translates to clinical responses.

Interestingly, even dendritic cells cultured with patient sera were able to generate minor responses and stable disease in a small series of patients [41].

18.12 Viral Vectors

Dendritic cells may also be modified by viral vectors in vivo to express certain tumor-associated antigens. This also offers the possibility to make these cells coexpress costimulatory molecules, as they are needed to prevent tolerance induction and to provoke an intense immune response. One such approach is in vitro vaccination of dendritic cells with a vaccinia based vector coding a carcinoembryonic antigen (CEA) peptide and the costimulatory molecules intercellular adhesion molecule (ICAM)-1, lymphocyte function-associated antigen (LFA)-3, and B7-1 [40,

46]. In 10 out of 12 patients there was an increase in CEA-associated T cell responses measured by ELISPOT. Minor responses and stable disease were noted as well. Further development of this vaccine led to inclusion of MUC-1 coding sequences into the vector and booster vaccination with fowlpox-based vaccines to prevent strong immune responses against the vector itself, which might prevent immune responses against the target antigens. Easier application by direct vaccination of the patients and therefore in vivo targeting of dendritic cells instead of more complicated in vitro processes is the theoretical advantage of such an approach [63, 64]. The vaccinations were accommodated by GM-CSF injections for better dendritic cells accrual. Used in a second-line setting for pancreatic cancer patients, a remarkably prolonged survival was noted in these phase I studies of 6.3 and 7.9 months under second line. Consequently, the given vaccine is currently being evaluated in a second-line phase III study.

Another approach that has so far only been used in a mouse model is to induce increased immunogenicity of tumors in vitro by vaccination with a IL-12 and B7.1 costimulatory molecule coding adenoviral vector that is injected directly into the tumor. This approach led to high response rates of about 80% in the treated animals [50].

18.13 Toll-Like Receptors

Toll-like receptors form a phylogenetically old mechanism of defense against microbes and are part of the innate immune system. At least ten different receptors can be distinguished, and every receptor recognizes certain antigens characteristic for bacterial or viral infections, but also signatures of cancer cells [54]. The receptors are expressed on many different cells such macrophages, dendritic cells, neutrophils, epithelial cells, and endothelial cells. Activation of these receptors leads via NF-kappa B to release of inflammatory cytokines, proteins involved in microbial killing and changes in the expression of endothelial adhesion molecules.

In cancer therapy, topical administration of toll-like receptor 7 and 8 agonists had been used for a while in benign and malignant skin tumors with some success [83].

Interestingly, in a mouse model, synergy between activation of TLR9, which is expressed on pancreatic tissue, by CpG repeats and gemcitabine has been reported [49].

In mice, it was also shown that Toll-like receptor (TLR)2 and -8 may downregulate Treg cells [12, 36, 45, 71]. Furthermore, generation of CTL could be enhanced by TLR3 and -7 activation [78]. Thus, activation of these receptors may be useful in overcoming tumor-induced immunosuppression and in generating a strong vaccine response. In pancreatic cancer, no studies have so far addressed toll-like receptor targeting in humans, but there are early trials with double-stranded (ds)RNA in breast cancer where TLR3 activation can trigger apoptosis [56]. Trials addressing TLR activation have been addressed in a breast cancer adjuvant trial [2] and in lung cancer (TLR-9) [34], and trials in solid tumors (TLR7) are ongoing [11] with reported responses. In lung cancer, the combination of chemotherapy and a TLR9 agonist showed markedly increased response rates in a phase II setting [34].

18.14 Immunocytokines

Another approach currently under development in solid tumors comprises immunocytokines. These consist of an antibody against a tumor-associated antigen coupled with a cytokine. An example for such a molecule is huKS-IL-2, an IL-2-linked epithelial cell adhesion molecule (EPCAM) antibody that is under development in prostate cancer [28] but has not yet been tested in pancreatic cancer, which expresses EPCAM as well.

18.15 CTLA-4 Antagonists

CTLA-4 or CD 152 is a accessory surface molecule that limits activation of T cells after antigen exposure. It prevents autoimmune reactions and is expressed in a later stage of antigen exposure. CTLA-4 blockage may therefore prevent tolerance induction, and CTLA-4 antibodies such as ipilimumab (MDX010) are under clinical evaluation in pancreatic cancer; another such antibody has been evaluated in melanoma [52]. The main toxicities are so-called immune breakthrough reactions linked to autoimmune disease, and in trials with prostate and renal cancer as well as melanoma, tumor regressions and tumor marker responses have been reported [39].

18.16 CCR-4 Blockage

Another approach in overcoming tumor-induced immunosuppression caused by accumulation of Treg cells in the tumor, which are partly attracted by chemokine receptor (CCR)-4 ligands, is to block this chemoattractant and thus prevent the homing of Treg cells in the tumor tissue. This approach is currently being evaluated in a phase I trial in leukemia patients in Japan, but no such experience in pancreatic cancer patients has been published so far [21].

18.17 Summary

With enhanced understanding of the regulation of the immune system, novel targets have been identified in the field of antitumor immunity. Many trials have shown immunologic responses, and some have also shown improved survival or response rates. Larger phase III trials with several agents are ongoing. Immunotherapy cannot yet replace chemotherapy, but it may in the future be an additional approach in fighting cancer and eradicating tumor stem cells.

References

1. Al-Hajj M, Becker MW, Wicha M, Weissman I, Clarke MF (2004) Therapeutic implications of cancer stem cells. Curr Opin Genet Dev 14:43–47
2. Andre F, Massard C, Assi H, Besse B, Sabourin J, Zitvogel L (2006) Toll like receptor 3 expression and efficacy of adjuvant treatment with polyadenylic-polyuridylic acid in patients with axillary node positive breast cancer: results from two randomized trials. 2006 ASCO Annual Meeting
3. Bang S, Kim HS, Choo YS, Park SW, Chung JB, Song SY (2006) Differences in immune cells engaged in cell-mediated immunity after chemotherapy for far advanced pancreatic cancer. Pancreas 32:29–36
4. Bernhardt SL, Gjertsen MK, Trachsel S, Moller M, Eriksen JA, Meo M, Buanes T, Gaudernack G (2006) Telomerase peptide vaccination of patients with non-resectable pancreatic cancer: a dose escalating phase I/II study. Br J Cancer 95:1474–1482
5. Brett BT, Smith SC, Bouvier CV, Michaeli D, Hochhauser D, Davidson BR, Kurzawinski TR, Watkinson AF, Van Someren N, Pounder RE, Caplin ME (2002) Phase II study of anti-gastrin-17 antibodies, raised to G17DT, in advanced pancreatic cancer. J Clin Oncol 20:4225–4231
6. Carbone DP, Ciernik IF, Kelley MJ, Smith MC, Nadaf S, Kavanaugh D, Maher VE, Stipanov M, Contois D, Johnson BE, Pendleton CD, Seifert B, Carter C, Read EJ, Greenblatt J, Top LE, Kelsey MI, Minna JD, Berzofsky JA (2005) Immunization with mutant p53- and K-ras-derived peptides in cancer patients: immune response and clinical outcome. J Clin Oncol 23:5099–5107
7. Chang DZ, Abou-Alfa GK, O'Reilly EM, Schwartz GK, Neville D, Siegel E, Levin A, Chapman PB (2003) Vaccination of pancreatic cancer patients against mutated K-ras. 2003 ASCO Annual Meeting
8. Cloosen S, Thio M, Vanclee A, van Leeuwen EB, Senden-Gijsbers BL, Oving EB, Germeraad WT, Bos GM (2004) Mucin-1 is expressed on dendritic cells, both in vitro and in vivo. Int Immunol 16:1561–1571
9. Crane CH, Ellis LM, Abbruzzese JL, Amos C, Xiong HQ, Ho L, Evans DB, Tamm EP, Ng C, Pisters PW, Charnsangavej C, Delclos ME, O'Reilly M, Lee JE, Wolff RA (2006) Phase I trial evaluating the safety of bevacizumab with concurrent radiotherapy and capecitabine in locally advanced pancreatic cancer. J Clin Oncol 24:1145–1151
10. Dauer M, Herten J, Bauer C, Renner F, Schad K, Schnurr M, Endres S, Eigler A (2005) Chemosensitization of pancreatic carcinoma cells to enhance T cell-mediated cytotoxicity induced by tumor lysate-pulsed dendritic cells. J Immunother 28:332–342
11. Dudek AZ, Yunis C, Kumar S, Harrison LI, Hawkinson RW, Miller JS (2005) Immune response activation by a Toll-like receptor 7 agonist: results of a phase 1 study. 2005 ASCO Annual Meeting
12. El Andaloussi A, Sonabend AM, Han Y, Lesniak MS (2006) Stimulation of TLR9 with CpG ODN enhances apoptosis of glioma and prolongs the survival of mice with experimental brain tumors. Glia 54:526–535

13. Elnemr A, Ohta T, Yachie A, Kayahara M, Kitagawa H, Fujimura T, Ninomiya I, Fushida S, Nishimura GI, Shimizu K, Miwa K (2001) Human pancreatic cancer cells disable function of Fas receptors at several levels in Fas signal transduction pathway. Int J Oncol 18:311–316
14. Gold DV, Modrak DE, Ying Z, Cardillo TM, Sharkey RM, Goldenberg DM (2006) New MUC1 serum immunoassay differentiates pancreatic cancer from pancreatitis. J Clin Oncol 24:252–258
15. Goldman MA (2003) The role of telomeres and telomerase in cancer. Drug Discov Today 8:294–296
16. Graeven U, Kremer B, Sudhoff T, Killing B, Rojo F, Weber D, Tillner J, Unal C, Schmiegel W (2006) Phase I study of the humanised anti-EGFR monoclonal antibody matuzumab (EMD 72000) combined with gemcitabine in advanced pancreatic cancer. Br J Cancer 94:1293–1299
17. Hamanaka Y, Suehiro Y, Fukui M, Shikichi K, Imai K, Hinoda Y (2003) Circulating anti-MUC1 IgG antibodies as a favorable prognostic factor for pancreatic cancer. Int J Cancer 103:97–100
18. Hassan R, Bera T, Pastan I (2004) Mesothelin: a new target for immunotherapy. Clin Cancer Res 10:3937–3942
19. Hassan R, Laszik ZG, Lerner M, Raffeld M, Postier R, Brackett D (2005) Mesothelin is overexpressed in pancreaticobiliary adenocarcinomas but not in normal pancreas and chronic pancreatitis. Am J Clin Pathol 124:838–845
20. Hemmati HD, Nakano I, Lazareff JA, Masterman-Smith M, Geschwind DH, Bronner-Fraser M, Kornblum HI (2003) Cancerous stem cells can arise from pediatric brain tumors. Proc Natl Acad Sci U S A 100:15178–15183
21. Ishida T, Ueda R (2006) CCR4 as a novel molecular target for immunotherapy of cancer. Cancer Sci 97:1139–1146
22. Jaffee EM, Hruban RH, Biedrzycki B, Laheru D, Schepers K, Sauter PR, Goemann M, Coleman J, Grochow L, Donehower RC, Lillemoe KD, O'Reilly S, Abrams RA, Pardoll DM, Cameron JL, Yeo CJ (2001) Novel allogeneic granulocyte-macrophage colony-stimulating factor-secreting tumor vaccine for pancreatic cancer: a phase I trial of safety and immune activation. J Clin Oncol 19:145–156
23. Jang JY, Kim SW, Ku JL, Park YH, Park JG (2005) Presence of CCK-A, B receptors and effect of gastrin and cholecystokinin on growth of pancreatobiliary cancer cell lines. World J Gastroenterol 11:803–809
24. Kim R, Emi M, Tanabe K, Arihiro K (2006) Tumor-driven evolution of immunosuppressive networks during malignant progression. Cancer Res 66:5527–5536
25. Kindler HL, Friberg G, Singh DA, Locker G, Nattam S, Kozloff M, Taber DA, Karrison T, Dachman A, Stadler WM, Vokes EE (2005) Phase II trial of bevacizumab plus gemcitabine in patients with advanced pancreatic cancer. J Clin Oncol 23:8033–8040
26. Kindler HL, Niedzwiecki D, Hollis D, Oraefo E, Schrag Hurwitz H, McLeod HL, Mulcahy MF, Schilsky RL, Goldberg RM (2007) A double-blind, placebo-controlled, randomized phase III trial of gemcitabine (G) plus bevacizumab (B) versus gemcitabine plus placebo (P) in patients (pts) with advanced pancreatic cancer (PC): a preliminary analysis of Cancer and Leukemia Group B (CALGB) 80303. ASCO 2007 Gastrointestinal Cancers Symposium, Orlando
27. Knaebel HP, Marten A, Schmidt J, Hoffmann K, Seiler C, Lindel K, Schmitz-Winnenthal H, Fritz S, Herrmann T, Goldschmidt H, Mansmann U, Debus J, Diehl V, Buchler MW (2005) Phase III trial of postoperative cisplatin, interferon alpha-2b, and 5-FU combined with external radiation treatment versus 5-FU alone for patients with resected pancreatic adenocarcinoma—CapRI: study protocol [ISRCTN62866759]. BMC Cancer 5:37
28. Ko YJ, Bubley GJ, Weber R, Redfern C, Gold DP, Finke L, Kovar A, Dahl T, Gillies SD (2004) Safety, pharmacokinetics, and biological pharmacodynamics of the immunocytokine EMD 273066 (huKS-IL2): results of a phase I trial in patients with prostate cancer. J Immunother 27:232–239
29. Kontani K, Taguchi O, Ozaki Y, Hanaoka J, Sawai S, Inoue S, Abe H, Hanasawa K, Fujino S (2003) Dendritic cell vaccine immunotherapy of cancer targeting MUC1 mucin. Int J Mol Med 12:493–502
30. Krempien R, Muenter MW, Huber PE, Nill S, Friess H, Timke C, Didinger B, Buechler P, Heeger S, Herfarth KK, Abdollahi A, Buchler MW, Debus J (2005) Randomized phase II—study evaluating EGFR targeting therapy with cetuximab in combination with radiotherapy and chemotherapy for patients with locally advanced pancreatic cancer—PARC: study protocol [ISRCTN56652283]. BMC Cancer 5:131

31. Laheru D, Biedrzycki B, Thomas AM, Jaffee EM (2005) Development of a cytokine-modified allogeneic whole cell pancreatic cancer vaccine. Methods Mol Med 103:299–327
32. Laheru D, Jaffee EM (2005) Immunotherapy for pancreatic cancer—science driving clinical progress. Nat Rev Cancer 5:459–467
33. Laheru D, Yeo C, Biedrzycki B, Solt S, Lutz E, Onners B, Tartakovsky I, Hruban R, Piantadosi S, Jaffee E (2007) A safety and efficacy trial of lethally irradiated allogeneic pancreatic tumor cells transfected with the GM-CSF gene in combination with adjuvant chemoradiotherapy for the treatment of adenocarcinoma of the pancreas. 2007 Gastrointestinal Cancers Symposium, Orlando, Florida
34. Leichman G, Gravenor D, Woytowitz D, Mezger J, Albert G, Schmalbach T, Al-Adhami M, Manegold C (2005) CPG 7909, a TLR9 agonist, added to first line taxane/platinum for advanced non-small cell lung cancer, a randomized, controlled phase II study. 2005 ASCO Annual Meeting
35. Li C, Heidt DG, Dalerba P, Burant CF, Zhang L, Adsay V, Wicha M, Clarke MF, Simeone DM (2007) Identification of pancreatic cancer stem cells. Cancer Res 67:1030–1037
36. Liu H, Komai-Koma M, Xu D, Liew FY (2006) Toll-like receptor 2 signaling modulates the functions of CD4+ CD25+ regulatory T cells. Proc Natl Acad Sci U S A 103:7048–7053
37. Liyanage UK, Goedegebuure PS, Moore TT, Viehl CT, Moo-Young TA, Larson JW, Frey DM, Ehlers JP, Eberlein TJ, Linehan DC (2006) Increased prevalence of regulatory T cells (Treg) is induced by pancreas adenocarcinoma. J Immunother 29:416–424
38. Liyanage UK, Moore TT, Joo HG, Tanaka Y, Herrmann V, Doherty G, Drebin JA, Strasberg SM, Eberlein TJ, Goedegebuure PS, Linehan DC (2002) Prevalence of regulatory T cells is increased in peripheral blood and tumor microenvironment of patients with pancreas or breast adenocarcinoma. J Immunol 169:2756–2761
39. Maker AV, Phan GQ, Attia P, Yang JC, Sherry RM, Topalian SL, Kammula US, Royal RE, Haworth LR, Levy C, Kleiner D, Mavroukakis SA, Yellin M, Rosenberg SA (2005) Tumor regression and autoimmunity in patients treated with cytotoxic T lymphocyte-associated antigen 4 blockade and interleukin 2: a phase I/II study. Ann Surg Oncol 12:1005–1016
40. Morse M, Clay T, Hobeika A, Osada T, Panicali D, Lyerly HK (2004) Phase I study of immunization with dendritic cells (DC) modified with recombinant fowlpox encoding carcinoembryonic antigen (CEA) and the triad of costimulatory molecules CD54, CD58, and CD80 (rF-CEA(6D)-TRICOM) in patients with advanced malignancies. 2004 ASCO Annual Meeting
41. Nesselhut T, Chang R, Matthes C, Marx D, Lorenzen DR, Cillien N, Martin M, Gorter R, Peters JH (2004) Cancer therapy with unloaded monocyte-derived dendritic cells in patients with inoperable pancreatic and gall bladder cancer. 2004 ASCO Annual Meeting
42. Ohm JE, Carbone DP (2001) VEGF as a mediator of tumor-associated immunodeficiency. Immunol Res 23:263–272
43. Ohta T, Elnemr A, Kitagawa H, Kayahara M, Takamura H, Fujimura T, Nishimura G, Shimizu K, Yi SQ, Miwa K (2004) Fas ligand expression in human pancreatic cancer. Oncol Rep 12:749–754
44. Pecher G, Haring A, Kaiser L, Thiel E (2002) Mucin gene (MUC1) transfected dendritic cells as vaccine: results of a phase I/II clinical trial. Cancer Immunol Immunother 51:669–673
45. Peng G, Guo Z, Kiniwa Y, Voo KS, Peng W, Fu T, Wang DY, Li Y, Wang HY, Wang RF (2005) Toll-like receptor 8-mediated reversal of CD4+ regulatory T cell function. Science 309:1380–1384
46. Petrulio CA, Kaufman HL (2006) Development of the PANVAC-VF vaccine for pancreatic cancer. Expert Rev Vaccines 5:9–19
47. Picozzi VJ, Kozarek R, Jacobs AD, Boone-Hill NK, Traverso LW (2003) Adjuvant therapy for resected pancreas cancer (PC) using alpha-interferon (IFN)-based chemoradiation: completion of a phase II trial. 2003 ASCO Annual Meeting
48. Plate JM, Plate AE, Shott S, Bograd S, Harris JE (2005) Effect of gemcitabine on immune cells in subjects with adenocarcinoma of the pancreas. Cancer Immunol Immunother 54:915–925
49. Pratesi G, Petrangolini G, Tortoreto M, Addis A, Belluco S, Rossini A, Selleri S, Rumio C, Menard S, Balsari A (2005) Therapeutic synergism of gemcitabine and CpG-oligodeoxynucleotides in an orthotopic human pancreatic carcinoma xenograft. Cancer Res 65:6388–6393
50. Putzer BM, Rodicker F, Hitt MM, Stiewe T, Esche H (2002) Improved treatment of pancreatic cancer by IL-12 and B7. costimulation: antitumor efficacy and immunoregulation in a nonimmunogenic tumor model. Mol Ther 5:405–412

51. Ramanathan RK, Lee KM, McKolanis J, Hitbold E, Schraut W, Moser AJ, Warnick E, Whiteside T, Osborne J, Kim H, Day R, Troetschel M, Finn OJ (2005) Phase I study of a MUC1 vaccine composed of different doses of MUC1 peptide with SB-AS2 adjuvant in resected and locally advanced pancreatic cancer. Cancer Immunol Immunother 54:254–264
52. Reuben JM, Lee BN, Li C, Gomez-Navarro J, Bozon VA, Parker CA, Hernandez IM, Gutierrez C, Lopez-Berestein G, Camacho LH (2006) Biologic and immunomodulatory events after CTLA-4 blockade with ticilimumab in patients with advanced malignant melanoma. Cancer 106:2437–2444
53. Ribas A (2005) Genetically modified dendritic cells for cancer immunotherapy. Curr Gene Ther 5:619–628
54. Romagne F (2007) Current and future drugs targeting one class of innate immunity receptors: the Toll-like receptors. Drug Discov Today 12:80–87
55. Ryschich E, Notzel T, Hinz U, Autschbach F, Ferguson J, Simon I, Weitz J, Frohlich B, Klar E, Buchler MW, Schmidt J (2005) Control of T-cell-mediated immune response by HLA class I in human pancreatic carcinoma. Clin Cancer Res 11:498–504
56. Salaun B, Coste I, Rissoan MC, Lebecque SJ, Renno T (2006) TLR3 can directly trigger apoptosis in human cancer cells. J Immunol 176:4894–4901
57. Saleh F, Renno W, Klepacek I, Ibrahim G, Dashti H, Asfar S, Behbehani A, Al-Sayer H, Dashti A (2005) Direct evidence on the immune-mediated spontaneous regression of human cancer: an incentive for pharmaceutical companies to develop a novel anti-cancer vaccine. Curr Pharm Des 11:3531–3543
58. Salem ML, Kadima AN, El-Naggar SA, Rubinstein MP, Chen Y, Gillanders WE, Cole DJ (2007) Defining the ability of cyclophosphamide preconditioning to enhance the antigen-specific CD8+ T-cell response to peptide vaccination: creation of a beneficial host microenvironment involving type I IFNs and myeloid cells. J Immunother 30:40–53
59. Schmidt J, Jager D, Hoffmann K, Buchler MW, Marten A (2007) Impact of interferon-alpha in combined chemoradioimmunotherapy for pancreatic adenocarcinoma (CapRI): first data from the immunomonitoring. J Immunother 30:108–115
60. Schmidt J, Ryschich E, Sievers E, Schmidt-Wolf IG, Buchler MW, Marten A (2006) Telomerase-specific T-cells kill pancreatic tumor cells in vitro and in vivo. Cancer 106:759–764
61. Schmitz-Winnenthal FH, Escobedo LV, Beckhove P, Schirrmacher V, Bucur M, Ziouta Y, Volk C, Schmied B, Koch M, Antolovic D, Weitz J, Buchler MW, Z'Graggen K (2006) Specific immune recognition of pancreatic carcinoma by patient-derived CD4 and CD8 T cells and its improvement by interferon-gamma. Int J Oncol 28:1419–1428
62. Schmitz-Winnenthal FH, Volk C, Z'Graggen K, Galindo L, Nummer D, Ziouta Y, Bucur M, Weitz J, Schirrmacher V, Buchler MW, Beckhove P (2005) High frequencies of functional tumor-reactive T cells in bone marrow and blood of pancreatic cancer patients. Cancer Res 65:10079–10087
63. Schuetz T, Marshall J, Kaufman HL, Safran H, Panical D (2004) Two phase I studies of prime-boost vaccinations with vaccinia-fowlpox vaccines expressing CEA, MUC-1, and TRICOM costimulatory molecules (B7.1/ICAM-1/LFA-3) in patients with advanced pancreatic cancer. 2004 ASCO Annual Meeting
64. Schuetz T, Kaufman HL, Marshall JL, Safran H (2005) Extended survival in second-line pancreatic cancer after therapeutic vaccination. 2005 ASCO Annual Meeting
65. Schulenburg A, Ulrich-Pur H, Thurnher D, Erovic B, Florian S, Sperr WR, Kalhs P, Marian B, Wrba F, Zielinski CC, Valent P (2006) Neoplastic stem cells: a novel therapeutic target in clinical oncology. Cancer 107:2512–2520
66. Shapiro J, Marshall J, Karasek P, Figer A, Oettle H, Couture F, Jeziorski K, Broome P, Hawkins R (2005) G17DT+gemcitabine [Gem] versus placebo+Gem in untreated subjects with locally advanced, recurrent, or metastatic adenocarcinoma of the pancreas: results of a randomized, double-blind, multinational, multicenter study. 2005 ASCO Annual Meeting
67. Sindelar WF, Maher MM, Herlyn D, Sears HF, Steplewski Z, Koprowski H (1986) Trial of therapy with monoclonal antibody 17-1A in pancreatic carcinoma: preliminary results. Hybridoma 5 [Suppl 1]:S125–S132
68. Singh SK, Clarke ID, Terasaki M, Bonn VE, Hawkins C, Squire J, Dirks PB (2003) Identification of a cancer stem cell in human brain tumors. Cancer Res 63:5821–5828

69. Singh SK, Hawkins C, Clarke ID, Squire JA, Bayani J, Hide T, Henkelman RM, Cusimano MD, Dirks PB (2004) Identification of human brain tumour initiating cells. Nature 432:396–401
70. Stift A, Friedl J, Dubsky P, Bachleitner-Hofmann T, Benkoe T, Brostjan C, Jakesz R, Gnant M (2003) In vivo induction of dendritic cell-mediated cytotoxicity against allogeneic pancreatic carcinoma cells. Int J Oncol 22:651–656
71. Sutmuller RP, den Brok MH, Kramer M, Bennink EJ, Toonen LW, Kullberg BJ, Joosten LA, Akira S, Netea MG, Adema GJ (2006) Toll-like receptor 2 controls expansion and function of regulatory T cells. J Clin Invest 116:485–494
72. Suzuki E, Kapoor V, Jassar AS, Kaiser LR, Albelda SM (2005) Gemcitabine selectively eliminates splenic Gr-1+/CD11b+ myeloid suppressor cells in tumor-bearing animals and enhances antitumor immune activity. Clin Cancer Res 11:6713–6721
73. Ueda M, Miura Y, Kunihiro O, Ishikawa T, Ichikawa Y, Endo I, Sekido H, Togo S, Shimada H (2005) MUC1 overexpression is the most reliable marker of invasive carcinoma in intraductal papillary-mucinous tumor (IPMT). Hepatogastroenterology 52:398–403
74. Ungefroren H, Voss M, Bernstorff WV, Schmid A, Kremer B, Kalthoff H (1999) Immunological escape mechanisms in pancreatic carcinoma. Ann N Y Acad Sci 880:243–251
75. Ungefroren H, Voss M, Jansen M, Roeder C, Henne-Bruns D, Kremer B, Kalthoff H (1998) Human pancreatic adenocarcinomas express Fas and Fas ligand yet are resistant to Fas-mediated apoptosis. Cancer Res 58:1741–1749
76. Vafa O, Kharki S, Vielmetter J, Chamberlain A, Hammond P, Dang W, Carmichael D, Kunkel L, Barbosa M, Desjarlais J (2006) Anti-EpCAM XmAb antibodies with improved cytotoxicity. 2006 ASCO Annual Meeting
77. Wadle A, Kubuschok B, Imig J, Wuellner B, Wittig C, Zwick C, Mischo A, Waetzig K, Romeike BF, Lindemann W, Schilling M, Pfreundschuh M, Renner C (2006) Serological immune response to cancer testis antigens in patients with pancreatic cancer. Int J Cancer 119:117–125
78. Warger T, Osterloh P, Rechtsteiner G, Fassbender M, Heib V, Schmid B, Schmitt E, Schild H, Radsak MP (2006) Synergistic activation of dendritic cells by combined Toll-like receptor ligation induces superior CTL responses in vivo. Blood 108:544–550
79. Watson SA, Gilliam AD, Grimes S, Broome P, Michaeli D (2002) Enhanced inhibition of pancreatic cancer by combination of the G17DT immunogen and gemcitabine. 2002 ASCO Annual Meeting
80. Weiner LM, Harvey E, Padavic-Shaller K, Willson JK, Walsh C, LaCreta F, Khazaeli MB, Kirkwood JM, Haller DG (1993) Phase II multicenter evaluation of prolonged murine monoclonal antibody 17–1A therapy in pancreatic carcinoma. J Immunother 13:110–116
81. Wierecky J, Mueller M, Brossart P (2006) Dendritic cell-based cancer immunotherapy targeting MUC-1. Cancer Immunol Immunother 55:63–67
82. Wobser M, Keikavoussi P, Kunzmann V, Weininger M, Andersen MH, Becker JC (2006) Complete remission of liver metastasis of pancreatic cancer under vaccination with a HLA-A2 restricted peptide derived from the universal tumor antigen survivin. Cancer Immunol Immunother 55:1294–1298
83. Woodmansee C, Pillow J, Skinner RB Jr (2006) The role of topical immune response modifiers in skin cancer. Drugs 66:1657–1664
84. Xiong HQ, Rosenberg A, LoBuglio A, Schmidt W, Wolff RA, Deutsch J, Needle M, Abbruzzese JL (2004) Cetuximab, a monoclonal antibody targeting the epidermal growth factor receptor, in combination with gemcitabine for advanced pancreatic cancer: a multicenter phase II Trial. J Clin Oncol 22:2610–2616
85. Yamamoto K, Ueno T, Kawaoka T, Hazama S, Fukui M, Suehiro Y, Hamanaka Y, Ikematsu Y, Imai K, Oka M, Hinoda Y (2005) MUC1 peptide vaccination in patients with advanced pancreas or biliary tract cancer. Anticancer Res 25:3575–3579
86. Yanagimoto H, Mine T, Yamamoto K, Satoi S, Honma S, Mizoguchi J, Yamada A, Oka M, Kamiyama Y, Itoh K, Takai S (2006) Immunological evaluation of personalized peptide vaccination with gemcitabine for advance pancreatic cancer patients. 2006 ASCO Annual Meeting
87. Z'graggen K, Post S, Scheithauer W, van Laethem J, Levy P, Buchner-Moell D, Finke L, Buechler M (2000) RAS peptide vaccination is a safe and immunologically effective treatment in patients with unresectable pancreatic cancer: results of a phase II study. 2000 ASCO Annual Meeting

88. Bellone G, Carbone A, Smirne C, Scirelli T, Buffolino A, Novarino A, Stacchini A, Bertetto O, Palestro G, Sorio C, Scarpa A, Emanuelli G, Rodeck U (2006) Cooperative induction of a tolerogenic dendritic cell phenotype by cytokines secreted by pancreatic carcinoma cells. J Immunol 1177:3448–3460
89. Nakatsura T, Senju S, Yamada K, Jotsuka T, Ogawa M, Nishimura Y (2001) Gene cloning of immunogenic antigens overexpressed in pancreatic cancer. Biochem Biophys Res Commun 9281:936–944
90. Philip PA, Benedetti J, Fenoglio-Preiser C, Zalupski M, Lenz H, O'Reilly E, Wong R, Atkins J, Abruzzese J, Blanke C (2007) Phase III study of gemcitabine [G] plus cetuximab [C] versus gemcitabine in patients [pts] with locally advanced or metastatic pancreatic adenocarcinoma [PC]: SWOG S0205 study. 2007 ASCO Annual Meeting Proceedings Part I. J Clin Oncol 5:[June Suppl]:18S LBA4509

19 Src Kinase and Pancreatic Cancer

A. Hilbig

Recent Results in Cancer Research, Vol. 177

Abstract

The c-Src non-receptor tyrosine kinase is overexpressed in a large number of human malignancies. It is linked to tumour development and progression to distant metastases by promoting cell proliferation, invasion, and motility. Recently, promising anticancer therapeutics targeting c-Src have been developed that are under clinical investigation.

19.1 Introduction and Historical Review

The non-receptor tyrosine kinase c-Src is one of the longest known proto-oncogenes. It has been shown to be overexpressed in various human malignancies, and its activity has been associated with the development of tumors and their progression to distant metastasis by promoting invasion and motility of tumor cells. Even though it is one of the most extensively studied oncogenes, its precise function in cancer is not fully understood.

In 1911 Peyton Rous was the first to describe a virus with the ability to cause transmissible tumor growth in chickens (Rous 1911a, b), a finding that was confirmed 40 years later when it was shown that a tumor induced by the Rous sarcoma virus (RSV) produced infected tumor cells (Rubin 1955). In the 1960s Huebner and Todaro (1969) postulated the existence of viral oncogenes as determinants for the development of cancer. The viral Src-gene (v-Src), which was identified in the viral genome in the 1970s (Czernilofsky et al. 1980; Takeya and Hanafusa 1982; Takeya et al. 1982), was shown to be conserved in the vertebrate genome, which indicated its origin from a normal human gene that had been incorporated into RSV. v-Src differs in sequence from human cellular Src (c-Src) in carboxy-terminal deletions and in point mutations throughout the gene. Because v-Src lacks the negative-regulatory C-terminal domain of human c-Src, the transforming capacity of v-Src is more pronounced than that of c-Src. The mechanism of action was further investigated by studies with different mutants of v-Src. It could be shown that various mutations altered the transformation potential, morphology, and the host range of the gene. A mutant found by Varmus et al., for example, was defective in transforming rat cells, but was able to transform embryonic fibroblasts (Varmus et al. 1981). Even though it is known that the human c-Src kinase gene plays a significant role in the development of numerous human cancers, it was not possible to derive a v-Src-transformed human fibroblast cell line.

19.2 Mechanisms of c-SRC Regulation and Activation

Human c-Src is a 60-kDa nonreceptor tyrosine kinase of a nine-member family (including FYN, YES, BLK, YRK, FGR, HCK, LCK, and LYN) of which c-Src is the one most often implicated in human cancer. It plays a critical role in regulation of proliferation, differentiation, migration, adhesion, invasion, angiogenesis, and immune function. All Src family kinases are composed of four Src homology (SH) domains (Brown and Cooper 1996): an amino-terminal membrane localization signal, known as Src homology 4 domain (SH4), a SH3 and SH2 domain, a tyrosine kinase domain (SH1) and a regulatory sequence.

The SH1 kinase domain contains the autophosphorylation site that is important for full Src activation, and the SH2 domain interacts with the negative-regulatory Tyr527 and binds to platelet-derived growth factor receptor (PDGFR) (Mori et al. 1993). The SH3 domain promotes intramolecular contact with the kinase domain in the inactive form of the protein, and the SH4 domain contains the myristoylation site that is important for membrane localization.

Src kinase family members are kept inactive through a negative regulation by interaction of the C-terminal tail and the SH2 and SH3 domains, which restricts the accessibility of the kinase domain site for ATP and substrates. In crystallographic studies it was shown that this interaction causes the c-Src molecule to form a closed configuration that covers the kinase domain (Yamaguchi and Hendrickson 1996). When the C-terminal tyrosine (position 527 in v-Src and 530 in c-SRC) is phosphorylated, Src is inactive; when it is dephosphorylated Src is active with the potential for autophosphorylation and for downstream interactions via phosphorylation of Src substrates. v-Src, unlike c-Src, lacks the regulatory carboxy-terminal tail and therefore is constitutively active and transformation-competent.

c-Src is regulated in terms of both protein levels and levels of activity by different mechanisms. The c-SRC tyrosine kinase (CSK) and its homolog c-Src kinase homologous kinase (CHK) inactivate c-Src by phosphorylation of the conserved tyrosine residue in the c-Src carboxy-terminal domain (Tyr530), which results in conformation change to the closed inactivated form (Cooper et al. 1986). Activation of c-Src via dephosphorylation of the C-terminal phosphate is executed by several protein phosphatases such as protein tyrosine phosphatase-α (PTPα), PTP1, SHP1 (SH2-containing phosphatase 1), and SHP2 (Zheng et al. 1992; Jung and Kim 2002).

Binding of focal-adhesion kinase (FAK) or its molecular counterpart CRK-associated substrate (CAS) to the SH2 and SH3 domains of c-Src also results in activation by displacement of intramolecular interactions that maintain the closed configuration (Thomas et al. 1998). Furthermore c-Src is activated via interaction with ligand-activated receptor tyrosine kinases, e.g., epidermal growth factor receptor (EGFR), PDGFR, human epidermal growth factor receptor (HER)2/neu, fibroblast growth factor receptor (FGFR), colony-stimulating factor-1, and hepatocyte growth factor, also leading to a disruption of inhibiting intramolecular interactions (Tice et al. 1999; Muthuswamy et al. 1994; DeMali et al. 1999; Bowman et al. 2001; Landgren et al. 1995; Courtneidge et al. 1993).

Another activation mode is the natural occurrence of mutational events, leading to truncated point mutation of c-Src just C-terminal to the regulatory Tyr530, resulting in c-Src activation, which is reported in colon and endometrial cancer (Irby et al. 1999).

Degradation of c-Src performed by the proteasome is regulated via ubiquitylation by the Casitas B-lymphoma (CBL) ubiquitin ligase (Kim et al. 2004). This degradation pathway seems to be deregulated in cancer cells leading to c-Src activation.

19.3 Intracellular Localization and Molecular Mechanisms of c-Src

For complete expansion of its transforming activity, the intracellular localization of c-Src seems to be essential. The highest level of transforming activity results from contact with the plasma membrane and subsequent autophosphorylation of Tyr419, which is enabled by interactions with activated receptor tyrosine kinases (Nigg et al. 1982; Johnson et al. 1996). Upon activation the SH3 domain c-Src becomes indirectly associated with actin, and subsequently activated c-Src is translocated to sites of cell adhesion in the periphery where the myristoylated SH4 domain attaches to the inner surface of the cell membrane (Sefton et al. 1982).

19.3.1 Adhesion, Motility, Invasion, and Angiogenesis

From transfection studies the role of c-Src in regulating proliferation has been well established. Furthermore, there is accumulating evidence that c-Src also affects adhesion, invasion, and motility—events that represent a prerequisite in tumor progression and metastasis (Frame 2002). Focal adhesion and adherens junctions are the subcellular structures responsible for the regulation of cell–matrix and cell–cell interactions (Sastry and Burridge 2000; Jamora and Fuchs 2002), and both are regulated by c-Src. Focal adhesions represent dynamic structures that assemble to allow cells to adhere to the extracellular matrix (ECM) and disband when the cell needs to move along or away from the ECM. This procedure is regulated by integrins and other cell surface molecules such as cadherins, selectins, syndecans, G protein-coupled receptors, receptor tyrosine kinases, and the actin cytoskeleton. In the end of the cascade stands Ras-homologous A (RHOA), a small guanosine triphosphate (GTP)-binding protein that regulates actin cytoskeletal organization, and its activation is an indispensable prerequisite for this process.

c-Src accounts for disassembly of focal adhesions, a process that occurs during normal cellular migration and mitosis leading to increased motility because the cells lose their matrix attachment. This mechanism seems to contribute to increased metastasis, as impaired adhesion is required for enhanced cell motility and invasion. It could be shown that c-Src-family kinases have a key role in focal adhesion disassembly and turnover by inhibiting downstream signaling of RHOA through activation of p190 RHO-GTPase activating protein (RHOGAP), which ultimately leads to disruption of focal adhesions (Chang et al. 1995).

The disruption of adherens junctions is also driven by c-Src via inhibition of E-cadherin localization and function at these cell-to-cell contact points promoting the release of cells from each other. Furthermore, c-Src and other tyrosine kinases induce the tyrosine phosphorylation and ubiquitylation of the E-cadherin-complex, which leads to degradation via endocytosis of E-cadherin (Fujita et al. 2002).

Motility of cells is a highly regulated, well-orchestrated, multistep process that requires formation of cellular protrusions such as lamellipodia and filopodia, their attachment to the ECM, and disassembly of focal adhesions and adherens junctions, as described above, to release cells from the EMC and from each other. This course of events leading to enhanced cell motility is called adhesion turnover (Laukaitis et al. 2001) and is regulated by several signaling molecules such as different catenins, vinculin, talin, and paxillin, integrin-matrix contacts, and cytoskeleton actin polymerization, all of which is influenced by the activity of c-Src.

Disruption of adherens junctions and focal adhesion due to c-Src activity are countered by cellular defects such as E-cadherin loss, leading to increased cell motility and also facilitating invasion of cells. In studies with transgenic mice, E-cadherin has been shown to act as an invasion suppressor (Frixen et al. 1991), and overexpression of E-cadherin can reduce the invasive phenotype of cells (Perl et al. 1998). In addition, c-Src has been shown to affect the invasion potency of cells via interaction with matrix metalloproteinases and tissue inhibitors of matrix metalloproteinases (Noritake et al. 1999).

Influencing another important mechanism leading to tumor progression, Src activity seems to regulate molecules associated with angiogenesis. Upon activation of signal transducer and activator of transcription 3 (STAT3), v-Src has been shown to induce expression of vascular endothelial factor (VEGF). In addition c-Src is required for hypoxia-induced VEGF production, and VEGF expression is inhibited by antisense c-Src. Furthermore, development of characteristic signs of angiogenesis such as formation of cord-like structures and sprouting was suppressed in endothelial cells expressing kinase inactive c-Src (Kilarski et al. 2003).

19.4 Src Phenotype

After transfection of normal fibroblasts with v-Src, the cells round up, disaggregate, and start to float in the culture medium because of loss of intercellular, integrin-based cytoskeletal attachments that normally hold them in an ordered monolayer. In addition, the transformed cells become more motile and lose their density inhibition, representing the main feature of cancer cells, leading them to form clumps of cells that are referred to as foci. Furthermore, v-Src-transfected cells show increased proliferation rates with reduced doubling times and increased nutrient requirement in vitro. Transfected cells in vivo show a rapid growth and form visible tumors within days of injection that are capable of local invasion and metastasis to distant sites, probably due to affection of cell adherence, motility, and invasion by Src kinase activity. Consistent with this, overexpression of Csk, a negative modulator of Src, suppresses metastasis in mouse models (Nakagawa et al. 2000).

19.5 Src Kinase and Pancreatic Cancer

Members of the Src kinase family are frequently overexpressed in a variety of epithelial tumors, mostly in colon and breast but also in pancreatic cancer (Summy and Gallick 2003), with c-Src being the most prevalent representative. c-Src overexpression was found in all of 13 analyzed human pancreatic cancer specimens compared with none of 6 normal pancreatic tissues. Furthermore, c-Src activity was shown to be increased in 14 of 17 pancreatic tumor cell lines (Lutz et al. 1998). The extent of c-Src expression seems to correlate with malignant potential and patient survival. Moreover, in vitro studies have shown that activated c-Src expression in pancreatic cancer cells resulted in upregulation of insulin-like growth factor (IGF-1) receptor expression, reduced expression of E-cadherin, and increased production of interleukin (IL)-8 and VEGF, leading to increased cell proliferation, decreased cell–cell adhesion, enhanced migration, and increased angiogenesis.

Given that Src kinase activity influences a plethora of mechanisms that allow tumor cells to proliferate and migrate, strategies to target Src kinase activity alone and in combination with cytotoxic drugs have been developed and might prove effective in cancer therapy.

19.5.1 Different Inhibitors of Src Kinase

19.5.1.1 Pyrazolopyrimidines PP1 and PP2

Two synthetic and cell-permeable pyrazolopyrimidines named PP1 and PP2 (Calbiochem/Merck AG) were shown to inhibit Src family kinases. PP1 is more selective for mutant Src compared to wild-type Src and also inhibits FYN, whereas PP2 inhibits LCK, FYN and HCK. Ito et al. treated pancreatic cancer cell lines (BxPC-3, MiaPaCa-2, and PANC-1) in vitro with PP1 and observed complete inhibition of Src phosphorylation and significantly reduced activity of matrix metalloproteinases (MMP2 and MMP9) which resulted in a growth inhibition of 50% and suppression of cellular invasion by up to 90% in all cell lines (Ito et al. 2003). In a pancreatic tumor cell line resistant to gemcitabine (PANC-1 GemRes) described by Duxbury et al., a higher level of Src expression, phosphorylation, and activity in comparison to original PANC-1 cells was shown. After treatment with PP2, chemosensitivity to gemcitabine was increased and expression of the putative chemoresistance enzyme RRM2 was suppressed as compared to cells with constitutively activated Src kinase (Duxbury et al. 2004a).

19.5.1.2 Anilinoquinazoline AZM475271

The anilinoquinazoline AZM475271 (AstraZeneca) is an orally active inhibitor of c-Src. Its antiproliferative and antimetastatic activity was tested in nude mice by orthotopic implantation of human pancreatic cancer. After treatment with AZM475271 a tumor reduction of 40% was seen and tumor cell proliferation and angiogenesis decreased, whereas apoptosis of tumor cells increased. When AZM475271 was combined with chemotherapeutic drugs such as gemcitabine, the tumor volume could be reduced by 90%, which could be explained by a chemosensitizing effect of AZM475271 to the cytotoxic effect of gemcitabine. Furthermore, no metastatic spread could be detected (Yezhelyev et al. 2004).

19.5.1.3 Other Inhibitors of Src-Kinase Activity (AP23846, SKI-606, AZD05230, siRNA)

AP23846 is an ATP-based c-Src kinase inhibitor which reduces cellular migration, VEGF expression, and IL-8 expression in pancreatic cancer cells (L3.6pl) in vitro. Its activity was shown to be nearly tenfold higher in solid tumor cells than that of the pyrazolopyrimidine PP2 (Summy et al. 2005).

SKI-606 that inhibits kinase activity of both Src and Abl inhibited Src autophosphorylation and tyrosine phosphorylation of FAK. It also showed inhibition of colony formation, proliferation, and tumor growth in experimental colon cancer and chronic myeloid leukemia (CML) (Golas et al. 2003, 2005). There are no published data available concerning SKI-606 activity in pancreatic tumors.

Duxbury et al. observed an increased gemcitabine-induced, caspase-mediated apoptosis and decreased AKT kinase activity using a c-Src-specific siRNA (Duxbury et al. 2004b).

19.5.2 Clinical Application of Src Kinase Inhibitors

To date one Src family kinase inhibitor has entered a clinical phase I/II multicenter trial. AZD0530, a novel, selective, and orally active Src kinase inhibitor that has been shown to inhibit tumor cell adhesion, migration, and invasion (Green et al. 2004) is currently being evaluated in combination with gemcitabine for the treatment of patients with unresectable or metastatic pancreatic carcinoma.

19.6 Future Perspectives and Conclusion

c-Src is one of the oldest and best-studied proto-oncogenes, and even though its role in the development of cancer is not yet fully understood, there is clear evidence for its participation in normal cell proliferation, maintenance of intercellular contacts, and cell motility. Upon activation, c-Src leads to a transformed cell phenotype with increased cellular proliferation, invasion, and motility, as well as decreased intercellular and cell-matrix adhesion. Because c-Src activation is found in many solid tumor types and due to the increased understanding of the mechanistic links of c-Src to processes promoting tumor progression, there has developed a clear rationale for targeting c-Src in cancer therapy. In the past decade, an enormous amount of knowledge has accumulated for the rational design of such molecular cancer therapies.

References

Bowman T, Broome MA, Sinibaldi D, Wharton W, Pledger WJ, Sedivy JM, Irby R, Yeatman T, Courtneidge SA, Jove R (2001) Stat3-mediated Myc expression is required for Src transformation and PDGF-induced mitogenesis. Proc Natl Acad Sci USA 98:7319–7324

Brown MT, Cooper AJ (1996) Regulation, substrates and functions of src. Biochim Biophys Acta 1287:121–149

Chang JH, Gill S, Settleman J, Parsons S (1995) c-Src regulates the simultaneous rearrangement of actin cytoskeleton, p190RhoGAP, and p120rasGAP following epidermal growth factor stimulation. J Cell Biol 130:355–368

Cooper JA, Gould KL, Cartwright CA, et al. (1986) Tyr527 is phosphorylated in pp60c-src: implications for regulation. Science 231:1431–1434

Courtneidge SA, Dhand R, Pilat D, Twamley GM, Waterfield MD, Roussel MF (1993) Activation of Src family kinases by colony stimulating factor-1, and their association with its receptor. EMBO J 12:943–950

Czernilofsky AP, Levinson AD, Varmus HE, Bishop JM, Tischer E, Goodman HM (1980) Nucleotide sequence of an avian sarcoma virus oncogene (src) and proposed amino acid sequence for gene product. Nature 287:198–203

DeMali KA, Godwin SL, Soltoff SP, et al. (1999) Multiple roles for Src in a PDGF-stimulated cell. Exp Cell Res 253:271–279

Duxbury MS, Ito H, Zinner MJ, et al. (2004a) Inhibition of SRC tyrosine kinase impairs inherent and acquired gemcitabine resistance in human pancreatic adenocarcinoma cells. Clin Cancer Res 10:2307–2318

Duxbury MS, Ito H, Zinner MJ, et al. (2004b) siRNA directed against c-Src enhances pancreatic adenocarcinoma cell gemcitabine chemosensitivity. J Am Coll Surg 198:953–959

Frame MC (2002) Src in cancer: deregulation and consequences for cell behaviour. Biochim Biophys Acta 1602:114–130

Frixen UH, Behrens J, Sachs M, Eberle G, Voss B, Warda A, Löchner D, Birchmeier W (1991) E-cadherin-mediated cell-cell adhesion prevents invasiveness of human carcinoma cells. J Cell Biol 113:173–185

Fujita Y, Krause G, Scheffner M, Zechner D, Leddy HE, Behrens J, Sommer T, Birchmeier W (2002) Hakai, a c-Cbl-like protein, ubiquitinates and induces endocytosis of the E-cadherin complex. Nat Cell Biol 4:222–231

Golas JM, Arndt K, Etienne C, et al. (2003) SKI-606, a 4-anilino-3-quinolinecarbonitrile dual inhibitor of Src and Abl kinases, is a potent antiproliferative agent against chronic myelogenous leukemia cells in culture and causes regression of K562 xenografts in nude mice. Cancer Res 63:375–381

Golas JM, Arndt K, Etienne C, et al. (2005) SKI-606, a Src/Abl inhibitor with in vivo activity in colon tumor xenograft models. Cancer Res 65:5358–5364

Green TP, Fennel M, Whittaker R, et al. (2004) Preclinical activity of AZD0530, a novel oral potent and selective inhibitor of Src family kinases. Eur J Cancer 2:A361

Huebner RJ, Todaro GJ (1969) Oncogenes of RNA tumor viruses as determinants of cancer. Proc Natl Acad Sci USA 64:1087–1094

Irby RB, Mao W, Coppola D, Kang J, Loubeau JM, Trudeau W, Karl R, Fujita DJ, Jove R, Yeatman TJ (1999) Activating SRC mutation in a subset of advanced human colon cancers. Nat Genet 21:187–190

Ito H, Gardner-Thorpe J, Zinner MJ, et al. (2003) Inhibition of tyrosine kinase Src suppresses pancreatic cancer invasiveness. Surgery 134:221–226

Jamora C, Fuchs E (2002) Intercellular adhesion, signalling and the cytoskeleton. Nat Cell Biol 4: E101–E108

Johnson LN, Noble ME, Owen DJ (1996) Active and inactive protein kinases: structural basis for regulation. Cell 85:149–158

Jung EJ, Kim CW (2002) Interaction between chicken protein tyrosine phosphatase 1 (CPTP1)-like rat protein phosphatase 1 (PTP 1) and p60(v-src) in v-src transformed Rat-1 fibroblasts. Exp Mol Med 34:476–480

Kilarski WW, Jura N, Gerwins P (2003) Inactivation of Src family kinases inhibits angiogenesis in vivo: implications for a mechanism involving organization of the actin cytoskeleton. Exp Cell Res 291:70–82

Kim M, Tezuka T, Tanaka K, et al. (2004) Cbl-c suppresses v-Src induced transformation through ubiquitin-dependent protein degradation. Oncogene 23:1645–1655

Landgren E, Blume-Jensen P, Courtneidge SA, Claesson-Welsh L (1995) Fibroblast growth factor receptor-1 regulation of Src family kinases. Oncogene 10:2027–2035

Laukaitis CM, Webb DJ, Donais K, Horwitz AF (2001) Differential dynamics of α-actinin during formation of disassembly of adhesions in migrating cells. J Cell Biol 153:1427–1440

Lutz MP, Esser IB, Flossmann-Kast BB, et al. (1998) Overexpression and activation of the tyrosine kinase Src in human pancreatic cancer. Biochem Biophys Res Commun 243:503–508

Mori S, Rönnstrand L, Yokote K, Engström A, Courtneidge SA, Claesson-Welsh L, Heldin CH (1993) Identification of two juxtamembrane autophosphorylation sites in the PDGFβ-receptor; involvement in the interaction with Src family tyrosine kinases. EMBO J 12:2257–2264

Muthuswamy SK, Siegel PM, Dankort DL, et al. (1994) Mammary tumors expressing the neu proto-oncogene possess elevated c-Src tyrosine kinase activity. Mol Cell Biol 14:735–743

Nakagawa T, Tanaka S, Suzuki H, Takayanagi H, Miyazaki T, Nakamura K, Tsuruo T (2000) Overexpression of the csk gene suppresses tumor metastasis in vivo. Int J Cancer 88:384–391

Nigg EA, Sefton BM, Hunter T, et al. (1982) Immunofluorescent localization of the transforming protein of Rous sarcoma virus with antibodies against a synthetic src peptide. Proc Natl Acad Sci USA 79:5322–5326

Noritake H, Miyamori H, Goto C, et al. (1999) Overexpression of tissue inhibitor of matrix metalloproteinases-1 (TIMP-1) in metastatic MDCK cells transformed by v-src. Clin Exp Metastasis 17:105–110

Perl AK, Wilgenbus P, Dahl U, et al. (1998) A causal role for E-cadherin in the transition from adenoma to carcinoma. Nature 392:190–193

Rous PA (1911a) Transmission of a malignant new growth by means of a cell-free filtrate. JAMA 56:198

Rous PA (1911b) A sarcoma of the fowl transmissible by an agent separable from the tumor cells. J Exp Med 13:397–411

Rubin H (1955) Quantitative relations between causative virus and cell in the Rous No. 1 chicken sarcoma. Virology 6:669–688

Sastry SK, Burridge K (2000) Focal adhesions: a nexus for intracellular signaling and cytoskeletal dynamics. Exp Cell Res 261:25–36

Sefton BM, Trowbridge IS, Cooper JA, Scolnick EM (1982) The transforming proteins of Rous sarcoma virus, Harvey sarcoma virus and Abelson virus contain tightly bound lipid. Cell 31:465–474

Summy JM, Gallick GE (2003) Src family kinases in tumor progression and metastasis. Cancer Metastasis Rev 22:337–358

Summy JM, Trevino JG, Lesslie DP, et al. (2005) AP23846, a novel and highly potent Src family kinase inhibitor, reduces vascular endothelial growth factor and interleukin-8 expression in human solid tumor cell lines and abrogates downstream angiogenic processes. Mol Cancer Ther 4:1900–1911

Takeya T, Hanafusa H (1982) DNA sequence of the viral and cellular src gene of chickens. 2. Comparison of the src genes of two strains of avian sarcoma virus and of the cellular homolog. J Virol 44:12–18

Takeya T, Feldman RA, Hanafausa H (1982) DNA sequence of the viral and cellular src gene of chickens. 1. Complete nucleotide sequence of an EcoRI fragment of recovered avian sarcoma virus which codes for gp37 and pp60src. J Virol 44:1–11

Thomas JW, Ellis B, Boerner RJ, Knight WB, White GC, Schaller MD (1998) SH2- and SH3-mediated interactions between focal adhesion kinase and Src. J Biol Chem 273:577–583

Tice DA, Biscardi JS, Nickles AL, Parsons SJ (1999) Mechanism of biological synergy between cellular Src and epidermal growth factor receptor. Proc Natl Acad Sci USA 96:1415–1420

Varmus HE, Quintrell N, Wyke J (1981) Revertants of an ASV-transformed rat cell line have lost the complete provirus or sustained mutations in src. Virology 108:28–46

Yamaguchi H, Hendrickson WA (1996) Structural basis for activation of human lymphocyte kinase Lck upon tyrosine phosphorylation. Nature 384:484–489

Yezhelyev MV, Koehl G, Guba M, et al. (2004) Inhibition of SRC tyrosine kinase as treatment for human pancreatic cancer growing orthotopically in nude mice. Clin Cancer Res 10:8028–8036

Zheng XM, Wang Y, Pallen CJ (1992) Cell transformation and activation of pp60c-src by overexpression of a protein tyrosine phosphatase. Nature 359:336–339

Printing: Krips bv, Meppel, The Netherlands
Binding: Stürtz, Würzburg, Germany